"With his deep and comprehensive knowledge of classic and contemporary sociology, Cockerham provides a clear, historically tied explanation of the roots and contributions of medical sociology."

Bernice Pescosolido, Distinguished Professor of Sociology and Director of the Indiana Consortium for Mental Health Services Research at Indiana University

"Bill Cockerham has added a unique and valuable contribution to medical sociology. His book shows the utility of sociological theory to medical sociology and, in turn, the contributions of medical sociological work to social theory. Readers will find new connections here."

Peter Conrad, Harry Coplan Professor of Social Sciences, Emeritus, Brandeis University

Sociological Theories of Health and Illness

Sociological Theories of Health and Illness reviews the evolution of theory in medical sociology beginning with the field's origins in medicine and extending to its present-day standing as a major sociological subdiscipline. Sociological theory has an especially important role in the practice of medical sociology because its theories distinguish the subdiscipline from virtually *all* other scientific fields engaged in the study of health and illness. The focus is on contemporary theory because it applies to contemporary conditions; however, since theory in sociology is often grounded in historical precedents and classical foundations, this material is likewise included as it relates to medical sociology today.

This book focuses on the most commonly used sociological theories in the study of health and illness, illustrating their utility in current examples of empirical research on a wide range of topics. The qualitative or quantitative research methods applicable to specific theories are also covered. Distinctions between macro- and micro-levels of analysis and the relevance of the agency–structure dichotomy inherent in all theories in sociology are discussed. Beginning with classical theory (Durkheim, Weber, and Marx) and the neglected founders (Gilman, Martineau, and Du Bois), along with symbolic interaction (Mead, Strauss) and labeling theory (Becker), and poststructuralism and postmodernism (Foucault), coverage is extended to contemporary medical sociology. Discussion of the stress process model (Pearlin) is followed by the social construction of gender and race and intersectionality theory (Collins), health lifestyle theory (Cockerham), life course theory (Elder), fundamental cause theory (Link and Phelan), and theories of the medical profession (Freidson), medicalization and biomedicalization (Conrad, Clarke), and social capital (Bourdieu, Putnam, and Lin).

William C. Cockerham is Distinguished Professor of Sociology and Chair Emeritus at the University of Alabama at Birmingham and Research Scholar of Sociology at the College of William and Mary. Currently a Deputy Editor of the *Journal of Health and Social Behavior*, he has served on the editorial board of several journals, including the *American Sociological Review* and *Society and Mental Health*. He is author of *Medical Sociology*, 15th ed. (Routledge 2021) and *Sociology of Mental Disorder*, 11th ed. (Routledge 2021).

Sociological Theories of Health and Illness

William C. Cockerham

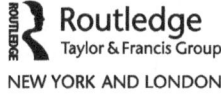
Routledge
Taylor & Francis Group

NEW YORK AND LONDON

First published 2021
by Routledge
52 Vanderbilt Avenue, New York, NY 10017

and by Routledge
2 Park Square, Milton Park, Abingdon, Oxon, OX14 4RN

Routledge is an imprint of the Taylor & Francis Group, an informa business

Library of Congress Cataloging-in-Publication Data
Names: Cockerham, William C., author.
Title: Sociological theories of health and illness / William C. Cockerham.
Description: New York, NY : Routledge, 2020.
Identifiers: LCCN 2020001489 (print) | LCCN 2020001490 (ebook) |
ISBN 9780367469108 (hardback) | ISBN 9780367469085 (paperback) |
ISBN 9781003046165 (ebook)
Subjects: LCSH: Social medicine. | Sociology.
Classification: LCC RA418 .C659 2020 (print) |
LCC RA418 (ebook) | DDC 362.1–dc23
LC record available at https://lccn.loc.gov/2020001489
LC ebook record available at https://lccn.loc.gov/2020001490

ISBN: 978-0-367-46910-8 (hbk)
ISBN: 978-0-367-46908-5 (pbk)
ISBN: 978-1-003-04616-5 (ebk)

Typeset in Bembo
by Newgen Publishing UK

To the memory of my parents Carl R. and Eva Louise, brother Paul, and son Bruce.

Contents

Chapter 1

Medical Sociology and Sociological Theory

The purpose of this book is to describe, discuss, and provide examples of the *major* theories commonly used in medical sociology or what is sometimes called health sociology or the sociology of health.[1] The focus is on contemporary theory because it applies to contemporary conditions; however, since theory in sociology is often grounded in historical precedents and classical foundations, this material is likewise included here as it relates to present-day medical sociology. Sociological theory has an especially important role in the practice of medical sociology because its theories distinguish the subdiscipline from virtually *all* other scientific fields engaged in the study of health and illness. It is not that these other fields are theoryless; rather, it is a sociological perspective, as exemplified by its theoretical viewpoints, which gives medical sociology its unique outlook in investigating and explaining health and illness. Consequently, a mastery of theory is a critical skill for its practitioners.

At the outset, it should be noted that "theory is in the eye of the beholder." What is meant by this is that theory is unsettled in sociology as various sociologists have their favorite theorists and theoretical perspectives and can be passionate advocates of their position, yet other sociologists and sociological theorists may disagree in part or in whole with that viewpoint. This is not necessarily a bad thing because debate can lead to the demise of out-of-date or weak theories, improvements in others, and the appearance of new ones more applicable to current conditions. It is up to the reader to look at the various theories to be discussed and decide for him or herself about the quality, validity, and utility of a particular theory.

A sociological perspective is the awareness or recognition that society and its various components have a reality above and beyond that of the individual that affects a person's behavior and way of life. This reality is not real in a material sense, but it nonetheless is a reality that exists in the mind as society's imprint on us and others. So while people usually choose their behavior, there are social structures in their lives that influence, shape, and give meaning to what they do. Even though such structures are "imagined," they have an "empirical" or real world existence in the way they affect social behavior. This is seen in the fact that families, groups, organizations, communities, social classes, nation-states, societies, and other social entities, along with various institutions such as religion, medicine, and the law—all have standards or norms of behavior, values, and customs that people who are associated with these entities are socialized to model their behavior after and accept as their own. Some people may deviate from what is considered socially acceptable behavior, but the reality of the existence of social entities beyond the individual and their influence still remains. Sociology's "gaze," however, looks not only at the impact of that reality upon individual and group behavior, but also at the social structures and conditions caused by an awareness of it. Sociology therefore helps us to understand the social forces at work in particular situations and the patterns of behavior that emerge from it.

When it comes to health and longevity, the social context of a person's life is particularly important because it determines the risk of exposure, susceptibility, and often the course and outcome of a health abnormality, regardless of whether it is infectious, metabolic, genetic, malignant, degenerative (Holtz et al. 2006), or mental (Cockerham 2017). A person's social circumstances, however, can also affect an individual's physical and/or mental health in positive, not just negative ways. Consequently, the "social" can be determining factors in the quality of a person's health and how long that individual lives. Such factors can determine not only whether or not a person becomes sick or stays healthy, but also how illness is experienced and the pattern of a population's level of health. Thus it is not surprising that social factors have become recognized as fundamental causes of health and mortality (Link and Phelan 1995; Phelan and Link 2013), and a sociological perspective is an important analytic tool in recognizing this.

As the late British historian Roy Porter (1997) pointed out many years ago, medicine can no longer be preoccupied with focusing on biological abnormalities and be indifferent as to how they got there. Medicine has to consider, among other things, wider questions of living conditions, lifestyle, diet, work situations, education, and family structure in meeting the challenges in treating the health problems of the "whole" person existing outside of a doctor's office in the real world. "Disease," according to Porter (1997:634), "became conceptualized after 1900 as a social no less than a biological phenomenon, to be understood statistically, sociologically, and psychologically—even politically."

Recognition of the connection between social conditions and health led to the development of medical sociology as a major subdiscipline within general sociology. Medical sociology focuses on the social causes and consequences of health and illness. It brings sociological perspectives, theories, and methods to the study of the social facets of health and illness behavior and the social determinants of health. Areas of investigation also include the social causes of health disparities, the social function of health care providers, the social organization and delivery of health care services, and the social aspects of health policy and its politics. The role of theory in this enterprise is particularly important, as will be seen.

Epidemiologic Transition Theory

It should be noted before continuing that medical sociology has become increasingly important in the study of health and disease, which is significant for the status of theory in the subdiscipline. The value of medical sociology for medicine, public health, and other health sciences becomes obvious when the epidemiological transition of diseases over the course of human history is considered. Epidemiologic transition theory, a theory in epidemiology (the science of epidemics), provides a framework for illustrating this outcome. Epidemiologic transition theory was originally formulated in 1971 by Abdel Omran who observed that some diseases were more prevalent in particular historical periods than others, a fact that led him to organize the major causes of mortality into three distinct stages:

1. The "Age of Pestilence and Famine" in which infectious and parasitic diseases are the major causes of death from the earliest times until the 1800s.
2. The "Age of Receding Epidemics," a transitional stage during which infectious and parasitic diseases are brought under control by improved hygiene, sanitation, nutrition, public health measures, higher standards of living, and medical advances featuring mass immunizations, antibiotics, and other innovations from the early 1800s to about 1960.
3. The "Age of Degenerative and Man-Made Diseases" in which noncommunicable or chronic diseases, such as cardiovascular disease and cancer, emerge as the dominant causes of mortality beginning around 1960.

Omran further notes that not all of the world undergoes a transition in diseases at the same time. Changes occur first in the most advanced countries, while developing countries slowly catch up as they experience varying degrees of modernization over the years. This theory seemed a reasonable summary of epidemiological trends until the 1970s and 1980s. But then there was a surprisingly rapid decline in deaths from cardiovascular disease (Bongaarts 2014), followed shortly thereafter by the arrival of new infectious diseases such as West Nile disease, SARS, and Ebola in the late 1990s and early 2000s (Armelagos and Harper 2016), along with the coronavirus (COVID-19) in 2019–2020. This development led some to propose further changes in the theory. These changes include adding newly emerging infectious diseases to the third stage as these diseases had made an unexpected and deadly appearance, or alternatively creating a new fourth stage:

4.   The "Age of Delayed Degenerative Diseases" in which chronic diseases like heart disease and cancer do not result in death until increasingly older ages due to further advances in medicine (Olshansky and Ault 1986), or the "Hybristic [or Mixed] Age" in which individual behaviors and lifestyles are added to heart disease and cancer as another major cause of mortality significantly affecting the other causes (Rodgers and Hackenberg 1987), or the "Age of the Cardiovascular Revolution" during which improvements in medicine pertaining to heart disease continue to reduce mortality and improve life expectancy (Meslé and Vallin 2006).

The title and contents of a new fourth stage are yet to be fully determined or agreed upon. The devastating effects of COVID-19 on the world brings back the first stage of the "Age of Pestilence," which turns epidemiologic transition theory back on its head and needs to be accounted for in devising a fourth stage. The addition of newly emerging infectious diseases in which a primary means of halting infections is "social distancing" and "stay-at-home" policies again points toward the relevance of the "social" in relation to disease. When the transition of diseases is viewed over time from the past to the present it is apparent that social behavior and conditions have gained in importance as causal factors in disease transmission. Stage 1 features infectious and parasitic diseases related to human migration, the transition from hunting and gathering societies to agricultural settlement, and the rise of trade and urban living. Stage 2 reflects the lessened prevalence of epidemics associated not just with medical advances but with better living conditions and improved normative behavior with respect to hygiene, sanitation, diet, and the like. In Stage 3, the connections between health lifestyles, stress, and other social factors with health become particularly obvious with respect to heart disease (Cockerham, Hamby, and Oates 2017) and cancer (Hiatt and Breen 2008).

And in a yet to be formulated Stage 4, social factors are especially relevant regardless of whether it is a case of (1) "delayed degenerative diseases" in which the biological effects of aging or the physical "weathering" of the body caused by social stress and the consequences of unhealthy lifestyle practices—are postponed as life expectancy increases, or (2) the "cardiovascular revolution" where health lifestyles are again paramount in mortality outcomes because of their close association with heart disease, or, what seems the best choice, (3) "hybristic (mixed) causes" in which risky behaviors (i.e., lifestyles) are recognized as a major cause of death for both chronic and infectious diseases, including the relevance of "social distance" as a causal factor in epidemics and pandemics. In this new fourth stage, smoking, obesity, and unhealthy behavior, along with the addition of climate change and newly emerging diseases, will be essential. What is obvious is that this current stage of epidemiological transition takes cognizance of the fact that health improvement requires behavioral changes. However, throughout each and every stage, social–class position has universally demarcated the rich from the poor in terms of who is the most healthy and who is least healthy in a consistent trend over centuries.

What is Theory?

Turning now to sociological theory, an initial step is to define it. There are varying definitions of theory, but one definition consistent with the way in which sociologists and other scientists generally understand and use the term is as follows: "a *theory* is a set of explicit, abstract, general, logically related statements formulated to explain phenomena in the natural world" (Webster and Markovsky 2007:4987). Sociological theories are similar to theories in other fields, including the physical sciences upon which scientific theories are often modeled, in that they likewise consist of a set of interrelated propositions that describe causal processes. That is, they are statements or propositions claiming that one class or type of phenomenon is connected in some way to another class of phenomenon invariably producing or causing a certain condition, behavior, or outcome.

Theories thus organize and categorize variables, explain past and present outcomes, predict future outcomes, and provide understanding about what causes those outcomes (Reynolds 2007). A major difference, however, between theories in the physical sciences and sociological theories is that physical science theories deal with events occurring in nature and the cosmos, whereas sociological theories explain human social behavior that is motivated. As Neil Smelser (1994:21) once explained about sociological theory:

> Every item of empirical research in the field, however narrowly defined and circumscribed, is rooted in general propositions about human beings and society and contains the seeds of abstract reasoning and normative evaluation. These elements are implicit but never absent. For this reason, theory should be regarded as an integral *aspect* of sociological inquiry rather than something separate from it. In another sense,

however, theory is distinguishable. It is legitimate to consider the relations among the general elements in their own right; in doing so, we enter the realm of sociological theory.

Theory is critically important to every scientific discipline because it provides a conceptualization about how sets of phenomena or a particular phenomenon operate in the empirical world. As Austrian-British philosopher Karl Popper pointed out long ago in *The Logic of Scientific Discovery* ([1934] 1992:59), theories are "nets" that allow us to catch what we call the world in order to understand and explain it, and we endeavor to make the net's mesh ever finer and finer. Theories in sociology provide definitions and sets of propositions explaining some facet or facets of social reality. Usually these propositions are testable, so the validity of the theory can be either confirmed, modified, or rejected (falsified). Therefore, as German medical sociologist Johannes Siegrist (2014:1637) observes, every theory needs to be tested and therefore it is essential that theoretical hypotheses and propositions are expressed in ways that allow for their rejection if found to be unsubstantiated or false. Over time, theories may be discarded as social conditions change or more informative theories emerge; consequently, theoretical work is continually ongoing and evolving.

Theoretical Levels

Theories in sociology explain social phenomena at three distinct levels: (1) micro, (2) meso/middle range, and (3) macro/grand. *Micro-level* theories explain patterns of face-to-face social interaction that regularly takes place between individuals and within small groups. Typically such theories are derived from relatively small samples of people (possibly 30 or less) whose social behavior can be directly observed and subjectively analyzed by a researcher using one or more qualitative methods, such as participant observation, in-depth interviews, focus groups, unobtrusive measures (i.e., analyzing public and private records, biographies and life histories, perhaps simple observations of what people are wearing or where they are standing in a room, physical trace analyses of activities like souvenirs purchased or even garbage left behind), ethnographies, and situational analysis consisting of mapping the positions, situations, and social worlds of those being studied (Clarke, Friese, and Washburn 2018; Denzin 2017; Denzin and Lincoln 2018; Guest, Tolley, and Wong 2014). Some qualitative researchers use *mixed methods*—such as conducting both observations and interviews in the same study—to ensure the reliability of their findings if each method confirms the findings of the other method. Or a small sample can be examined qualitatively within a much larger sample in a quantitative study for the same reason.

Qualitative (non-numerical) methods are generally used in micro-level studies because the small number of participants is usually too few for meaningful quantitative (numerical/statistical) analyses. Although qualitative findings cannot be proven or disproven mathematically, they can be systematically evaluated for their (1) *credibility* (substantiated by data), (2) *dependability* (by using established research techniques), (3) *confirmability* (confirmed by other researchers), and (4) *transferability* (conceptually representative of similar study populations) in order to negate subjective bias or misinterpretation (Guest, Tolley, and Wong 2014). Qualitative studies also may utilize *analytic induction*, which is a method of discovery and verification that requires a researcher to search for negative cases that provide contradictory evidence and, if found, formulate a new hypothesis that is fully corroborated by the data (Denzin 2017).

Qualitative research and the micro-level theories that result from it can provide insightful data on face-to-face social interaction and small-group relationships and circumstances. This is because this type of research takes one directly into the social world of the people being studied and obtains their view of that world in their own words, perspectives, and actions. As I have stated elsewhere: "It puts a human face on what would otherwise be only a narrative of numbers" (Cockerham 2013a:26). However, qualitative approaches that concentrate on what individuals say or do are nevertheless constrained by their small scale. That is, there are limits to what can be achieved by micro-level methods in that such methods are not equipped theoretically or methodologically to explain or measure the dynamics of higher-level (meso and macro) social phenomena or interaction between such larger-scale phenomena (Sibeon 2004).

Meso-level/middle-range theories lie between the micro and macro levels. Meso-level theories focus on explaining the behavior and social conditions generated by social structures just above individuals and small groups, such as large groups, communities, formal organizations, institutions, social movements, political parties, and the like. Such collectivities have their own norms, values, and behavioral settings that influence the behavior of the people that are part of them. Medical personnel can interact routinely with their particular set of colleagues and have a shared small-group perspective at a micro level, but their views can also be shaped by the normative atmosphere of the larger health care delivery system within which they all participate, which can be studied at a meso level.

Also at a level above the micro, are theories of the *middle-range* that address specific topics or areas of investigation such as medicalization, health lifestyles, or health disparities. The concept of theories of the middle range was advanced by Robert Merton (1957) who rejected grandiose and abstract theorizing as a standard for sociology, as well as micro-level theories of limited scope, in favor of what he called "substantive theories" of the middle range based on empirical research and data. These mid-level theoretical approaches typically utilize quantitative methods featuring various types of statistical analysis. Data supporting or rejecting meso-level and middle-range theories usually come from social surveys based on representative samples of large populations.

This approach is preferred when an overall or more general assessment of social phenomena beyond the micro level is needed and reliance on in-depth information obtained from a few individuals is insufficient. Sociologists had turned to the use of statistics between 1890 and 1915 in order to demonstrate that sociology followed established scientific procedures and at the same time develop their own modes of statistical analysis to differentiate their discipline from other, less quantitative sciences (Camic and Xie 1994). Large data sets more readily lent themselves to statistical analyses in which the scientific "truth" of theories can be proven or disproven. Not only can statistics analyze a large amount of information, but also depict how the world is organized and structured beyond individuals and small groups so that theories can be constructed to accurately account for the social processes representative of larger social entities (Babbie, Wagner, and Zaino 2019; Ritchey 2009; Wagner and Gillespie 2019).

Therefore, as British sociologist David Rose and his colleagues (Rose, Harrison, and Pevalin 2010:28, original emphasis) make clear: "most importantly, *we have to think theoretically before we think statistically.*" What this means is that a causal or explanatory narrative (a theory) is needed that can be formed into a testable hypothesis before a statistical test can be applied. That is, clear causal narratives theoretically explaining *social relationships* between variables need to be constructed prior to testing and statistical validation.

Finally, there are *macro-level/grand* theories at the societal level that model large-scale social processes within or between whole societies. Macro-level theories theorize about social processes involving national or even global systems of social stratification, culture, religion, politics, economies, and the like. These are theories about how entire societies and social systems operate. A problem, however, with many theories at the macro level is that they are difficult if not impossible to test because their scope covers such large phenomena. In one sense, they tell us everything, but at the same time they also tell us nothing that can be verified.

This category of theory also includes *grand theories* that attempt to explain the totality of social structures and social behavior in large, sweeping abstract generalizations about society (Sibeon 2004). While some of these theories still exist (e.g., classical Marxism), they are also typically quantitatively and qualitatively untestable and, as noted by British sociologist Roger Sibeon (2004:9), "bear little relation to concrete empirical happenings in particular times and particular places." They also tend to be inconclusive and, as Greek-British sociologist Nicos Mouzellis (2008) adds, even trivial if their universal scope does not consider the historical and cultural contexts in which all large-scale social phenomena are embedded. "On the other hand," says Mouzellis (2008:218),

> when universal theories manage to avoid such trivialities and tell us something interesting, i.e. something we did not know about the social world, they are wrong; their universal and countless scope does not allow specification of the conditions in which the statements put forward are valid and those in which they are not.

Consequently, in medical sociology, as well as in contemporary sociology generally, virtually all theoretical work is either micro or meso/middle range. They are typically evidence-based.

Agency versus Structure

Before examining the major theories in medical sociology in the chapters to come, it is relevant to discuss the agency–structure interface which will be on view in each theory discussed. One way to depict structure is as the skeleton of a body or the framework of a house, and agency as the processes taking place within that body or house (Stones 2018). Each can have an effect upon the other. This circumstance becomes a concern in constructing theory in sociology because some theories favor the constraining and enabling role of structure and others emphasize the choice and creativity of individual agency. According to British social theorist Margaret Archer (1995), the agency–structure issue has been *the* central sociological question since the beginning of sociology. As Archer (1995:1) puts it: "The vexatious task of understanding the linkage between 'structure and agency' will always retain this centrality because it derives from what society intrinsically is."

Stated simply, people exercise choice (or agency) and therein become the "agent" of their behavior, but that behavior typically falls within the parameters or behavioral boundaries set by the social structures (i.e., families, groups, professions, social-class positions) in their lives that have the normative influence or power to shape decision-making. *Agency* is a sociological term referring to the ability of the individual to select his or her behavior, while social *structures* produce regularities in social interaction (by way of socially prescribed norms, roles, and institutions), systematic social relationships (such as kinship, group affiliations, social class, gender, and other forms of stratification), and the resources that are available. Social structures channel behavior in particular directions as opposed to others that might be taken. While most theories recognize that agency and structure are both important in some way, debate centers over the extent to which one or the other is dominant in determining social behavior and identifying the social situations in which that dominance occurs.

Agency is formally defined as the process by which individuals, influenced by their past but also oriented toward the future (as a capacity to imagine alternative possibilities) and the present (as a capacity to consider both past habits and future situations within the contingencies of the moment), critically evaluate and choose their course of action (Emirbayer and Mische 1998:963).

Agency thus refers to an actor's ability to (1) initiate self-chosen actions and (2) act independently of structural influences (Campbell 2009), especially in regard to achieving positive future outcomes (Hitlin and Johnson 2015). Advocates of agency-oriented theories in sociology invariably accentuate the ability of individuals to choose their behavior regardless of structural influences or constraints. However, agency theories that underemphasize the effects of structure on the individual run the danger of engaging in what Archer (1995:4) calls "upwards conflation" which is a term she assigns to theories whose behavioral models give so much causal power to individuals that it acts in a one-way, upward direction to create structure and does not seem capable of allowing structure to act back on individuals.

Alternately, proponents of structurally oriented theories emphasize the power of structures to contour individual dispositions and behaviors along socially prescribed lines. Structures, according to William Sewell (1992:19), are "sets of mutually sustaining schemas and resources that empower or constrain social action and tend to be reproduced by that social action." Schemas are defined as rules or procedures applied to the enactment of social life, while resources are either human (i.e., physical strength, dexterity, knowledge) or nonhuman (naturally occurring or manufactured) that can be used to enhance or maintain power. Sewell equates resources with the power to influence action consistent with British sociologist Anthony Giddens' (1984) concept of the duality of structure, which depicts structure as having the potential to *either* constrain or enable action. The enabling function suggests resources increase the range and style of options from which the actor can choose, but constraint means that resources invariably limit choices to what is possible. Although the enabling/constraining functions of social structures might seem contradictory, in fact, social reality is like this in the empirical world in that an individual's resources may allow them to achieve their choices fully or partially, or be so inadequate that choices are impossible to realize.

In the case of theoretical models in which structure is overwhelmingly dominant, Archer (1995:3) says such theories reflect "downwards conflation" in that they overstate the causal power of structure to the extent that individuals lack behavioral creativity and choice. Rather, individual choices in behavior are determined more or less exclusively by the social structures in a person's life; for example, upper-class people usually act in an upper-class manner and lower-class individuals will invariably act in lower-class ways because of the norms and values inherent in their respective class positions. Agency theorists, however, maintain that agency will never be completely determined by structure, but conversely it is also clear that "there is no hypothetical moment in which agency actually gets 'free' of structure; it is not, in other words, some pure … [form of] free will" (Emirbayer and Mische 1998:1004).

So while agency is important, structure is always there in the background. This is because, as Polish-British sociologist Zygmunt Bauman (1999) observes, individual choices in *all* circumstances are confined by two sets of constraints: (1) choosing from among what is available and (2) social rules or codes telling the individual the rank order and appropriateness of preferences. People do have the capability to act independently of the social structures in their lives, but the occasions on which they do so may be rare because of the constraining and enabling qualities of structures. Nevertheless, there may be situations in which agency is dominant and others in which structure is stronger, yet both are present in all social settings and the quality of a theory rests upon its capacity to distinguish the extent of their relative influence.

The Status of Theory in Early Medical Sociology

Medical sociology was initially a field whose work was largely applied or pragmatic, not theoretical (Cockerham 1983; Scambler 1987). In fact, medical sociology had been characterized in the 1970s and 1980s as "theoretically impoverished" (Johnson 1975; Scambler 1987). It had emerged in the late 1940s and 1950s as a promising new sociological subdiscipline because it had the potential to align itself with medicine in its efforts to provide comprehensive patient care (Simmons and Wolff 1954). Alvin Gouldner (1970:345), in his book, *The Coming Crisis of Western Sociology*, widely read by sociologists in the 1970s, had called attention to post-World War II efforts to finance the social sciences to help solve the problems of industrial societies and welfare states. What this meant for the fledgling science of medical sociology was a demand for applied and policy-oriented research, as the field appeared to be a prototypical social science along the lines exactly described by Gouldner.

While this was one way to use medical sociology, there was not much in medical sociology to use. The field barely existed. A few studies on the patient-physician relationship and the social ecology of mental illness, along with early essays and books written about medical sociology, had been published almost entirely by physicians. This body of work had not provided the critical mass needed to establish a sociological subdiscipline (Bloom 2002).

Nevertheless, public awareness and common sense that socially and economically disadvantaged people had shorter life spans and more health problems than the affluent, aroused interest in the subdiscipline as Western governments turned their attention from fighting a world war to rebuilding society. A field like medical sociology seemed to be a potentially promising ally for improving population health. Postwar government and private foundation funding thus provided the catalyst for the emergence of a new sociological specialty that could potentially inform medical practice and policy. It was primarily through the stimulus of this external funding that sociologists and health professionals adopted medical sociology as a career field (Claus 1982; Cockerham 1983). Some participants, especially in Europe, had no training whatsoever in medical sociology or had not even taken a class in sociology at a university, but were attracted to the field because of the availability of jobs and financial support for research in a new and potentially interesting health-oriented subdiscipline (Claus 1982; Illsley 1975).

In the United States, where medical sociology developed more extensively than anywhere else in the world, its emergence was stimulated by the expansion of the National Institutes of Health (NIH) in the late 1940s. Particularly important, according to August Hollingshead (1973), a medical sociologist who participated in some of the early research programs, was the establishment of the National Institute of Mental Health (NIMH) that was instrumental in both encouraging and funding joint sociological and medical projects. The NIMH accomplished this by bringing sociologists and medical people together to discover their common interests, then plan and engage in cooperative research. "It was through the impetus provided by this money," noted British sociologist Malcolm Johnson (1975:89), "that sociologists and medical [personnel] changed their affiliations and embraced the field of medical sociology." Samuel Bloom (2002:156) describes this situation in his authoritative book on the history of American medical sociology this way:

> Although private sources of support remained important, medical sociology's development at this stage was closely associated with the NIMH, then the newest federal institute.
>
> In my opinion, NIMH, created in 1946, was the single institution that more than any other, was responsible for the emergence of medical sociology as we now know it. In the background there was, of course, the postwar increase of the government's role in all of science in the United States, and medical sociology was part of that process.

Under the auspices of NIMH, medical sociology's initial alliance with medicine was in psychiatry. A basis for cooperation existed because of earlier research in Chicago in 1939 on urban mental health, conducted by Robert Faris (a sociologist) and H. Warren Dunham (a psychiatrist). A particularly significant cooperative effort that followed led to the publication in 1958 of *Social Class and Mental Illness: A Community Study* by Hollingshead (a sociologist) and Frederick Redlich (a psychiatrist). This landmark research, conducted in New Haven, Connecticut, produced important evidence that social factors could be correlated with different types of mental disorders and the way in which people received psychiatric care. Persons in the most socially and economically disadvantaged segments of society were found to have the highest rates of mental disorder in general and excessively high rates of schizophrenia—the most disabling mental illness—in particular. This study attracted international attention and is considered one of the most important studies ever of the relationship between mental disorder and social class. The study played a key role in the debate during the 1960s, leading to the establishment of community mental health centers in the United States, as did other significant joint projects involving sociologists and psychiatrists, such as the Midtown Manhattan study in New York City conducted by Leo Srole and his colleagues (1962).

Psychiatry began moving away from sociology and talking therapies like psychoanalysis in the 1960s toward a focus on the use of psychopharmaceuticals to control abnormal behavior (Cockerham 2017). However, funding from federal and private organizations also helped stimulate cooperation between sociologists and other physicians with regard to physical health. In 1949, the Russell Sage Foundation funded a program to improve the utilization of social science research in medical practice. One result was the publication of *Social Science in Medicine* in 1954 by Leo Simmons (a sociologist) and Harold Wolff (a neurologist) with a particular focus on the link between socially induced stresses and disease. Other work sponsored by the Sage Foundation came later, including Edward Suchman's book on *Sociology and the Field of Public Health* (1963).

Since funding agencies were not interested in theoretical work on the part of medical sociologists, they sponsored and favored sociological research on health that had practical utility. Theory was absent in these early research efforts oriented toward helping solve clinical problems or address policy issues, rather than developing or testing theory and utilizing it as a tool to enhance understanding. Studies on patient attributes, attitudes, and behavior (Gold 1977), along with their utilization of medical services, were common. Gouldner (1970) pointed out that this situation always pressures theory to be practical as well. And the few theories that were developed during this period tended to be utilitarian, as seen, for example, in Suchman's (1965) model describing the five probable stages of a sick person's illness experience.[2]

As Gouldner (1970:82) stated:

> Social theory "for its own sake" or "pure" theory, is always vulnerable and of challengeable legitimacy in a utilitarian culture. Insofar as "theory" is regarded as the least practical aspect of social science—that is, as "mere" theory—the social science of a utilitarian culture always tends toward a theoryless empiricism, in which the conceptualization of problems is secondary and energies are instead given over to questions of measurement, research or experimental design, sampling or instrumentation. A conceptual vacuum is thus created, ready to be filled in by the common-sense concerns and practical interests of clients, sponsors, and research funders; in this way sociology is made useful to their interests.

In the case of medical sociology, the subdiscipline is useful to the interests of medicine, various other health-related professions, and policymakers seeking sociological insights about the relationship between social behaviors and conditions relevant to health. In this circumstance, applied research is essential, as medical sociology would not be important if it was not useful in helping people and societies to be healthy as a central contribution of its research orientation.

Nevertheless, by the twenty-first century medical sociology had evolved into more of an independent partnership with medicine in many institutional settings than simply serving as a subordinate area of research. Several factors were important in this development. First, physicians are not trained in medical sociology and therefore generally lack the background to conduct research requiring a sociological perspective and methodologies. They rely on medical sociologists for this expertise. Conversely, medical sociologists are not clinicians. So the grounds exist for a partnership, as each jointly brings his or her particular professional skills to the research enterprise. This is especially the case if the sociologist is a colleague with shared leadership responsibilities in the design and implementation of research rather than a subordinate employee.[3] Second, medical sociologists began examining the field of medicine itself as a social institution. This was primarily seen in the United States, where the medical profession became an object of critical study, as medical sociologists focused objectively on its relationships with patients and other health care providers and on the organizational structure of health care delivery systems (Bloom 2002). The medical profession's weak professional sanctions for medical mistakes and malpractice, the plight of the poor and medicine's opposition to national health insurance, and a decline in professional autonomy were all researched critically in the latter part of the twentieth century (see, for example, Hafferty and McKinlay 1993; Light 1993; Ritzer and Walczak 1988; Starr 1982).

While such research could seem hostile to medicine, Brazilian medical sociologist Everado Nunes (2014) states that physicians and medical sociologists nevertheless work well together if a critical role is perceived as objective and constructive, rather than antagonistic. And third, medical sociologists started investigating questions of sociological interest in medical settings, not just those determined by physicians. They independently brought their own topics to the study of health, such as social stress, medicalization, women's health issues, gender roles in medical practice, neighborhood health disadvantages, health lifestyles, social capital, health disparities, and other questions best answered by a sociological perspective.

As medical sociology was establishing a more solid professional footing, the use of theory became more common. Medical sociologists generally have the same or similar training in research methods and theory. Such training typically emphasizes that empirical research and theory are joint aspects of the same investigative activity (Denzin 2017). Consequently, the appearance of theory at some point should have been a predictable outcome. While some scholars may favor one endeavor as more important than the other, *both* are nonetheless central to the research enterprise. As German sociologist Richard Münch (1994:7) succinctly observed some years ago: "A scientific discipline does not make progress by accumulating large mountains of data if they have no relation to theoretical questions."

Consequently, research in empirical settings is one of the two primary analytical pillars of medical sociology. The other is sociological theory. The interrelationship between empirical research and sociological theory is extremely close by necessity. Empirically grounded research is needed to verify or disprove theory, while theory is required to give a shape or form, as well as insight, to empirical findings. According to Aage Sorensen (2009:369):

> The integration [of social theory and empirical research] comes about by two activities, theory development and gathering of evidence, inspiring and reinforcing each other: research improves theory and theory improves research. More precisely, evidence produced by research using appropriate methodology, ... speaks to the validity and usefulness of theory, while theory inspires procedures and questions for the research enterprises.

Theoretical knowledge, as Münch (1994:4) reminds us, is explanatory in character; however, theory does not simply describe what happened in the past or happens in the present but explains *why* things happen the way they do or will happen when certain conditions exist. The conceptual framework provided by theory is the medium through which reality is explained and understood. As symbolic interactionist theorist Herbert Blumer (1931:515) commented about theory in the 1930s, which remains relevant today: "To speak of a science without concepts suggests all sorts of analogies—a carver without tools, a railroad without tracks, a mammal without bones, a love story without love."

The Status of Theory in Medical Sociology Today

As will be discussed in the forthcoming chapters, medical sociology has moved from being an atheoretical subdiscipline to a field in which theory has become a significant vehicle for expressing its findings and conclusions. While medical sociology had acquired a reputation for being atheoretical that persisted for decades, even after it was no longer true, considerable theoretical work in the field had nevertheless been taking place (Cockerham 2005, 2013a, 2013b, 2013c; Cockerham, Hamby, and Oates 2017; Cockerham and Scambler 2016; Collyer 2015; Conrad 2007, 2013; De Maio 2010; Link and Phelan 1995; McDonnell et al. 2009; Phelan and Link 2013; Scambler 2012, 2018). Much of it occurred in sociology departments in American universities, as medical sociology matured as a subdiscipline and became more closely aligned with general sociology through their commonalities— namely mutual theories and research methods. Contemporary medical sociology came to have a theoretically rich and abundant literature with its own theories specific to the subdiscipline, some of which are based on perspectives shared with sociology at large and others that are unique to its subject matter.

The result is that medical sociologists are making greater use of sociological theory than ever before to amplify the explanatory power of their empirical findings. Theory is typically required to be utilized in research papers submitted for publication in medical sociology's scientific journals. A common question for the reviewers of such papers judging their quality pertains to whether or not the paper uses or contributes to theory. This situation clearly indicates that the use of theory is a general requirement for success in publishing research findings in medical sociology. It also suggests that through theory medical sociology is improving its connection to general sociology, as sociology increasingly recognizes that considerations of health are evident in the everyday social lives of people and medical sociology has the capacity for explaining it. Medical sociology has, in fact, taken the lead in developing its own theories rather than relying on general sociology to produce relevant theories. Evidence for this is found in the current upsurge of theoretical work in medical sociology, marking the field today as a highly theoretically engaged sociological subdiscipline, which is the subject matter of this book.

Summary

As noted in the beginning of this chapter, the purpose of this book is to describe, discuss, and provide examples of the major theories commonly used in medical sociology with a focus on contemporary theory. A central theme of the chapter has been to illustrate the important role that sociological theory has in the practice of medical sociology. This is because its theories distinguish the subdiscipline from virtually all other scientific fields engaged in the study of health and illness. Such theories provide a sociological perspective or gaze on medical care, disease, health disparities, and other facets of the "social" in relation to health. A mastery of theory is a critical skill for medical sociologists.

As for medical sociology, its importance becomes particularly obvious when epidemiologic transition theory, a theory based in epidemiology, depicts the manner in which the major causes of mortality have changed over time. The theory maintains that infectious and parasitic diseases were prevalent in causing mortality in Stage 1, receded in Stage 2, and were largely replaced by chronic diseases, namely heart disease and cancer, in Stage 3. However, this typology was subject to change again when deaths from cardiovascular diseases abruptly declined after 1960, leading to suggestions that newly emerging infectious diseases be added to Stage 3 or a new Stage 4 be created that recognized the cardiovascular revolution, or the degenerative diseases of aging or hybristic (a mixture) diseases that includes risky behavior and behavioral features of pandemics. Social causes gain in significance in each stage.

A theory is a set of statements or propositions claiming that one class or type of phenomenon is connected in some way to another class of phenomenon that produces a certain condition, behavior, or outcome. Theories explain and provide understanding about what causes something to invariably happen in the way that it does. In sociology, there are three levels of theoretical explanation: (1) the micro, (2) the meso/middle range, and (3) the macro/grand. Virtually all sociological theories today are in the micro or meso/middle range in order to be tested with empirical data so it can be determined whether their conclusions are valid or false. Macro and grand theories make sweeping generalizations about large-scale social phenomena that cannot be tested empirically. They tell us everything about something but nothing that can be verified with certainty since their propositions are too general to be validated with scientific accuracy.

There is also the agency–structure interface in which some theories emphasize agency, a term referring to the ability of individuals to act independently as their own agents in choosing their behavior. Other theories are instead oriented toward explaining the effects of social structures on channeling individual behavior down particular pathways as opposed to others that might be taken. While most theories recognize that agency and structure are both important, there is debate over the extent to which one or the other is dominant in determining social behavior and the social situations in which that dominance occurs.

As for the status of sociological theory in medical sociology, the subdiscipline was one-sidedly atheoretical in its early development. Funding agencies, such as the NIMH, which were instrumental in sponsoring initial research in the field, were not interested in theoretical work on the part of medical sociologists. Rather, they favored research on health that had practical utility by way of helping to solve clinical problems or provide policy recommendations. This situation changed, however, as medical sociology evolved into a highly theoretically engaged specialty.

Guide to Critical Thinking

1. What is a sociological perspective and how would it apply to analyzing health problems?
2. How does epidemiologic transition theory illustrate the increasing importance of medical sociology in the study of health and disease?
3. Define theory and explain its use in research.
4. Describe the different levels of theory in sociology and their characteristics.
5. Define agency and structure in sociological theory. What types of social phenomena do they represent? Explain their relationship.
6. Why did the use of theory in medical sociology become commonplace?

Notes

1   Because of space limitations, not all of the many theories in medical sociology can be included in these pages but only those that are currently most prominent and for whom a sizeable body of literature exists.
2   According to Suchman (1965), the illness experience consists of (1) symptom experience (feels sick), (2) assumption of the sick role (acts sick), (3) medical care contact (sees a doctor), (4) dependent-patient role (becomes a patient), and (5) recovery and rehabilitation (gets well). Even though the illness experience may not involve all five of the stages and can be terminated at any stage, the model depicts the types of decisions and actions patients take over the course of an illness.
3   For example, medical sociologists partnered with physicians and other health scientists in a study of African American health funded by the National Institute of Minority Health and Health Disparities (NIMHD) in 2012–2017 as part of

the Mid-South Transdisciplinary Collaborative Center for Health Disparities Research in the Division of Preventive Medicine at the University of Alabama at Birmingham (UAB) School of Medicine (see the January 2017 special issue of the *American Journal of Preventive Medicine*, co-edited by Mona Fouad, William Cockerham, and Mario Sims).

Suggested Reading

Cockerham, William C. (ed.). 2021. *The New Blackwell Companion to Medical Sociology*. Oxford: Wiley Blackwell.
Contains chapters providing an overview of medical sociology, including theory, by an international group of authors who are specialists in their fields.

References

Archer, Margaret. 1995. *Realist Social Theory: The Morphogenetic Approach*. Cambridge: Cambridge University Press.

Armelagos, George J. and Kristin N. Harper. 2016. "Emerging Infectious Diseases, Urbanization, and Globalization in the Time of Global Warning," in William Cockerham (ed.), *The New Blackwell Companion to Medical Sociology*. Oxford: Wiley-Blackwell, pp. 291–311.

Babbie, Earl, William E. Wagner III, and Jeannie Zaino. 2019. *Adventures in Social Research*, 10th ed. Thousand Oaks, CA: Sage.

Bauman, Zygmunt. 1999. *In Search of Politics*. Stanford, CA: Stanford University Press.

Bloom, Samuel W. 2002. *The Word as Scalpel: A History of Medical Sociology*. New York: Oxford University Press.

Blumer, Herbert. 1931. "Science Without Concepts." *American Sociological Review* 36(January):515–33.

Bongaarts, John. 2014. "Trends in Causes of Death in Low-Mortality Countries: Implications for Mortality Projections." *Population and Development Review* 40(2):189–212.

Camic, Charles and Yu Xie. 1994. "The Statistical Turn in American Social Science: Columbia University, 1890–1915." *American Sociological Review* 59(5):773–805.

Campbell, Colin. 2009. "Distinguishing the Power of Agency from Agentic Power: A Note on Weber and the 'Black Box' of Personal Agency." *Sociological Theory* 27(4):407–18.

Clarke, Adele E., Carrie Friese, and Rachel Washburn. 2018. *Situational Analysis*, 2nd ed. Thousand Oaks, CA: Sage.

Claus, Lisbeth M. 1982. *The Growth of a Sociological Discipline*, Vol. I. Leuven, Belgium: Katholieke Universiteit Leuven.

Cockerham, William C. 1983. "The State of Medical Sociology in the United States, Great Britain, West Germany, and Austria: Applied vs Pure Theory." *Social Science & Medicine* 17:1313–27.

Cockerham, William C. 2005. "Health Lifestyle Theory and the Convergence of Agency and Structure." *Journal of Health and Social Behavior* 46(1):51–67.

Cockerham, William C. 2013a. *Social Causes of Health and Disease*, 2nd ed. Cambridge: Polity.

Cockerham, William C. (ed.). 2013b. *Medical Sociology on the Move: New Directions in Theory*. Dordrecht: Springer.

Cockerham, William C. 2013c. "Sociological Theory in Medical Sociology in the Early Twenty-First Century." *Social Theory & Health* 11(3):241–55.

Cockerham, William C. 2017. *Sociology of Mental Disorder*, 10th ed. London: Routledge.

Cockerham, William C. and Graham Scambler. 2016. "Medical Sociology and Sociological Theory," in William Cockerham (ed.), *The New Blackwell Companion to Medical Sociology*. Oxford: Wiley-Blackwell, pp. 3–26.

Cockerham, William C., Shawn Bauldry, Bryant W. Hamby, James M. Shikany, and Sejong Bae. 2017. "A Comparison of Black and White Racial Differences in Health Lifestyles and Cardiovascular Disease." *American Journal of Preventive Medicine* 52:S56–S62.

Cockerham, William C., Bryant W. Hamby, and Gabriela Oates. 2017. "The Social Determinants of Chronic Disease." *American Journal of Preventive Medicine* 52:S5–S12.

Collyer, Fran (ed.). 2015. *The Palgrave Handbook of Social Theory in Health, Illness and Medicine*. Basingstoke: Palgrave Macmillan.

Conrad, Peter. 2007. *The Medicalization of Society*. Baltimore, MD: Johns Hopkins University Press.

Conrad, Peter. 2013. "Medicalization: Changing Contours, Characteristics, and Contexts," in William Cockerham (ed.), *Medical Sociology on the Move: New Directions in Theory*. Dordrecht: Springer, pp. 195–214.

De Maio, Fernando. 2010. *Health and Social Theory*. Basingstoke: Palgrave Macmillan.

Denzin, Norman K. 2017. *The Research Act*. New York: Routledge.

Denzin, Norman K. and Yvonna S. Lincoln (eds.). 2018. *The Sage Handbook of Qualitative Research*, 5th ed. Thousand Oaks, CA: Sage.

Emirbayer, Mustafa and Ann Mische. 1998. "What is Agency?" *American Journal of Sociology* 103(4):962–1023.

Faris, Robert E. and H. Warren Dunham. 1939. *Mental Disorders in Urban Areas*. Chicago, IL: University of Chicago Press.

Giddens, Anthony. 1984. *The Constitution of Society: Outline of a Theory of Structuration*. Berkeley, CA: University of California Press.

Gold, Margaret. 1977. "A Crisis of Identity: The Case of Medical Sociology." *Journal of Health and Social Behavior* 18(June):160–8.

Gouldner, Alvin W. 1970. *The Coming Crisis of Western Sociology*. New York: Avon.

Guest, Greg, Elizabeth E. Tolley, and Christina M. Wong. 2014. "Qualitative Research Methods," in William C. Cockerham, Robert Dingwall, and Stella Quah (eds.), *The Wiley Blackwell Encyclopedia of Health, Illness, Behavior, and Society*, Vol. IV. Oxford: Wiley Blackwell, pp. 1947–52.

Hafferty, Frederic W. and John B. McKinlay (eds.). 1993. *The Changing Medical Profession: An International Perspective*. New York: Oxford University Press.

Hiatt, Robert A. and Nancy Breen. 2008. "The Social Determinants of Cancer: A Challenge for Transdisciplinary Science." *American Journal of Preventive Medicine* 35:S141–S150.

Hitlin, Steven and Monica Kirkpatrick Johnson. 2015. "Reconceptualizing Agency within the Life Course: The Power of Looking Ahead." *American Journal of Sociology* 120(5):1429–72.

Hollingshead, August B. 1973. "Medical Sociology: A Brief Review." *Milbank Memorial Fund Quarterly* 51(Fall):531–42.

Hollingshead, August B. and Frederick C. Redlich. 1958. *Social Class and Mental Illness: A Community Study*. New York: Wiley.

Holtz, Timothy H., Seth Holmes, Scott Stonington, and Leon Eisenberg. 2006. "Health is Still Social: Contemporary Examples in the Age of Genome." *PLoS Medicine* 3:e419–25.

Illsley, Raymond. 1975. "Promotion to Observer Status." *Social Science & Medicine* 9:63–7.

Johnson, Malcolm. 1975. "Medical Sociology and Sociological Theory." *Social Science & Medicine* 9:227–32.

Light, Donald W. 1993. "Countervailing Power: The Changing Character of the Medical Profession in the United States," in Fred Hafferty and John McKinlay (eds.), *The Changing Medical Profession: An International Perspective*. New York: Oxford University Press, pp. 69–79.

Link, Bruce G. and Jo C. Phelan. 1995. "Social Conditions as Fundamental Causes of Disease." *Journal of Health and Social Behavior* 36(extra issue):80–94.

McDonnell, Orla, Maria Lohan, Abbey Hyde, and Sam Porter. 2009. *Social Theory, Health and Healthcare*. Basingstoke: Palgrave Macmillan.

Merton, Robert K. 1957. *Social Theory and Social Structure*. Glencoe, IL: Free Press.

Meslé, France and Jacques Vallin. 2006. "The Health Transition: Trends and Prospects," in Graziella Caselli, Jacques Vallin, and Guillaume Wunsch (eds.), *Demography: Analysis and Synthesis*, Vol. 2. Cambridge, MA: Academic Press, pp. 247–66.

Mouzellis, Nicos R. 2008. *Modern and Postmodern Social Theorizing*. Cambridge: Cambridge University Press.

Münch, Richard. 1994. *Sociological Theory*, Vol. 1. Chicago, IL: Nelson-Hall.

Nunes, Everardo Duarte. 2014. "A construção teórica na sociologia da saúde: uma reflexão sobre a sua trajetória." [Theoretical Construction in the Sociology of Health: A Reflection on its Trajectory] *Ciência e Saúde Coletiva* [*Science and Public Health*] 19(4):1007–18.

Olshansky, S. Jay and A. Brian Ault. 1986. "The Fourth Stage of the Epidemiologic Transition: The Age of Delayed Degenerative Diseases." *The Milbank Quarterly* 64(3):355–91.

Omran, Abedl R. 1971. "The Epidemiological Transition: A Theory of the Epidemiology of Population Change." *Milbank Memorial Fund Quarterly* 49(5): 509–38.

Phelan, Jo C. and Bruce G. Link. 2013. "Fundamental Cause Theory," in William Cockerham (ed.), *Medical Sociology on the Move: New Directions in Theory*. Dordrecht: Springer, pp. 105–26.

Popper, Karl. [1934] 1992. *The Logic of Scientific Discovery*. London: Routledge.

Porter, Roy. 1997. *The Greatest Benefit to Mankind: A Medical History of Humanity*. New York: W.W. Norton.

Reynolds, Paul Davidson. 2007. *A Primer in Theory Construction*. Boston, MA: Allyn and Bacon.

Ritchey, Ferris E. 2009. *The Statistical Imagination*, 2nd ed. New York: McGraw-Hill.

Ritzer, George and David Walczak. 1988. "Rationalization and the Deprofessionalization of Physicians." *Social Forces* 67(1):1–22.

Rodgers, Richard G. and Robert Hackenberg. 1987. "Extending Epidemiologic Transition Theory: A New Stage." *Social Biology* 34(3–4):234–43.

Rose, David, Eric Harrison, and David Pevalin. 2010. "The European Socio-economic Classification: A Prolegomenon," in David Rose and Eric Harrison (eds.), *Social Class in Europe: An Introduction to the European Socio-economic Classification*. London: Routledge, pp. 3–38.

Scambler, Graham (ed.). 1987. *Sociological Theory and Medical Sociology*. London: Tavistock.

Scambler, Graham (ed.). 2012. *Contemporary Theorists for Medical Sociology*. London: Routledge.

Scambler, Graham. 2018. *Sociology, Health and the Fractured Society*. London: Routledge.

Sewell, William H. 1992. "A Theory of Structure: Duality, Agency, and Transformation." *American Sociological Review* 98:1–2.

Sibeon, Roger. 2004. *Rethinking Social Theory*. London: Sage.

Siegrist, Johannes. 2014. "Middle-Range Theory," in William C. Cockerham, Robert Dingwall, and Stella Quah (eds.), *The Wiley Blackwell Encyclopedia of Health, Illness, Behavior, and Society*, Vol. IV. Oxford: Wiley Blackwell, pp. 1636–9.

Simmons, Leo W. and Harold G. Wolff. 1954. *Social Science in Medicine*. New York: Russell Sage Foundation.

Smelser, Neil J. 1994. *Sociology*. Cambridge, MA: Blackwell.

Smelser, Neil J. 1997. *Problematics of Sociology*. Berkeley, CA: University of California Press.

Sorensen, Aage B. 2009. "Statistical Models and Mechanisms of Social Processes," in Peter Hedström and Björn Wittrock (eds.), *Frontiers of Sociology*. Leiden: Brill, pp. 369–99.

Srole, Leo, T. S. Langner, S. T. Michael, M. K. Opler, and T. A. C. Rennie. 1962. *Mental Health in the Metropolis: The Midtown Manhattan Study*, Vols. 1 and 2. New York: McGraw-Hill.

Starr, Paul. 1982. *The Social Transformation of American Medicine*. New York: Basic Books.

Stones, Rob. 2018. "Agency and Structure," in Bryan S. Turner (ed.), *The Wiley-Blackwell Encyclopedia of Social Theory*. Oxford: Wiley-Blackwell, pp. 20–4.

Suchman, Edward A. 1963. *Sociology and the Field of Public Health*. New York: Russell Sage Foundation.

Suchman, Edward A. 1965. "Social Patterns of Illness and Medical Care." *Journal of Health and Human Behavior* 6(Spring):2–16.

Wagner, William E. III and Brian J. Gillespie. 2019. *Using and Interpreting Statistics in the Social, Behavioral, and Health Sciences*. Thousand Oaks, CA: Sage.

Webster, Murray, Jr. and Barry Markovsky. 2007. "Theory Construction," in George Ritzer (ed.), *The Blackwell Encyclopedia of Sociology*, Vol. X. Oxford: Blackwell, pp. 4987–93.

Chapter 2

Origin of Medical Sociology

Medical sociology's origins are completely unlike those of other major socio-logical subdisciplines in that it did not evolve directly out of nineteenth- and early twentieth-century social thought, and, moreover, another discipline (medicine) initially sponsored its birth. Consequently, medical sociology came about through the convergence of two branches of learning, medicine and sociology, with very different histories and orientations. This circum-stance, in turn, had a significant effect on the early formulation and utiliza-tion of sociological theory by those working in the field.

Medical Sociology's Origins in Medicine

German Influences

Medical sociology's origins are somewhat amorphous as its beginnings as something called "medical sociology" was not at the hands of sociologists. Rather, physicians were the *first* to point out the relevance of the field in their efforts to develop a comprehensive understanding of health and dis-ease. It was a German physician, Rudolf Virchow (1821–1902), known for his significant discoveries in cellular pathology and experimental physiology, and a dominant figure in biomedical research in Berlin for some 50 years, who famously pointed out in 1848 that "medicine is a social science" (Porter 1997:643). This statement was made after Virchow investigated the breakout of a typhus epidemic in 1847 in the Prussian province of Upper Silesia where he determined that an improvement in social conditions for a suppressed Polish minority would produce a more rapid, successful, and longer-lasting cure than medicine; there are times, said Virchow, when a physician's respon-sibility was to serve as an "attorney for the poor" (Porter 1997:415). He argued that the poor should have quality medical care and a free choice of physicians, with improved medical treatment joining with better social con-ditions as the key to achieving the best health possible for the impoverished.

Virchow's contention, however, that adverse social conditions were the cause of many health problems was rejected for political reasons by the Imperial Prussian government who did not want to be held responsible for an epidemic, and he fell into disfavor among the ruling authorities.

Despite his continued eminence in medical science, Virchow's perspective on the social causes of disease was neglected by many in the medical profession as well. Physicians in the 1800s, just as they are today, were primarily focused on treating patients and improving their care, not social reform. The French scientist Louis Pasteur (1822–1896) had demonstrated the effectiveness of his germ theory of disease in 1885 that maintained infections had a specific pathogenic cause (bacteria) that could be treated successfully within a biomedical framework. Robert Koch (1843–1910) in Germany and others in bacteriological research decisively confirmed the germ theory and uncovered the causes of multiple diseases, including typhoid, tetanus, and diphtheria, along with the vaccines providing immunity. Medicine's thinking was dominated by a search for drugs as "magic bullets" that could kill disease (DuBos 1959). Microbiology and physiology were the major areas of research in medicine at this time.

Yet Virchow's calls for giving attention to social conditions were not entirely unheeded, as other physicians likewise found connections between social factors and health (Porter 1997:643). For example, another Berlin physician, Salomon Neumann (1819–1908), supported Virchow's view by arguing that medicine was at its core a social science when he observed the link between poverty and poor health in 1862 (Bloom 2002). To him, poverty and poor health went hand-in-hand. Next was Alfred Grotjahn (1869–1931) who undertook his medical education at the University of Berlin where "Virchow was virtual ruler of the medical faculty as professor of pathological anatomy" (Rabson 1936:47). Grotjahn had spent his first year of medical training at the University of Kiel where he also signed up for a sociology course with the noted German sociologist Ferdinand Tönnies (1855–1936), author of the classic work *Gemeinschaft und Gesellschaft* [Community and Society] published in 1887. Apparently Tönnies was not a good lecturer and so he and Grotjahn, along with the only other student in the class, roamed the city discussing sociology while observing social conditions in person. After he received his medical degree, Grotjahn went into general practice in Berlin where:

> Meanwhile he was busy with his work in sociology and in what he was to found as a distinct branch of medicine, social hygiene. He was one of the founders of the German Sociology Association, taking part in the various seminars. The first monograph to appear, 1902, was on changes in popular nutrition in which comparison was made between the diet

of rural populations with its marked local character and that of industrial populations with monetary payments.

(Rabson 1936:48)

Grotjahn also published a book with the title *Social Pathology*, appearing
first in 1912 and culminating in a third edition in 1923, that presented a
pathology of human diseases from a social perspective and linked various
social conditions to specific ailments. Similarly, by the 1920s in Britain,
the Medical Research Council (MRC) not only promoted randomized
clinical trials for testing drugs but also the development of "social medicine" as a scientific discipline utilizing statistical analysis and the social
sciences in the prevention of disease. According to Carl Binger (Porter
1997:528), an American physician, there had been a shift in emphasis
in medicine in the first decades of the twentieth century away from a
reliance on autopsies to more of a focus on laboratory research to the
extent that:

> in the clinic a brilliant and correct diagnosis (sometimes, to be sure, only
> corroborated at post-mortem examination) was no longer the supreme
> intellectual achievement. Insight and understanding of mechanisms and
> processes became increasingly important.

American Origins

When it came to gaining insight into processes that cause sickness, especially
the health problems of the "whole person" whose symptoms and complaints
extend into causal factors in the social environment, sociological knowledge was relevant. This was seen in the United States where John Shaw
Billings (1838–1913), organizer of the National Library of Medicine and
compiler of the *Index Medicus*, had written about hygiene and sociology
as early as 1879. The term "medical sociology," however, did not appear in
print until 1894 when another physician, Charles McIntire, used it in the
title of an article, "The Importance of the Study of Medical Sociology," that
was published in the *Bulletin of the American Academy of Medicine*. In introdu-
cing this topic, McIntire ([1894:423] 1991:30) asks: "A question then arises,
can there be a particular department of the science of sociology worthy the
name of Medical Sociology?" His answer is yes, there can be, and McIntire
([1894:426] 1991:31) goes on to say that:

> Medical Sociology then has a two-fold aspect. It is the science of the
> social phenomena of the physicians themselves, as a class apart and sep-
> arate; and the science which investigates the laws regulating the relations

between the medical profession and human society as a whole: treating of the structure of both, how the present conditions came about, what progress civilization has effected, and indeed everything relating to the subject.

McIntire depicted ways (i.e., vocabulary, customs, education) in which the medical profession was a distinct social entity. He claimed a close relationship between physicians and the problems of general sociology, thereby suggesting that sociology has questions which can only be solved from a medical standpoint—all of which constitutes a field of study that he was the first to name: "Medical Sociology." In the first textbook on medical sociology published in 1958 in the U.S., the author Norman Hawkins (1958:18) identified McIntire ([1894] 1991) as the founder of medical sociology, stating that:

> A careful and protracted search reveals no pronouncement on the subject prior to McIntire, and it is very unlikely that the term could have occurred much earlier, … In view of the social and medical climate then existing it is not surprising that McIntire's paper should have been written, nor that it should have been written by a physician.

McIntire's paper had previously been a keynote address given on June 3rd, 1893, to a meeting of the American Academy of Medicine in Milwaukee, Wisconsin. His talk, reported in an editorial in Volume 17 of the *American Lancet* (1893:269), was described as a highlight of the meeting and showed "very clearly that as a branch of general sociology the relations of medical men have a definite place not yet fully defined or carefully studied." The *Lancet* (1893:270) editorial went on to welcome medical sociology as an ally:

> It is clear that there is a way of action which will enable a doctor to accomplish the most good and the least harm as he is compelled to pursue an active career among the laity and the profession. The question arises: What is that way? To answer this, is the province of "Medical Sociology." We are aware that pirates exist, who want conflict in order that they may prey upon the spoils of the vanquished; that anarchists abound, who thrive upon the deeds of the lawless; but the mass of human beings, including the medical profession, prefer light to darkness, order to confusion, and would welcome any studies which would aid them in the peaceful pursuit of their calling to the best advantage of all concerned.

Moreover, from 1895 (Volume 1) to 1918 (Volume 19), the American Academy of Medicine published the *Journal of Sociologic Medicine* that focused on medical education, medical organizations and societies, professionalization, and various health topics, such as diet, sleep, and cancer. Financial problems and internal bickering over the journal's access to papers presented at its annual meeting ended its existence. In the meantime, Elizabeth Blackwell (1821–1910) overcame gender discrimination to become the first woman to graduate from an American medical school in 1849 at the now defunct Geneva Medical College in New York. She was admitted as a practical joke on a vote by the all-male student body after the faculty cowardly passed the decision on whether to admit her on to them. Blackwell was barred from viewing nudity in classroom settings and had some other restrictions, but she nevertheless ranked at the top of her class (Porter 1997:357). She went on to practice medicine in New York and later in her native England, and authored a book, self-published in 1899 and commercially published in 1902, with the title *Essays in Medical Sociology*. Her essays dealt with a Christian-oriented account of human sexuality, sexually transmitted (venereal) diseases, over-population, and the rescue of women from prostitution.

This was the first book with medical sociology included in the title ever published. Other relevant early work by physicians included James Warbasse (1866–1957) who published a book in 1909 called *Medical Sociology: A Series of Observations Upon the Sociology of Health and the Relations of Medicine* about physicians as a unique social class with its own characteristics. Warbasse also organized a Section on Sociology for the American Public Health Association which existed between 1909 and 1921 that lacked sociologists and was comprised almost entirely of physicians and social workers who focused their attention on the problems of female and child labor, immigration, and slum housing (Bloom 2002).

Where was Sociology?

Thus far in this account, medical sociology would appear to be created almost exclusively by the medical profession, as physicians drew upon concepts from a fledgling sociology and applied them to medicine to both construct and name a field of study that became medical sociology. Where was sociology as the science of society in all of this? We know from early histories of sociology that the discipline was undergoing its own formative years in the U.S. and Europe in the late 1800s and early 1900s and that medical sociology was not mentioned as one of its core areas of engagement (Barnes 1948; Bloom 2002; Bottomore and Nisbet 1979).

Sociology's Early Founders

The individual generally recognized in sociology as the first sociologist is a fourteenth-century Arab scholar, Ibn Khaldun (1332–1406), born in Tunisia, who eventually settled in Egypt where he worked as a teacher and judge. In his best-known book, *Al' Ibar*, Khaldun suggested the creation of a new science of civilization to explain the history and social dynamics of Arab society. He introduced a theory (*Al' Assabiyya*) of group or tribal social solidarity describing the close social bonds in nomadic tribes like the Bedouins of the Arabian Peninsula and the Berbers of North Africa (Alatas and Sinha 2017), and he also noted that the population density of large urban areas like Cairo and Fez explained the greater frequency of pestilences (epidemics) in those locales (Rosen 1979). Khaldun's theorizing is the first known to be conducted along sociological lines, but his ideas did not find their way into Western social thought until the late twentieth century nor lead to the establishment of sociology as a science.

The person generally credited as the founder of sociology is the French scholar Auguste Comte (1798–1857) who called for a science of society to study social processes and social change. He originally wanted to name this new science "social physics," but the term had already been used by a Belgian social statistician Adolphe Quetelet (1796–1874), inventor of the Quetelet Index, which is the present-day Body Mass Index (BMI) used to determine whether a person is over or underweight. Social physics was Quetelet's title for a potentially new academic field utilizing statistics to study society objectively that he discussed in an 1835 book, *Treatise on Man*. This meant Comte had to find another name. He decided on "sociology" which comes from Latin (*socius*—meaning companion) and Greek (*olgy*— the study of). Sociology thus literally means the study of companions. Since the term "sociology" was a hybrid of Latin and Greek, some language purists found it offensive but it remained as it was (Heilbron 2015).

Comte's major work was a six-volume treatise, *Cours de Philosophie Positive* [Course in Positivist Philosophy], published between 1830 and 1842. Positivism is a view in the philosophy of science that knowledge is valid only when it is based on scientific evidence, a position that has been subject to strong debate. Comte's book included many of the concepts originally expressed by Henri de Saint-Simon (1760–1825), for whom Comte had worked as a secretary, as well as other European theorists, such as David Hume (1711–1776) and Immanuel Kant (1724–1804). Comte integrated these ideas into a comprehensive and systematic positivist concept of society, which was not an easy task. Some of Comte's contributions were original, namely his theory of the law of three stages describing the evolution of the human mind from a primitive to a scientific level and the hierarchy of the sciences. The latter theory depicted scientific thought as an evolutionary process by which one science built on the accomplishments of its predecessors. Beginning with mathematics as the foundation, and proceeding upward through astronomy, physics, chemistry, and biology, and finally sociology which was to sit at the top of all sciences as the capstone, Comte argued that sociologists should form a "priesthood" to manage public education and direct social policy on the basis of scientific study. He did not, however, enjoy great personal or professional success and held a minor administrative post in a Paris school where he was appreciated by only a dwindling handful of disciplines, remaining a marginal figure in French academic circles.

Nevertheless, the potential utility of such a science was increasingly apparent in a Europe undergoing massive social change in the late eighteenth and the nineteenth centuries, and Comte had provided a rationale for it. The old traditional social structures of feudalism that had lasted centuries were either destroyed in the case of the French Revolution or dissolved by the twin processes of industrialization and urbanization unleashed by the Industrial Revolution. No longer did the majority of people live in rural villages within an extended kinship system and produce almost all of what they needed themselves in order to live. Peasants moved to cities to become workers in manufacturing firms. The rise of trade ended the subsistence economy of the medieval era and generated large towns which became economic and cultural centers. Political influence became vested in financial wealth instead of the ownership of land, and wealthy industrialists moved into the top rungs of society; the divine right to rule (handed down by God) attached by tradition to monarchs was replaced by rational-legal authority and representative government; the size of a middle class increased significantly; and a large working class emerged between the middle and lower classes. Western society underwent a dramatic social transformation.

Europe's modernization, however, also brought significant social problems. The cities and towns of the period were unprepared for the great influx of people who left the countryside to seek work in urban centers. Large sections of formerly medieval cities were transformed into sprawling, chaotic slums. Squalor, poor sanitation, long working hours, low wages, and child labor became commonplace as a rural peasant population evolved into an industrial working class. The impetus for the emergence of sociology as a scientific field originated in the social changes brought on by the modernization of Western Europe and the need to understand them. Sociology thus originates within a *European* historical context and it is this context that is the defining background for the discipline and its theories (Alatas and Sinha 2017).

What this means is that sociological theory is Western in origin and outlook, leaving the rest of the world with a general theoretical orientation that is geographically specific. This has been held as an example of the Global North colonizing the Global South by imposing its theories on the rest of the world without reciprocal dialogue (Connell 2007). However, theory today is what it is, and the West's head start in the social sciences and its more extensive development and discourse about theory allowed it to maintain its theoretical dominance in the absence of competing and generalizable non-Western theories.

Box 2.1 The Dominance of the English Language in Sociology

Language played a decisive role in the hegemony of the West in the social sciences, especially in sociology. Although sociology began in France, it spread quickly in Britain and had its greatest early success in the United States (Heilbron 2015). As the importance of English-language sociology increasingly moved to the forefront of the discipline, the requirement to read its literature and write in English to publish in sociological journals of significance became an essential skill. Unless translated, work published in languages other than English does not cross its national boundaries and has only local distribution. As Dutch sociologist Johan Heilbron (2015:2) explains:

> In contemporary social science, books and journals that are not available in English have become more or less invisible outside the language in which they have been published. The United States is the predominant power in international social science and English has become its lingua franca, but although French work has lost some of its standing, it at least has retained some of its originality.

Comte had promoted the idea of a sociological science in Europe and his work had been translated into English, but it remained for others to be more decisive in establishing sociology as an academic discipline and medical sociology as a sociological subdiscipline. One notable figure was the British sociologist Herbert Spencer (1820–1903) who promoted considerable interest in sociology because of his ideas and popularity as a writer. Spencer was home-schooled, but earned a scholarly reputation as an author. His books were considered essential reading by many intellectuals of the period (Barnes 1948; Coser 1977). Spencer is best known in sociology for his theory of social evolution or "Social Darwinism." He applied Charles Darwin's ideas about evolution (e.g., the "survival of the fittest") to the evolution of society that maintained stronger ("fit") societies prosper, while weaker ("unfit") ones decline and disappear. This thesis had great appeal for people in Britain and the United States because it emphasized progress and, on the whole, made their level of civilization at the time appear to be a great success.

But Spencer's ideas fell out of favor when severe economic downturns later caused widespread unemployment and social adversity, thereby demonstrating that progress could have setbacks. Fault was found with some of his other conclusions, such as the claim that technological development and moral improvement accompanied one another hand-in-hand. The more a society was technologically developed, the more moral it was supposed to be. Yet the disadvantaged circumstances of the new industrial working class (i.e., low wages, long working hours, unhealthy living conditions) was considered by social reformers of the period to be immoral rather than moral.

It was Émile Durkheim of France, along with Max Weber and Karl Marx of Germany, instead of Spencer, who emerged as the most influential classical theorists in the late nineteenth century. They are generally recognized as *the* central figures in the establishment of sociology as an academic discipline. Their contributions to theory that medical sociologists still draw from will be examined in chapters 4 and 5. While controversy arises about who else should be included as a founder, and there are other candidates, there is general agreement in the sociological literature today on the status of Durkheim, Weber, and Marx (Giddens et al. 2018; Henslin 2019; Macionis 2018; Ritzer and Murphy 2019; Ritzer and Stepnisky 2018).

The controversy about who else's work is of monumental significance (who should be canonized) in sociology besides the Durkheim–Weber–Marx trio is centered on correcting existing geographical (Europe), gender (male), and racial (white) imbalances (Alatas and Sinha 2017) and/or providing more recent candidates (Outhwaite 2009). A particular problem for non-Western theorists is that their work is non-Western and of limited applicability elsewhere, namely in the West, whereas the established canons in sociology, especially Weber, either include the non-Western world in their work or have had their views imposed on it. According to British sociologist William Outhwaite (2009:1036), these particular credentials (European, male, and white) are a "general feature of British sociology, that … remains particularly strong in the field of social theory and the philosophy of social science"; namely, that "the 'theory boys' tended to be … boys."

The same can be said of American sociology and sociology globally, as Singapore sociologists Farid Alatas and Vineeta Sinha (2017) observe that sociology is taught in universities in Africa and Asia much the same as it is in Britain and North America. They contend it is time to move on to consider non-European and women sociologists who are mentioned only in passing or have been ignored. Outhwaite (2009) suggests that the present-day originators of sociology will likely be only of historical interest at some point and perhaps it is now appropriate to consider late-twentieth-century theorists as canons, such as Zygmunt Bauman (Poland/Britain), Ulrich Beck (Germany), Pierre Bourdieu (France), and Anthony Giddens (Britain)—who are also

European, male, and white—but additionally consider the counter-example of adding a female, Margaret Archer (Britain), who has done fundamental work in critical realism.[1]

Even so, this potential line-up of major theorists remains as European and white in its entirety as its forerunners. As for most female theorists, Outhwaite notes that they have tended to focus on feminist theory, which to him has yet to become a core topic in sociology, and in his view canonization is best achieved by generalists, not specialists. Outhwaite (2009:1036) says:

> It is probably essential for canonical status to be categorized as a general theorist, rather than one specializing in class, gender, ethnicity or in a specialism such as work, education or medicine. But it may also be important to be more than just a theorist and to have some substantive work, such as Giddens's on the state or on self-identity, which readers without a taste for pure theory can latch onto.

Until such time as sociology's canons are changed or enlarged numerically, the views of Marx, Durkheim, and Weber remain foundational work. Most versions of medical sociology's origin, however, claim the field was ignored by the "big" three classical theorists (Cockerham 1983; Gerhardt 1989; Ruderman 1981; Williams 2003). The reason for this is that unlike modes of economic production, legal authority, religion, social stratification, and various other social processes and institutions, medicine did not influence the way societies were organized and structured, or shaped social behavior. Medicine's function was to combat disease, not influence societies to adopt particular social relationships and structural features.

Yet Australian medical sociologist Fran Collyer (2010) points out that Durkheim, Weber, and Marx did not ignore the subject of health altogether. They *did* refer to health and/or disease in some of their writings. For example, Collyer (2015:47) finds that Marx and his colleague Friedrich Engels in the 1840s "had quite a bit to say about illness and disease," which was not surprising "given the dreadful living conditions of the working class at that time" and perhaps Marx's own physical afflictions were made worse by smoking, eating poorly, and not exercising. However, there is no evidence that either Marx or Engels tried to establish medical sociology or promoted the initial use of sociological theory in a nonexistent subdiscipline or, for that matter, even thought about doing so.

Engels' ([1845] 1999) separate observations of English working-class life, published in 1845 under the title of *The Condition of the Working Class in England in 1844*, included descriptions of squalid and unhealthy living and work conditions linked to early industrialization. However, Engels was not a sociologist, and in this instance was a political activist writing about the plight of factory workers. He concluded that the working class was a "race" apart from the English bourgeoisie (middle and upper classes) because of their different dialect, customs, and religion (Catholicism), without noting that many of them were Irish immigrants, not English at all (McDonnell et al. 2009:41). Nevertheless, he found their lives characterized by hardship, accidents, exposure to toxic air, susceptibility to disease, alcoholism, sexual promiscuity, and lessened life expectancy, thereby locating the ultimate cause of their poor health and high mortality (what he called "murder") in their exploited status under capitalism.

Engels was far from being the only person disturbed by the appalling conditions faced by the English working class during early industrialization. William Blake, the famous English poet, for instance, referred to coal-burning and polluting factories as "these dark Satanic Mills" in his classic 1804 poem *Jerusalem*, while the French historian and journalist Alexis de Tocqueville ([1835] 1958:107), known for his commentaries on early nineteenth-century society in Europe and the United States, described the newly industrialized city of Manchester, England, this way:

> From this foul drain the greatest stream of human industry flows out to fertilize the whole world. From this filthy sewer pure gold flows. Here humanity attains its most complete development and its most brutish, here civilization works its miracles and civilized man is turned almost into a savage.

Another, slightly earlier study in Britain was that of Edwin Chadwick, a pioneer in public health, whose *Report of an Enquiry into the Sanitary Conditions of the Labouring Population of Great Britain* in 1842 also linked poverty and filthy living conditions to sickness. While the studies conducted by Engels and Chadwick were important pioneering efforts associating adverse social conditions with poor health, neither study was directly coupled theoretically, methodologically, or substantively at the time to sociology.

Weber's influence in medical sociology is derived from the use of his theories by medical sociologists and his direct comments about health are minimal. Weber mentions health once in his book *The Protestant Ethic and the Spirit of Capitalism* where he (Weber [1930] 1958:163) discusses the acquisition of wealth as a "calling" in the Protestant (Calvinist) faith and comments that: "To wish to be poor, it was often argued, the same as wishing to be unhealthy; it is objectionable as a glorification of works and derogatory to the glory of God."

He also criticized medicine by critiquing a major presupposition underlying its mission to extend life in his famous essay "Science as a Vocation" (Collyer 2010:93). While Weber ([1919] 1946:144) recognized the technical ability of medicine to prolong life and diminish suffering to the greatest degree possible in his day, he questioned whether it "ultimately makes sense to do so" in situations of continued suffering just because medical science makes it possible. As Weber ([1919] 1946:144) put it:

> By this means the medical man preserves the life of the mortally ill man, even if the patient implores us to relieve him of life, even if his relatives, to whom his life is worthless, and to whom the costs of maintaining his worthless life grow unbearable, grant his redemption from suffering.

But he adds that medicine is duty bound to do everything possible they can to keep a patient alive. Whether or not a life is *worth* living, says Weber, is not answered by medicine or the natural sciences, but the human sciences. In taking this position, Weber was protesting against the efforts of the physical sciences in Germany in the early twentieth century to try to marginalize human [social] sciences like sociology, history, law, political science, economics, and philosophy, even though these disciplines, in his view, have humane answers to problems that go beyond straightforward technical solutions.

Moreover, during World War I, for 14 months in 1914–1915, Weber served as a captain in the German army medical corps in Heidelberg as a hospital director and disciplinary officer for the staff. He gained practical experience in bureaucratic procedures useful in formulating what is still the most influential theory of bureaucracy in sociology. Weber was released from active duty at his request after a reorganization of hospital services in the city left him without a military assignment (Radkau 2009). Regardless of his hospital experience, Weber did not formulate theories unique to medical sociology or cause it to come into existence.

The only work of the classical theorists that can arguably be *directly* connected to medical sociology is Durkheim's ([1897] 1951) study of suicide. For this project, Durkheim discussed mental health, namely normal and psychopathic psychological states, along with determining social causes for suicide, classifying its social types, and explaining the nature of suicide as a social phenomenon. Yet his intent in doing so was to establish general sociology by applying scientific methods to the investigation of a social problem which, in this instance, happened to be suicide. Durkheim's practical goal was to demonstrate that sociology was an independent science capable of explaining such phenomena as differences in suicide rates which some scientists of the day thought to be purely psychological in origin or due to mental disease, not social factors.

This aim is seen in the comments of both of Durkheim's most authoritative biographers, Britain's Steven Lukes (1973:192) and Canada's Marcel Fournier (2013:229), who find that the subject of suicide offered itself as an opportunity to demonstrate the research principles expressed by Durkheim in his earlier book *The Rules of Sociological Method* ([1895] 1964). As Durkheim ([1897] 1951:36–8) himself notes in the preface to *Suicide: A Study in Sociology*: "Suicide has been chosen as its subject ... because it seemed to us to be particularly timely ... [and] by such concentration, real laws are discoverable which demonstrate the possibility of sociology better than any dialectical argument." Thus, it was not suicide per se that captured his attention but the fact that "suicide was peculiarly well suited to the task of establishing Durkheim's claims for sociology" (Lukes 1973:192–3). As Lukes (1973:194) explained:

> In the first place, it was on the face of it, the most private of acts— "an individual action affecting the individual only," which "must seemingly depend exclusively on individual factors, thus belonging to psychology alone." Explaining it, or more precisely explaining differential suicide rates sociologically, would be a singular triumph. In the second place, it had the most direct bearing on the initial question of Durkheim's sociological work—"what are the bonds which unite men with one another?"—for it offered the clearest case of the dissolution of those bonds.

In *Suicide*, Durkheim does not actually use the word "disease," rather he refers to "neurasthenia," a vaguely defined medical diagnosis popular in the 1800s that is no longer used in the U.S. It is a condition of excessive fatigue (i.e., chronic fatigue syndrome) accompanied by headaches, irritability, and depression. Durkheim ([1897] 1951:298) notes that suicide had been represented in his time as a product of neurasthenia but says: "Yet we have found no immediate and regular relationship between neurasthenia and the social suicide rate." When rates of neurasthenia were low, he found suicide rates were high, and when suicides were low, neurasthenia rates were high. Neurasthenia was therefore not the major cause of suicide. "The conclusion from all these facts," states Durkheim ([1897] 1951:299), "is that the social suicide-rate can be explained only sociologically." So Durkheim did not ignore mental health in his analysis of suicide, but he pursued its causes in different types of social integration or, most importantly, in the lack thereof.

Elsewhere, in *The Rules of Sociological Method*, Durkheim uses health as an example of "normal" and disease and crime as representative models of "pathological" processes. So Durkheim did refer to mental health and health generally in his writings. But did he establish medical sociology as a distinct sociological subdiscipline in doing so? The answer is no. In sum, it is correct to say the three leading classical theorists and founders of sociology— Durkheim, Weber, and Marx—did not formulate sociological theories of health and medicine, nor recognize medical sociology as a potential field of sociological inquiry, deliberately promote it, organize it, give it a name, or provide evidence they were even aware of it.

Sociology's Neglected Founders and Medical Sociology

Martineau. If the founders of sociology were not cognizant of the possibility of a sociological subdiscipline of medical sociology, what about the neglected founders? Harriet Martineau (1802–1876), an English woman, is sometimes depicted as a neglected founder of sociology and authored *Life in the Sick Room* in 1844. The book is about her personal experience with pain during a lengthy period when she was incapacitated and features practical recommendations and spiritual advice about how to cope with physically painful sensations. However, modern-day claims that her book is a precursor to a medical sociology that did not exist at that time or in the immediate future are highly questionable. The book is neither a sociological analysis of pain nor is there proof of its direct influence on the subsequent development of medical sociology. Since Martineau's pain caused a self-consciousness about her body that she said she might not have otherwise been aware, a better case might be made that this book was more important for forthcoming accounts of the experience of embodiment found in the future literature on the sociology of the body—although it was not cited in British sociologist Bryan Turner's seminal work in this field, *Body and Society* (1984).

Nonetheless, Martineau, who was self-educated and suffered the loss of most of her hearing as a young girl, was clearly an unusual person in that she acquired a reputation not only as a sociologist, but also as a political economist, journalist, anti-slavery abolitionist and feminist, as well as an author of novels, children's stories, and books and essays on travel, religion, matrimony, and other subjects (Annandale 2015; Hoecker-Drysdale 2011). As for sociology, she translated Comte's obtuse and difficult six-volume *Course in Positive Philosophy* ([1853] 1896) from French into English in 1853. She reduced it to three volumes in the process. Comte was so pleased with the translation that he requested it be retranslated from English back into French for republication. The book had little impact in England (Inglis 2006), although Martineau considered this translation to be possibly her best work ever (Hoecker-Drysdale 2011) and some sociologists subsequently found it to be the best source for understanding Comte's work (Coser 1977). Martineau, moreover, developed her own methodological framework for analyzing societies that consisted of investigating its politics, morals, economy, religion, agriculture, domestic life, civil liberties, status of women, and other indicators utilized in her anti-slavery book *Society in America* (1837).

She also wrote *How to Observe Morals and Manners* (1838) some 15 years before she translated Comte's volumes and almost 60 years before Durkheim ([1895] 1964) published *The Rules of Sociological Method*. Martineau does not appear to use the word "sociology" in this book, perhaps because it was not an established or well-known term in 1838 (Comte was inventing it during 1830 to 1840), but she does discuss social institutions and public records as the primary source of information on a society's morals and manners. In fact, she clearly favors such sources of information over anything individuals can provide. Martineau (1838:64) wrote:

> Though the facts sought by travellers relate to Persons, they may most readily be learned by Things. The eloquence of Institutions and Records, in which the action of the nation is embodied and perpetuated, is more comprehensive and faithful than that of any variety of individual voices. The voice of a whole people goes up in the silent workings of an institution; the condition of the masses is reflected from the surface of a record. The Institutions of a nation,—political, religious, or social—put evidence into the observer's hands as to its capabilities and wants which the study of individuals could not yield in a lifetime. The Records of any society, be they what they may, whether architectural remains, epitaphs, civic registers, national music, or any other manifestations of the national mind which may be found among every people, afford more information on Morals in a day than converse with individuals in a year.

Martineau's methodological emphasis on "things," not people, to determine a society's sociability was not out of line with Durkheim's ([1897] 1951) utilization of Western European suicide rates to study suicide (Annandale 2015). While her method would not be regarded as adequate today by sociologists engaging in survey research and conducting face-to-face interviews, or utilizing participant observation or focus groups to collect data directly from individuals, it nonetheless is an example of unobtrusive measures that shows a sociological perspective ahead of her time. Yet Martineau was not given high status as one of sociology's founders and was indeed neglected. Why? Some feminist scholars suggest it was because of the difficulty women had in being recognized for intellectual contributions in the nineteenth century and also that she might not have been considered a credible sociologist by some working in the discipline (Annandale 2015; Hoecker-Drysdale 2011). She lacked a formal education and published on a great variety of topics, including fiction, and sociology was just one of her varied interests.

Gilman. Another person mentioned as a possibility for initiating medical sociology in sociology is Charlotte Perkins Gilman (1860–1935), an American, who wrote a 13-page fictional short story called "The Yellow Wall-paper"

(1892) considered to be an important feminist account of male-centric attitudes toward the mental health of women in the nineteenth century (Allen 2011; Annandale 2015). The lead female character's loving, supportive, and caring physician husband and her physician brother in the story diagnose her symptoms as "temporary depression" or "hysteria." She is confined to an unstimulating upstairs bedroom with yellow wallpaper that takes on a symbolic meaning of its own as she becomes increasingly delusional and psychotic. The extent to which this short story promoted the inception of medical sociology has yet to become apparent. As for Gilman, she had studied art for two years, was self-educated in sociology and went on to become a novelist and short-story writer, as well as a sociologist. She joined the American Sociological Society (ASS), the forerunner to the American Sociological Association, in 1905 when it was first organized, and considered Lester Ward (1841–1913), the first president of ASS, a friend and mentor.

Her father, however, had abandoned his family after her mother's health precluded future pregnancies, leaving Gilman to become her mother's lifelong caretaker beginning as a young girl; her brother left for Utah when older where he married and divorced three times, and her first marriage to a sexually demanding and philandering artist was extremely unhappy (Allen 2011). Perhaps not surprisingly because of these experiences, her most noted publications in sociology were *Women and Economics* (1898) which is a feminist account of heterosexuality and marriage as sexual slavery for women and *The Man-Made World, or Our Androcentric Culture* (1911), a feminist critique of patriarchy, which she dedicated to Lester Ward. Gilman's publications seem largely applicable to feminist sociology rather than foundational works for medical sociology.

Du Bois. The other individual in the neglected founder category is William Edward Burghardt (W.E.B.) Du Bois (1868–1963). Du Bois was the first African American to earn a Ph.D. from Harvard, which he did in 1895 in history. Du Bois had also studied history, economics, and sociology at the University of Berlin and was exposed to the ideas of some of Germany's more innovative social scientists of the day, such as the historical economist Gustav von Schmoller (1838–1917) and the sociologist Georg Simmel (1858–1918). Du Bois emerged from his studies with extraordinary academic credentials in the late nineteenth century, which he intended to use to conduct research relevant to improving the social position of blacks in American society (Morris 2017; Taylor 2011; Wright 2016).

His first faculty position was at historically black Wilberforce University in Ohio (1894–1896) as a professor of ancient languages, followed by an appointment as an "assistant in sociology" at the University of Pennsylvania (1896–1897). While there he went directly into black neighborhoods, observing social conditions and interviewing some 5,000 individuals for his book, *The Philadelphia Negro* (1899). Organizing his analysis around the concept of heterogeneity, Du Bois determined that blacks were not a single, monolithic group in Philadelphia but a diverse population with distinct intraracial differences in social-class position (namely, families of undoubted respectability, the respectable working class, the poor, and criminals), as well as diversity in politics and church membership (Du Bois 1899; Hunter 2015). Black society, in Du Bois's (1968:206) view, was not locked into a fixed and rigid social structure, but was changing and evolving. He coined the term "the Talented Tenth" to describe the ten percent of blacks in his study qualifying as an intellectual elite whom he believed could serve as role models for achieving racial equality (Wright 2016).

Atlanta University, an historically black institution in the city of Atlanta, Georgia, offered Du Bois the opportunity in 1898 to establish an academic base to conduct a long-term study of black Americans, which he accepted to become a professor in history and economics and director of the Atlanta Sociological Laboratory. Earl Wright II (2016) calls this laboratory "The First American School of Sociology" in that it preceded the famous (in sociology) "Chicago School of Sociology" that dominated the discipline from 1915 to 1940. Despite problems in funding and other issues, Du Bois conducted a series of annual conferences and studies of urban blacks from 1898 to 1910. He continued to edit the lab's reports until 1913, three years after he had left Atlanta to become the Director of Publications and Research for the National Association for the Advancement of Colored People (NAACP).

One of these reports (Atlanta University Publication #11, 1906) was on "The Health and Physique of the Negro American." It was based on two centuries of data (1700–1900) from the U.S. Census, life insurance company reports, U.S. Surgeon General reports, various city records, reports from black hospitals, pharmacies, medical schools, and physicians, along with the physical measurements of 1,000 Hampton University student volunteers (Wright 2016:45–7). The study concluded that infant and overall mortality among blacks was decreasing, mortality from tuberculosis—a particularly deadly disease for blacks at the time—was declining, and no evidence was found that blacks were physically inferior to whites.

This report qualifies as the first academic study of physical health conducted by a sociologist *ever*. Not only was it the first such study of the health of blacks, it was the first sociological study of the physical health of anyone. But it was ignored. Why? Wright (2016:97–9) and others (Morris 2017) make the case that the university's marginalization and invisibility in the scientific world was due to racism as evidenced by a general lack of interest in what the Atlanta Laboratory was doing. Wright (2016:47) quotes E. Montague Cobb of Howard University School of Medicine, cited by Du Bois (1968:vi) in his autobiography, who claimed that neither the black medical profession nor the educational world were ready to receive such research at the time and whites were hostile to it; thus, Du Bois's only venture into health studies is depicted in American football terms as "an extraordinary forward pass heaved the length of the field, but there were no receivers."

Summary

Medical sociology came about through the convergence of two branches of learning, medicine and sociology, with very different histories and orientations. Neither the most important classical theorists in sociology—Durkheim, Weber, and Marx—nor the neglected founders established medical sociology. Rather, its origin was in medicine. Physicians, such as Virchow, Grotjahn, and Neumann in Germany, during the 1800s had observed and publicized the relationship between health and social conditions, while McIntire, Blackwell, and Warbasse in the U.S. in the early 1900s initiated discussions about the need for medical sociology, wrote about it, and McIntire named the field.

Guide to Critical Thinking

1. Is the origin of medical sociology in medicine or sociology? How did its origin affect the use of sociological theory among those working in the field?
2. Who gave medical sociology its name and why?
3. Which classical theorist is best connected to medical sociology? Explain.

Note

1 Critical realism is a theoretical perspective that emerged in Britain in the 1990s and is largely based on the work of the English philosopher Roy Bhaskar (1944–2014) and its subsequent application to sociology by Margaret Archer (1995, 2000, 2003). Briefly stated, a goal of critical realism is to connect agency and structure in a way that the distinguishing properties of both can be realistically explained. Consequently, critical realism treats agency and structure as fundamentally distinct but interdependent elements that need to be studied separately in order to understand their respective contributions to the conduct of social life. It takes the position that social systems are open to change and people in their role as agents have the critical reflexivity and creativity to shape structure, yet, in turn, are themselves shaped by structure through patterned forms of behavior in a dialectical process in which each acts upon the other. Structure, for its part, is relatively enduring, although it can be modified, and deep structures have generative mechanisms going beyond superficial observation that influence behavior. While the theory's propositions have considerable relevance for research in

medical sociology (see, for example, Scambler 2018), it has yet to be widely used and there is little applicable empirical data in support of the theory to date.

Suggested Reading

Alatas, Farid Syed and Vineeta Sinha. 2017. *Sociological Theory Beyond the Canon*. London: Palgrave Macmillan.
Reviews the sociological theories of Marx, Weber, and Durkheim as well as various non-Western and women theorists.

References

Alatas, Farid Syed and Vineeta Sinha. 2017. *Sociological Theory Beyond the Canon*. London: Palgrave Macmillan.
Allen, Judith A. 2011. "Charlotte Perkins Gilman," in George Ritzer and Jeffrey Stepnisky (eds.), *The Wiley-Blackwell Companion to Major Social Theorists*, Vol. I. Oxford: Wiley-Blackwell, pp. 283–304.
American Lancet. 1893. "Editorial." 17:269–70.
Annandale, Ellen. 2015. "Harriet Martineau and Charlotte Perkins Gilman: Forgotten Women in the Study of Health and Gender," in Fran Collyer (ed.), *The Palgrave Handbook of Social Theory in Health, Illness and Medicine*. Basingstoke: Palgrave Macmillan, pp. 19–34.
Archer, Margaret S. 1995. *Realist Social Theory: The Morphogenetic Approach*. Cambridge: Cambridge University Press.
Archer, Margaret S. 2000. *Being Human: The Problem of Agency*. Cambridge: Cambridge University Press.
Archer, Margaret S. 2003. *Structure, Agency and the Internal Conversation*. Cambridge: Cambridge University Press.
Barnes, Harry Elmer. 1948. *An Introduction to the History of Sociology*. Chicago, IL: University of Chicago Press.
Blackwell, Elizabeth. 1902. *Essays in Medical Sociology*. London: Ernest.
Bloom, Samuel W. 2002. *The Word as Scalpel: A History of Medical Sociology*. New York: Oxford University Press.
Bottomore, Tom and Robert Nisbet. 1979. *A History of Sociological Analysis*. London: Heinemann.
Cockerham, William C. 1983. "The State of Medical Sociology in the United States, Great Britain, West Germany, and Austria: Applied vs Pure Theory." *Social Science & Medicine* 17:1313–27.
Collyer, Fran. 2010. "Origins and Canons: Medicine and the History of Sociology." *History of the Human Sciences* 23:86–108.
Collyer, Fran. 2015. "Karl Marx and Frederich Engels: Capitalism, Health and the Healthcare Industry," in Fran Collyer (ed.), *The Palgrave Handbook of Social Theory in Health, Illness and Medicine*. Basingstoke: Palgrave Macmillan, pp. 35–58.
Comte, Auguste. [1853] 1896. *The Positive Philosophy of Auguste Comte*. London: Bell.
Connell, Raewyn. 2007. *Southern Theory: Social Science and the Global Dynamics of Knowledge*. Cambridge: Polity.

Coser, Lewis A. 1977. *Masters of Sociological Thought*, 2nd ed. New York: Harcourt Brace Jovanovich.

Du Bois, W. E. B. 1899. *The Philadelphia Negro: A Social Study*. Philadelphia, PA: University of Pennsylvania Press.

Du Bois, W. E. B. 1968. *The Autobiography of W. E. B. Du Bois: A Soliloquy on Viewing My Life from the Last Decade of Its First Century*. New York: International Publishers.

DuBos, René. 1959. *The Mirage of Health*. New York: Harper & Row.

Durkheim, Émile. [1895] 1964. *The Rules of Sociological Method*. Glencoe, IL: Free Press.

Durkheim, Émile. [1897] 1951. *Suicide: A Study in Sociology*. New York: Free Press.

Engels, Friedrich. [1845] 1999. *The Condition of the Working Class in England in 1844*. Oxford: Oxford University Press.

Fournier, Marcel. 2013. *Émile Durkheim*. Cambridge: Polity.

Gerhardt, Uta. 1989. *Ideas about Illness: An Intellectual and Political History of Medical Sociology*. London: Macmillan.

Giddens, Anthony, Mitchell Duneier, Richard P. Applebaum, and Deborah Carr. 2018. *Introduction to Sociology*, 10th ed. New York: W. W. Norton.

Gilman, Charlotte Perkins. 1892. "The Yellow Wall-paper." *New England Magazine* 5(January):647–56.

Gilman, Charlotte Perkins. 1898. *Women and Economics: A Study of the Economic Relation between Men and Women as a Factor in Social Evolution*. Boston, MA: Small, Maynard & Co.

Gilman, Charlotte Perkins. 1911. *The Man-Made World or, Our Androcentric Culture*. New York: Charlton.

Hawkins, Norman. 1958. *Medical Sociology*. Springfield, IL: Charles Thomas.

Heilbron, Johan. 2015. *French Sociology*. Ithaca, NY: Cornell University Press.

Henslin, James M. 2019. *Essentials of Sociology: A Down to Earth Approach*, 14th ed. Boston, MA: Sage.

Hoecker-Drysdale, Susan. 2011. "Harriet Martineau," in George Ritzer and Jeffrey Stepnisky (eds.), *The Wiley-Blackwell Companion to Major Social Theorists*, Vol. I. Oxford: Wiley-Blackwell, pp. 61–95.

Hunter, Marcus Anthony. 2015. "W.E.B. Du Bois and Black Heterogeneity: How *The Philadelphia Negro* Shaped American Sociology." *The American Sociologist* 46(2):219–33.

Inglis, David. 2006. "The Peculiarities of the British: Social Theory in the United Kingdom," in Gerard Delanty (ed.), *Handbook of Contemporary European Social Theory*. London: Routledge, pp. 82–94.

Lukes, Steven. 1973. *Émile Durkheim*. Harmondsworth: Penguin.

Macionis, John J. 2018. *Sociology*, 16th ed. Harlow: Pearson Education.

Martineau, Harriet. 1837. *Society in America*. New York: Saunders and Otley.

Martineau, Harriet. 1838. *How to Observe Morals and Manners*. London: C. Knight.

Martineau, Harriet. [1844] 2003. *Life in the Sick Room*. Orchard Park: Broadview Press.

McDonnell, Orla, Maria Lohan, Abbey Hyde, and Sam Porter. 2009. *Social Theory, Health and Healthcare*. Basingstoke: Palgrave Macmillan.

McIntire, Charles [1894] 1991. "The Importance of the Study of Medical Sociology." *Bulletin of American Academy of Medicine* 1:425–33. Reprinted in *Sociological Practice*

9(1):30–7, 1991. Available at: http://digitalcommons.wayne.edu/socprac/vol9/iss1/5.

Morris, Aldon. 2017. *The Scholar Denied: W.E.B. Du Bois and the Birth of Modern Sociology.* Berkeley, CA: University of California Press.

Ogburn, William Fielding. 1922. *Social Change with Respect to Culture and Original Nature.* New York: Huebsch.

Outhwaite, William. 2009. "Canon Formation in Late 20th-Century British Sociology." *Sociology* 43(6):1029–45.

Porter, Roy. 1997. *The Greatest Benefit to Mankind: A Medical History of Humanity.* New York: W.W. Norton.

Rabson, S. Milton. 1936. "Alfred Grotjahn, Founder of Social Hygiene." *Bulletin of the New York Academy of Medicine* 12(2):43–58.

Ritzer, George and Jeffrey Stepnisky. 2018. *Sociological Theory*, 10th ed. Los Angeles, CA: Sage.

Ritzer, George and Wendy A. Wiedenhoft Murphy. 2019. *Essentials of Sociology*, 3rd ed. Thousand Oaks, CA: Sage.

Rosen, George. 1979. "The Evolution of Social Medicine," in Howard E. Freeman, Sol Levine, and Leo G. Reeder (eds.), *Handbook of Medical Sociology*, 3rd ed. Englewood Cliffs, NJ: Prentice-Hall, pp. 23–50.

Ruderman, Florence. 1981. "What is Medical Sociology?" *Journal of the American Medical Association* 245:927–9.

Scambler, Graham. 2018. *Sociology, Health and the Fractured Society.* London: Routledge.

Taylor, Paul C. 2011. "William Edward Burghardt Du Bois," in George Ritzer and Jeffrey Stepanisky (eds.), *The Wiley-Blackwell Companion to the Major Social Theorists*, Vol. 1. Oxford: Wiley-Blackwell, pp. 426–47.

Tocqueville, Alexis de. [1835] 1958. *Journeys to England and Ireland.* New Haven, CT: Yale University Press.

Tönnies, Ferdinand. 1887. *Gemeinschaft und Gesellschaft [Community and Society].* Leipzig: Fues's Verlag.

Turner, Bryan S. 1984. *The Body and Society.* Oxford: Blackwell.

Warbasse, James P. 1909. *Medical Sociology: A Series of Observations Upon the Sociology of Health and the Relations of Medicine.* New York: Appleton.

Weber, Max. [1919] 1946. "Science as a Vocation," in H. Gerth and C. Wright Mills (eds. and trans.), *From Max Weber: Essays in Sociology.* New York: Oxford University Press, pp. 129–56.

Weber, Max. [1930] 1958. *The Protestant Ethic and the Spirit of Capitalism*, Talcott Parsons (trans.). New York: Scribner's.

Williams, Garteh. 2003. "The Determinants of Health: Structure, Context, and Agency." *Sociology of Health & Illness* 25:131–54.

Wright, Earl II. 2016. *The First American School of Sociology.* Farnham: Ashgate.

Chapter 3

Medical Sociology and the Rise of Theory

The evidence thus far shows medical sociology was initially created by medicine, but interest in it by sociologists began to surface. One of the first was Bernard Stern (1894–1956), a Jewish immigrant from Germany. In 1927, some twenty years after Du Bois's ground-breaking study of African American health, Stern published what appears to be the first book on health and medicine in the U.S. from a distinctly sociological perspective. Earlier, Michael Davis had published *Immigrant Health and the Community* in 1921, but on reading his book it is apparent that it is more applicable to social work than sociology. Stern's book, *Social Factors in Medical Progress*, was a Marxist interpretation of medical history. What made it sociological was that it applied William Ogburn's (1922) theory of social change to the historical evolution of medical science. Ogburn depicted technological development as the primary catalyst for change, which fit medicine's experience. This book was followed by another in 1941, *Society and Medical Progress*, in which Stern argued that social factors were important in successfully treating patients.

Stern had attended medical school in Austria for a year before dropping out because of ill health and instead earned a doctorate in social anthropology at Columbia University, to which he eventually returned as a faculty member in sociology. He turned his attention to the study of the role of medicine in society; in doing so he promoted the establishment in sociology of a "sociology of medicine" and criticized sociologists for not giving more attention to medical problems (Bloom 2002). He did this at a time when there was almost nothing on the topic in sociology as Du Bois's study was generally unknown.

In a presentation, with the title "Toward a Sociology of Medicine," at the annual meeting of the Eastern Sociological Society in 1951, Stern ([1959] 1991:40) contended that the moment had arrived for the sociology of medicine to separate from social medicine, a medical field which he considered vague, ill-defined, no longer a bold idea, and focused on specific diseases rather than the health problems of the "whole person" that required consideration of the social environment. In his view, a sociology of medicine was best equipped to research the latter topic. Stern's ([1959] 1991:40–2) argument for this field to have its own existence included the need for sociological research on chronic diseases, the status effects of medical specialization, the organization of the modern hospital, the aging of the population, the distribution of medical services to disadvantaged groups, and similar topics. As Stern ([1959] 1991:39) put it:

> The field of sociology of medicine offers a stimulating area of research for sociologists who accept this definition of the function of their discipline. Its problems are vital ones and its data are sufficiently capable of controlled observation to enable the sociologists to test the validity of current concepts and to permit the formulation of new principles. Its range of problems … in fact, … [run] the entire gamut of conventional topics under which sociologists are prone to classify their major interests. The sociology of medicine permits the fruitful marriage of theory and practice; it is both speculative and practical, analytical and constructive.

Despite his well-developed rationale for advancing the sociological study of medicine, Bloom (2002) notes that Stern's primary influence was on his students who went on to become medical sociologists. Stern ended his 25-year career at Columbia, just as he had started, as a lecturer, never advancing to a professorial rank. He edited a Marxist journal and held leftist political views which many of his contemporaries rejected, although his sociological work in relation to medicine did not overtly advocate a political agenda. Bloom (2002:100) states: "The irony for Stern was that despite his reasoned scholarship and the lack of dogmatism in his writings, he was during the last decade of life publicly judged mainly as a radical."

Medical Sociology's Emergence in Sociology

Nevertheless, Stern's call for the formation of a specialty in medical sociology in the U.S. came at a time when the number of sociologists showing an interest in health and medicine was growing and starting to teach medical sociology courses in medical schools and sociology departments in universities, as well as working on funded research. Medicine had opened the door to jobs in this field and many responded (Claus 1982; Cockerham 1983). In a significant development, Yale University reacted to this emerging interest by offering the first Ph.D. program in medical sociology in 1954, which signified that the field's academic legitimacy and potential for theoretical discourse had arrived.[1]

Earlier, in 1950, a group of social scientists interested in the study of health and medicine had met informally at the Society for Applied Anthropology meeting at Vassar College in New York (Wardwell 1982). The purpose of the meeting was to organize the interested parties into an identifiable professional group. Walter Wardwell (1982:565), a medical sociologist, who attended the meeting said that: "I recall no discussion of the boundaries of the field or of its central focus, or even whether a definition of the field was needed, which left each person to define the field at will." Perhaps because the majority of participants were sociologists, the "prevailing sentiment," says Wardwell, was that they align themselves with the American Sociological Society (ASS). The result of this meeting was the formation of a Committee for Medical Sociology that operated as an informal group in ASS beginning in 1955 under the leadership of August Hollingshead. When ASS became the American Sociological Association (ASA) in 1959, this committee petitioned ASA on September 3, 1959 to become a Section on Medical Sociology (Bloom 2002; Wardwell 1982).[2]

Medical sociology subsequently became one of the largest ASA sections (currently the third largest) and at times has been the largest. The effect of the affiliation with ASA was to strengthen the professional credentials of medical sociologists through a formal connection to academic sociology. As Wardwell (1982:565) pointed out, the establishment of medical sociology as a section of ASA (1) announced the field as part of sociology rather than some other social science; (2) signaled that the field was not to be limited to applications of social science to medicine, but would also include its own approaches toward understanding, analyzing, and verifying scientific hypotheses; and (3) making the field a subdivision of the principal academic society of sociologists which ensured that it could avoid potential domination by the medical profession.

Consequently, the 1950s were a watershed period for American medical sociology, which included the professionalization of the field and a foundation for the emergence of theory. Until this time medical sociology was unquestionably an applied atheoretical subdiscipline, but this was about to change. What turned out to be an important early step in the direction of theory begins with Lawrence J. Henderson's 1935 paper, "Physician and Patient as a Social System," which appeared in the *New England Journal of Medicine*. Henderson (1878–1942) was a physician and biochemistry professor at Harvard College, who became interested in sociological theory and changed careers to teach in the new social relations (sociology) department when it was formed in the early 1930s (Bloom 2002).

Henderson (1935a) drew from the natural sciences, specifically physics and physiology, to advance a theory in sociology that social relationships were social "systems" in that one relationship interacted with another in an interconnected state of mutual dependence. Henderson (1935b) illustrated this concept with his depiction of the interaction that takes place between doctors and their patients. Doctors needed patients in order to perform their role and patients likewise needed doctors. Henderson was a significant influence on Talcott Parsons, who was one of his students. In fact, Parsons (1951:vii) credited Henderson for identifying "the extreme importance of the concept of system in scientific theory." Not only did medical sociology originate in medicine, but a physician turned sociologist provided the foundation for the first major sociological theory in the subdiscipline.

Talcott Parsons and the Sick Role

The decisive event that oriented medical sociology toward theoretical concerns was the publication of Parsons' long anticipated book, *The Social System* (1951). This book solidified the author's reputation at the time as *the* dominant figure in American sociology and in sociology globally (Callinicos 2007; Gouldner 1970; Ritzer and Stepnisky 2018). Anything Parsons (1902–1979) published attracted attention because it was widely believed at the time that he and his students were devising the future direction for all of sociology (Johnson 1975:1). Parsons' reputation had been established with the publication of his book, *The Structure of Social Action* (1937), when he was an assistant professor at Harvard. This book had reviewed the theoretical reasoning of Alfred Marshall, Vilfredo Pareto, Émile Durkheim, and Max Weber and expressed the foundation of Parsons' own approach to structural logic. *The Structure of Social Action* also introduced the theories of Durkheim and Weber, neither of whom were particularly well-known internationally at the time (Johnson 1975).

The Social System, coming years later in 1951, presented a structural-functionalist model of society that contained Parsons' concept of the sick role. This was the first time any major sociological theorist had directly focused on the function of medicine in a concept of society.

Parsons' interest was in comparing the roles of professionals in capitalist and socialist societies. One of his examples was medical practice. "This field [medicine] has been a subject of long-standing interest on the author's part," wrote Parsons (1951:428–9) about himself, "as a result of which he has a greater command of the empirical material in this field than in most others." Parsons had participated in an incomplete field study of medical practice in the Boston area some years before and had access to the unpublished data; additionally, he had undergone training in psychoanalysis in the 1950s at the Boston Psychoanalytic Institute (Parsons 1951; Smelser 1998).

This latter experience, along with the recommendation of a colleague, had immersed him in the theories of the Austrian psychoanalyst Sigmund

Freud, who also became an important influence in his thinking (Parsons 1981). Moreover, Parsons had completed his doctoral studies in sociology and economics at Heidelberg University in Germany in 1927. While there, he participated in the "Weber Circle" that continued to meet regularly to discuss sociology after Weber's death with his widow, Marianne Weber, hosting the gatherings in her home. Parsons subsequently received her permission to translate Weber's book, *The Protestant Ethic and the Spirit of Capitalism* ([1930] 1958) from German into English, since no English translation was yet available. "The very fact that I later decided to translate it," said Parsons (1981:164), "is an index of its impact on me." Parsons went on to reintroduce the importance of both Weber and Durkheim to European sociologists through his publications and reputation after the disruption of World War II. This was a major contribution toward reestablishing sociology in Europe following the war. Parsons' concept of the sick role in *The Social System* (1951) is based on structural–functionalist theory, or simply functionalism, the seeds of which originated in Durkheim's *The Division of Labor in Society* ([1893] 1964). Briefly stated, the Parsonian version of functionalist theory maintains that social systems are composed of closely interconnected parts and that changes occurring in one part of the system inevitably affect to some degree all other parts of that system. This is because society exists in a state of equilibrium or balance in which its components operate in unison through a consensus of shared norms and values that are "functional" in that they produce stable and harmonious patterns of social life. These patterns counterbalance "dysfunctional" processes, such as sickness and crime that disrupt social order.

The tendency of a society to establish and maintain a state of equilibrium is similar to the biological concept of homeostasis, in which the human body attempts to regulate its physiological functioning within a relatively constant range. In fact, Henderson (1935b:46; Gerhardt 1989:xvi), a major influence on Parsons as previously noted, had claimed that physiological equilibrium is *logically* identical with social equilibrium. Consequently, a social system is viewed in a functionalist perspective as maintaining its ability to function by regulating its various parts within a relatively constant range of well-being. Dysfunctional processes are contained and isolated by institutions within the system, such as hospitals for the sick and prisons for criminals. A social system may have problems but still "function" because of its overall capacity to operate efficiently.

Sickness is accorded a deviant social status by Parsons and since the sick are often unable to take care of themselves, it is necessary for them to seek treatment from physicians in order to recover and, if necessary, be hospitalized. This behavior is predicated on the assumption that being sick is undesirable and the sick person wants to get well. Medical practice in this context is a mechanism by which a social system seeks to control the illnesses of its deviant sick by returning them to as normal a state of functioning as possible.

However, being sick, Parsons argues, is not just experiencing the physical condition of a sick state; rather, it constitutes a social role because it involves behavior based on institutional expectations and is reinforced by the norms of society corresponding to these expectations. Parsons' concept of the sick role consists of four basic propositions outlining the normative pattern for being sick in society:

- *The sick person is exempt from "normal" social roles.* An individual's illness is grounds for his or her exemption from normal roles and responsibilities. The degree of exemption is based on the nature and severity of the illness and requires legitimation by a physician as the authority on what constitutes sickness. Legitimation serves the social function of protecting society against malingering.
- *The sick person is not responsible for his or her condition.* An individual's illness is usually thought to be beyond his or her own control. Some curative process, apart from personal willpower or motivation, is needed to get well.
- *The sick person should try to get well.* The first two aspects of the sick role are conditional on the third, which is recognition by the sick person that being sick is undesirable. Exemption from normal responsibilities is temporary and conditional on the desire to regain normal health. Thus, the sick person has an obligation to get well.
- *The sick person should seek technically competent help and cooperate with the physician.* The obligation to get well involves a further obligation on the part of the sick person to seek technically competent help, usually from a physician. The sick person is also expected to cooperate with the physician in the process of trying to get well.

As noted earlier in this chapter, this was the first theoretical concept directly applicable to medical sociology. At the time, in the 1950s, when Parsons formulated the sick role, his view of functionalism was *the* leading theoretical perspective in all of sociology, and Parsons extended this dominance to medical sociology. His concept was recognized as "a penetrating and apt analysis of sickness from a distinctly sociological point of view" (Freidson 1970:228). Consequently, Parsons, more so than any other sociologist, ushered medical sociology into "academic respectability" by providing it with its inaugural theoretical orientation. Although Parsons' views were later subjected to severe criticism, this eventual outcome does not negate this significant contribution to medical sociology. He demonstrated that the topic of sickness could be an important area of sociological theorizing (Cockerham 2012).

Several follow-on studies were based on Parsons' sick role concept (for example, see Chalfant and Kurtz 1971; Cole and LeJeune 1972; Waitzkin 1971). Additionally, Merton and his colleagues extended the functionalist mode of analysis to the socialization of medical students in their book, *The Student Physician* (1957), with Renée Fox's chapter on training for uncertainty another noteworthy contribution to the literature. However, other major works in medical sociology grounded in a functionalist perspective were not forthcoming with the exception of Uta Gerhardt's defense of Parsons in her book *Ideas About Illness* (1989) and Fox's textbook, *The Sociology of Medicine* (1989) that had a special acknowledgment to Parsons who had introduced her to the field as a student.

Although once the dominant theory in all of sociology, we know now that Parsons was unsuccessful in providing the definitive theory of society and structural-functionalism is no longer an active theory. In fact, one of Parsons' most lasting contributions may have been to call attention to medical sociology as a fertile theoretical field and, in doing so, anoint it as an academic subdiscipline.

Oddly, the first textbook in the field in the U.S., *Medical Sociology: Theory, Scope and Methods* (1958) by Norman Hawkins, cited neither Parsons, nor the sick role. While this might be evidence that the sick role was not such a pivotal event in medical sociology, Hawkins was an *applied* medical sociologist at the University of Texas Medical Branch in Galveston. He approached medical sociology from what he described as a biocultural standpoint. "Most events of concern to medical sociology," said Hawkins (1958:68), "are reactions of systems composed of organisms and environments." Consequently, in his chapter on "The Matrix of Man," he presented a homeostatic (physiological/biological) theory of society as an "open system" very similar to that of Parsons (though citing neither Parsons nor Henderson), and did so in relation to an analysis of stress. Hawkins (1958:69) observed that his theory "embraces the chemical, physical, psychological, and cultural organization of humankind" and credits medical sociology as "not bound by historic trends in theory which tend to create vested interests," which allowed him to take an interdisciplinary approach. In this chapter, he also discusses "the culture of theory" that is largely a critique of the works of Darwin and Freud, and the need to test theories empirically. Otherwise, the textbook was about aging, applied science, community relations, and research methods. "Only a very conceited or very ignorant persons" said Hawkins (1958:xiii), "would expect the statements in this book to stand for any great span of time as an important contribution to learning." Which, indeed, was true.

Coincidentally or not, another medical sociology book came out the same year from the same department that nonetheless included an essay by Parsons (1958) and other papers by academic as well as applied medical sociologists. This was the first edition of E. Gartly Jaco's edited book, *Patients, Physicians, and Illness* (1958). Jaco was a member of the faculty in the same medical sociology department at the University of Texas Medical Branch at Galveston as Hawkins. Whether they ever discussed each other's books in detail with one another is not known, though one would think likely. Nonetheless, Jaco's book was decidedly different, in that his was an edited collection of readings with sociological theory. It included Parsons' paper, "Definitions of Health and Illness in Light of American Values and Social Structure," in all three editions, the last of which appeared in 1979 with half of the 27 chapters authored or co-authored by medical sociologists in sociology departments. Three chapters were on the sick role alone.

Another indicator of Parsons' impact on medical sociology is the prominence of his work in the first and subsequent editions of the *Handbook of Medical Sociology* (Freeman, Levine, and Reeder 1963); some 12 out of 19 substantive chapters in the initial edition cited his publications. In the many textbooks on medical sociology that appeared in the 1960s and 1970s, Parsons' theories were clearly prominent. This is seen in the first editions of David Mechanic's *Medical Sociology* (1968), Rodney Coe's *Sociology of Medicine* (1970), Leon Robertson and Margaret Heagarty's *Medical Sociology: A General Systems Approach* (1975), and Andrew Twaddle and Richard Hessler's *A Sociology of Health* (1977), which included a foreword written by Parsons.

The banner year for American textbooks in medical sociology was 1978 in which four such books were published—the second editions of Mechanic and Coe, John Denton's *Medical Sociology*, and the first edition of the author's *Medical Sociology* text (Cockerham 1978) that will appear in a fifteenth (2021) edition. Elsewhere, in Britain, the first medical sociology textbook was *Sociology in Medicine* (1962) by Mervyn Susser and William Watson, while in the former West Germany the first was *Lehrbuch der Medizinisichen Soziologie* [Textbook of Medical Sociology] (1974) by Johannes Siegrist and in communist East Germany it came much later in *Medizin Soziologie* [Medical Sociology] (1987) edited by Hannes Hüttner. The French, however, did not have a textbook until 1994 with the publication of *Sociologie de la maladie de la Medecine* [Sociology of Illness and Medicine] by Paul Adam and Claudine Herzlich. All of these books not only discussed Parsons, but they signaled the existence of a large market for such publications in the U.S. and Europe, in addition to providing evidence of an established, robust, and highly active sociological subdiscipline interested in health with a theoretical orientation.

Yet as Fran Collyer (2018:113) notes, even as Parsons' status reached its peak, criticisms of functionalist theory and of Parsons began. Four major shortcomings of the sick role were identified: (1) some sick people behaved differently than Parsons suggested; (2) the sick role did not necessarily apply to individuals with chronic diseases (i.e., heart disease) who could not be cured or returned to normal functioning; (3) was based on the interaction between doctors and patients in office settings that could differ elsewhere (i.e., emergency rooms, hospitals, public health campaigns); and (4) reflected a middle-class pattern of behavior not necessarily applicable to people with a lower socioeconomic status (SES) (see Burnham 2012; Cockerham 2017). "Unlike some sociologists," observed Benton Johnson (1975:1), "Parsons [did] not enjoy a fight."[3] And so he rarely responded to attacks. However, Parsons (1975) did respond to critiques of the sick role by pointing out that he never claimed his sick role concept explained all illness behavior; instead, it was an ideal-type model that could be used for comparative purposes and for analyzing physician–patient encounters in which the interaction is primarily guidance on the part of the physician in clinics or offices and cooperation by the patient.

Functionalism's period as the leading theoretical paradigm in sociology worldwide was short-lived. One problem is that the logic inherent in functionalism can be seen as *tautological,* a term which means repetitious or circular reasoning. As Ritzer and Stepnisky (2018:257) explain, functionalism defines a social system in terms of its parts and then defines the parts in terms of the system, and because "each is defined in terms of the other, neither the social system nor its parts are in fact defined at all." This criticism arises as a result of a vagueness or lack of specificity in the theory common in macro-level or "grand" theories that are so broad their generalizations cannot be tested empirically. Functionalism was also disparaged by various scholars for providing a static image of society highly resistant to change; moreover, its emphasis on value consensus, stability, social order, and balance seemed to justify the maintenance of the status quo that perpetuated social inequalities and the power of already existing elite groups. Sociologists who studied conflict found functionalism lacking because it did not adequately consider conflict as a source of social change, especially rapid and revolutionary change. Symbolic interactionists objected to the relegation of individuals to relatively passive roles in large social systems and the theory's disregard of creativity and innovation at the individual and small-group level. Some of this debate took place in medical sociology and stimulated the development of alternative theoretical views, especially from symbolic interaction.

Before the beginning of the twenty-first century, functionalism was a dead theory in both sociology and medical sociology, and virtually no sociologist today identifies as a functionalist. Ritzer and William Yagatich (2012:105) described functionalism, along with conflict theory and symbolic interaction, as a "zombie theory" existing with a bare minimum of life. That is, the theory exists and is oddly still featured as a major school of social thought in introductory textbooks, but for all practical purposes is "dead" and no longer used. An apt summary by Thomas Kemple (2006:10–11) states:

> The irony in Parsons's famous opening question [in *The Structure of Social Action*]—"Who now reads Spencer?"—lies … in the fact that Parsons's own work is now just as unlikely to be read or remembered, having supposedly been surpassed by later generations of … theorists.

The Schism Between Sociologists in Medicine and of Medicine

Following Parsons and the other developments previously discussed that took place in the 1950s, it was clear that medical sociology was firmly established in the U.S. more so than any other place in the world. The *Journal of Health and Social Behavior* followed in 1960 that became the leading academic journal in medical sociology and an official publication of ASA in 1966. The first edition of the *Handbook of Medical Sociology* (Freeman, Levine, and Reeder 1963) had been written because of the "phenomenal expansion of interest" in the study of health problems (Leavell 1963:ix). Medical sociology was evolving into a major field. The expansion in the U.S., unlike Europe, primarily came from academic medical sociologists with training and interest in theory (Cockerham 1983). On the academic side, theory was especially valued; on the medical side, practical application was paramount and therefore a division existed.

This situation escalated into friction between sociologists doing medical work in applied environments and those doing largely theoretical work, usually in nonmedical academic settings. This division of labor was reflected in Robert Straus's (1957) familiar observation that there was a sociology *of* medicine and a sociology *in* medicine. The dispute that developed was over whether the sociologists of medicine (theoretical) have more to contribute to sociology than the sociologists in medicine (applied). The former did work based on sociological definitions of a problem while the latter did the same based on medical definitions. While medical sociologists affiliated with departments of sociology in universities were in a stronger position to produce work that satisfies sociologists as good sociology, the sociologists in medical institutions had the advantage of participation in medicine and research opportunities unavailable to those outside medical practice.

Yet the requirement for medical sociologists in applied settings to produce work especially relevant to patient care, medical education, or health policy constrained their ability to contribute to sociology. This circumstance resulted in lessened professional status for applied sociologists, even though their work could be more medically meaningful. The applied medical sociologist was not usually also a physician and therefore an auxiliary to research projects in medicine, while regarded in sociology as a practitioner for hire producing less intellectual work. The key difference in the two medical sociologies was in the development, testing, and verification of theory. One group typically did it and the other did not.

The high importance that sociology has historically assigned to theory is the primary determinant in its allocation of status. According to Collyer (2012:160), despite "a pervasive ideology of camaraderie and democracy" among sociologists, the field is nonetheless "unmistakably hierarchical" with "the privileging of academic sociologists" relative to those working elsewhere and "the valuing of theoreticians above the methodologists and 'applied' sociologists." As British sociologist Gordon Horobin (1985:103) once observed: "Those who teach 'theory' enjoy high status in academic departments, while those who are actually engaged in theory building have the highest status of all." Consequently, theory has a high value in medical sociology. Studies combining theory with empirical data are the most highly regarded throughout sociology.

The schism between the two medical sociologies, however, never seriously developed outside the U.S. Medical sociology in Britain, for example, was first institutionalized in medicine as part of social medicine; academic sociology did not appear in most British universities until the 1960s or later. As Malcolm Johnson (1975:229) observed, "in Britain there is no tradition of the early scholarly kind and the grandparents of medical sociology here made their reputations through the medium of applied research within the medical setting." In Germany, sociology had been suppressed by the Nazis in the 1930s and did not reappear until after World War II. Medical sociology was not organized until 1970 and only then by federal legislation that mandatorily established the field in West German medical schools. In the Scandinavian countries, Finnish medical sociologist Elianne Riska (2003) found that the emergence and the development of medical sociology was influenced more by debates within medicine where most medical sociologists worked than by trends in sociology. And she adds that while Straus's distinctions between sociology in and sociology of medicine described the work of medical sociologists up to the 1970s, medical sociology went on to establish a character of its own and by the early 2000s was mostly pursued as sociology *with* medicine in medical schools and elsewhere.

By the end of the twentieth century, the schism had largely but not entirely disappeared in the U.S. Even though most research in medical sociology remains oriented toward practical problem solving, the use of sociological theory is now widespread. There has been a general evolution of work in medical sociology that combines both applied and theoretical approaches, with the utilization of theory becoming increasingly common throughout medical sociology as a framework for explaining or predicting health-related social behavior and social conditions. Medical sociologists in universities responded to funding requests for applied research, while some of their counterparts in medical institutions also did theoretical work. Anselm Strauss (1916–1996), for instance, on the faculty of the University of California at San Francisco School of Nursing, was a leading figure in symbolic inter-action theory in the 1960s and 1970s, and one of the most noted medical sociologists of all time. The schism has clearly shrunk. Wardwell (1982:571) perhaps said it best long ago, when he concluded:

> Why is it that the question of sociologists' independence has not been so acutely raised in other subfields of sociology? We no longer debate whether there should be a sociology *of* industry rather than a sociology *in* industry, ... a sociology *of* religion rather than a sociology *in* religion. Each research study is judged on its merits. Perhaps it is time to stop worrying over whether a medical sociologist's work is the sociology *of* medicine or the sociology *in* medicine.

As for medicine, it nurtured, funded, and sponsored medical sociology early in its development and continues to do so today. In fact, one could arguably state that medicine has been more supportive of medical sociology at various times in its history than sociology and, furthermore, that the origin of med-ical sociology is actually found in medicine, not sociology. Medicine rec-ognized its worth much earlier. Yet, beginning in the 1950s and continuing through the 1960s, medical sociology was embraced by general sociology. The field was becoming too large and important to disregard or relegate to the margins of the discipline. It became increasingly clear that a large group of sociologists worked in this area and that considerations of health permeate many aspects of social life and well-being. Theory and research methodology link medical sociology to the larger discipline of sociology more exten-sively than any other aspects of sociological practice and, as noted, theory is its most distinguishing characteristic in comparison to other health-related fields. The remaining chapters will discuss the major theories in medical sociology today.

Summary

While medicine applied some of the early thinking in sociology to medical problems and population health, the applied medical sociology that emerged in medical circles slowly blended into academic medical sociology as interest in the field increased. The academic side of medical sociology was signifi-cantly boosted by the appearance of Parsons' concept of the sick role which was the first theory advanced by a leading sociological theorist. Although Parsons' version of functionalist theory fell into disfavor, his concept of the sick role stimulated the rise of theory in medical sociology. As the use of sociological theory increased in importance, a schism began to grow in the U.S. between sociologists of medicine (who use theory) and sociologists in medicine (who do applied research) over whose work is the most important. The key difference between the two groups was the utilization of theory. In recent years this schism has declined in relevance as both groups of sociologists increasingly do the same type of work combining empirical research with theory.

Guide to Critical Thinking

1. Why was Parsons' concept of the sick role important?
2. What does the sick role explain?
3. What are the strengths of the sick role concept?
4. What are the weaknesses of the sick role concept?
5. Is the sick role concept still relevant today or should it be abandoned?

Notes

1   By 1965, some 15 university graduate programs listed medical sociology as a primary area of expertise, which increased to 39 by 1972, and leaping ahead to 2018 there were some 80 universities in the United States and four in Canada with this specialty. In 1994, the Department of Sociology at the University of Alabama at Birmingham (UAB) offered the first Ph.D. *in* medical sociology, rather than a doctorate in sociology with a specialization in medical sociology, with the UAB Department of Medicine a major sponsor. In 2017, a B.S. in medical sociology was added to prepare undergraduates for graduate work in medical sociology or for medical school.

2   ASA lists 1962 on its website as the official year the Medical Sociology Section was established, but this appears incorrect as it conflicts with the eyewitness accounts of Wardwell (1982) and Bloom (2002). A query to ASA by the author shows that in 1959 the ASA Council voted to accept the petition for a Section on Medical Sociology as proposed by Bloom (*American Sociological Review* 1959[24]:865). But it is not clear if this is the official founding since the Secretary's Report (*American Sociological Review* 1959[24]:869) states the Committee on Medical Sociology had obtained the required 200 members and *will* apply to the Council.

However, the Report on Activities of the Section on Medical Sociology (*American Sociological Review* 1960[25]:958) states that the ASA Council authorized the Section on Medical Sociology in 1959. Wardwell (1982:565) and Bloom (2002:217–20) say the Section was approved in 1959 with 230 members, grew to 407 members by January 1960 and had more than 700 members by April 1961. Wardwell was a participant at the ASA meeting in 1959, while Bloom was also there as the secretary of the Committee on Medical Sociology (1957–1959) and reappointed by the new Section on Medical Sociology beginning in 1959. He was responsible for keeping the records. Why ASA uses an official date of 1962 is unknown and likely wrong.

3   Other sociologists like a good fight. Pierre Bourdieu (1930–2002), for example, the influential French social theorist whose work is often cited in medical sociology, was featured in a 2001 film with the apt title "Sociology is a Martial Art," which showed him explaining and defending publicly some of his ideas.

Suggested Reading

Bloom, Samuel W. 2002. *The Word as Scalpel: A History of Medical Sociology.* New York: Oxford University Press.
Although outdated, Bloom's book remains an informative history of the early development of American medical sociology.
Cockerham, William C. 2013. "Sociological Theory in Medical Sociology in the Early Twenty-first Century." *Social Theory & Health* 11(3):241–55.
A review of contemporary theory in medical sociology.

References

Adam, Paul and Claudine Herzlich. 1994. *Sociologie de la maladie et de la Medecine* [*Sociology of Illness and Medicine*]. Paris: Nathan.
Bloom, Samuel W. 2002. *The Word as Scalpel: A History of Medical Sociology.* New York: Oxford University Press.
Burnham, John C. 2012. "The Death of the Sick Role." *Social History of Medicine* 25(4):761–76.
Callinicos, Alex. 2007. *Social Theory*, 2nd ed. Cambridge: Polity.
Chalfant, H. Paul and Richard Kurtz. 1971. "Alcoholics and the Sick Role: Assessments by Social Workers." *Journal of Health and Social Behavior* 12(March):66–72.
Claus, Lisbeth M. 1982. *The Growth of a Sociological Discipline*, Vol. I. Leuven, Belgium: Katholieke Universiteit Leuven.
Cockerham, William C. 1978. *Medical Sociology*. Englewood Cliffs, NJ: Prentice-Hall.
Cockerham, William C. 1983. "The State of Medical Sociology in the United States, Great Britain, West Germany, and Austria: Applied vs Pure Theory." *Social Science & Medicine* 17:1313–27.
Cockerham, William C. 2012. "Current Directions in Medical Sociology," in George Ritzer (ed.), *The Wiley-Blackwell Companion to Sociology*. Oxford: Wiley-Blackwell, pp. 385–401.
Cockerham, William C. 2017. *Medical Sociology*, 14th ed. New York: Routledge.
Coe, Rodney. 1970. *Sociology of Medicine*. New York: McGraw-Hill.
Cole, Stephen and Robert LeJeune. 1972. "Illness and the Legitimation of Failure." *American Sociological Review* 37(June):347–56.
Collyer, Fran. 2012. *Mapping the Sociology of Health and Medicine: America, Britain and Australia Compared*. Basingstoke: Palgrave Macmillan.

Collyer, Fran. 2018. "Envisaging the Healthcare Sector as a Field: Moving from Talcott Parsons to Pierre Bourdieu." *Social Theory & Health* 16(2):111–26.

Davis, Michael. 1921. *Immigrant Health and the Community*. New York: Harper.

Denton, John. 1978. *Medical Sociology*. Boston, MA: Houghton Mifflin.

Durkheim, Émile. [1893] 1964. *The Division of Labor in Society*. New York: Free Press.

Fox, Renée C. 1989. *The Sociology of Medicine*. Englewood Cliffs, NJ: Prentice-Hall.

Freeman, Howard E., Sol Levine, and Leo G. Reeder (eds.). 1963. *Handbook of Medical Sociology*. Englewood Cliffs, NJ: Prentice-Hall.

Freidson, Eliot. 1970. *Profession of Medicine*. New York: Dodd, Mead.

Gerhardt, Uta. 1989. *Ideas about Illness: An Intellectual and Political History of Medical Sociology*. London: Macmillan.

Gouldner, Alvin W. 1970. *The Coming Crisis of Western Sociology*. New York: Avon.

Hawkins, Norman. 1958. *Medical Sociology*. Springfield, IL: Charles Thomas.

Henderson, Lawrence J. 1935a. "Physician and Patient as a Social System." *New England Journal of Medicine* 212(May 2):819–23.

Henderson, Lawrence J. 1935b. *Pareto's General Sociology: A Physiologist's Interpretation*. Cambridge, MA: Harvard University Press.

Horobin, Gordon. 1985. "Medical Sociology in Britain: True Confessions of an Empiricist." *Sociology of Health & Illness* 7(1):94–107.

Hüttner, Hannes (ed.). 1987. *Medizin Soziologie [Medical Sociology]*. Berlin: Verlag Volk und Gesundheit.

Jaco, E. Gartly (ed.). 1958. *Patients, Physicians, and Illness: A Source Book in Behavioral Science and Health*. New York: Free Press.

Johnson, Benton. 1975. *Functionalism in Modern Sociology: Understanding Parsons*. Morristown, NJ: General Learning Press.

Johnson, Malcolm. 1975. "Medical Sociology and Sociological Theory." *Social Science & Medicine* 9:227–32.

Kemple, Thomas M. 2006. "Founders, Classics, and Canons in the Formation of Social Theory," in Gerard Delanty (ed.), *Handbook of Contemporary European Social Theory*. London: Routledge, pp. 3–13.

Leavell, Hugh R. 1963. "Introduction," in Howard Freeman, Sol Levine, and Leo G. Reeder (eds.), *Handbook of Medical Sociology*. Englewood Cliffs, NJ: Prentice-Hall, pp. ix–xii.

Mechanic, David. 1968. *Medical Sociology*. New York: Free Press.

Merton, Robert K., George Reader, and Patricia L. Kendall (eds.). 1957. *The Student Physician*. Cambridge, MA: Harvard University Press.

Ogburn, William Fielding. 1922. *Social Change with Respect to Culture and Original Nature*. New York: Huebsch.

Parsons, Talcott. 1937. *The Structure of Social Action*. New York: McGraw-Hill.

Parsons, Talcott. 1951. *The Social System*. New York: Free Press.

Parsons, Talcott. 1958. "Definitions of Health and Illness in Light of American Values and Social Structure," in E. Gartly Jaco (ed.), *Patients, Physicians, and Illness*. New York: Free Press, pp. 165–87.

Parsons, Talcott. 1975. "The Sick Role and the Role of the Physician Reconsidered." *Milbank Memorial Fund Quarterly* 53:257–78.

Parsons, Talcott. 1981. "Revisiting the Classics throughout a Long Career," in Buford Rhea (ed.), *The Future of the Sociological Classics*. London: George Allen & Unwin, pp. 183–94.

Riska, Elianne. 2003. "Developments in Scandinavian and American Medical Sociology." *Scandinavian Journal of Public Health* 31:389–94.

Ritzer, George and Jeffrey Stepnisky. 2018. *Sociological Theory*, 10th ed. Los Angeles, CA: Sage.

Ritzer, George and William Yagatich. 2012. "Contemporary Sociological Theory," in George Ritzer (ed.), *The Wiley-Blackwell Companion to Sociology*. Oxford: Wiley-Blackwell, pp. 98–118.

Robertson, Leon and Margaret Heagarty. 1975. *Medical Sociology: A General Systems Approach*. Chicago, IL: Nelson-Hall.

Siegrist, Johannes. 1974. *Lehrbuch der Medizinischen Soziologie* [*Textbook of Medical Sociology*]. Munich: Urban & Schwarzenberg.

Smelser, Neil J. 1998. *The Social Edges of Psychoanalysis*. Berkeley, CA: University of California Press.

Stern, Bernhard J. 1927. *Social Factors in Medical Progress*. New York: Columbia University Press.

Stern, Bernhard J. 1941. *Society and Medical Progress*. Princeton, NJ: Princeton University Press.

Stern, Bernhard J. [1959] 1991. "Toward a Sociology of Medicine." *Sociological Practice* 9(1):38–42.

Straus, Robert. 1957. "The Nature and Status of Medical Sociology." *American Sociological Review* 22:200–4.

Susser, Mervyn W. and William Watson. 1962. *Sociology in Medicine*. London: Oxford University Press.

Twaddle, Andrew C. and Ricard M. Hessler. 1977. *A Sociology of Health*. St. Louis, MO: Mosby.

Waitzkin, Howard. 1971. "Latent Functions of the Sick Role in Various Settings." *Social Science & Medicine* 5:45–75.

Wardwell, Walter I. 1982. "The State of Medical Sociology—A Review Essay." *Sociological Quarterly* 23(4):563–71.

Chapter 4

Classical Theory
Durkheim and Weber

A "canon" is a set of exemplary texts that defines a field. The three established canons in sociology are found in the work of Émile Durkheim, Max Weber, and Karl Marx (Connell 1997; Ritzer and Stepnisky 2018; Royce 2015). While there are other candidates from sociology's classical era, these three have stood the test of time. They did not appear together as the most important canons of sociology in English-language introductory textbooks until the 1970s, but once it happened, their status has continued to the present day (see, for example, Giddens et al. 2018; Henslin 2019; Macionis 2018; Ritzer and Murphy 2019). While there is an inconclusive debate mentioned in the last chapter about who else's work should be canonized, there is general agreement about these three scholars from sociology's classical period (Royce 2015). Many classical theorists are, of course, only of historical interest since they no longer apply to our time; however, some of the theories of Durkheim, Weber, and Marx have persisted as authoritative sources for present-day theorizing in medical sociology.

As will be seen in later chapters, theory construction in sociology tends to be cumulative and the classics provide building blocks and legitimacy for many current theories (Baert 2007), including those in medical sociology (Cockerham 2013c). As Patrick Baert (2007) points out, sociology takes its founders very seriously. Consequently, theory formation often proceeds in a cumulative fashion with present work building on the past. In this regard, sociology is much like the practice of case law in which the precedence set by prior court decisions is taken into account in determining present-day legal verdicts. Since Talcott Parsons, sociologists in all specialties have used the classics as authoritative foundations for new theories. "Underlying this intellectual genre," states Baert (2007:121), "is the assumption that the classics need to be consolidated, combined, recycled and built upon—as if sociologists have taken on board Newton's aphorism that 'if I have seen farther, it is by standing on the shoulders of giants.'"

It is therefore pertinent to review the work of the canonized theorists before jumping ahead to the present because their influence remains. This chapter reviews the theories of Émile Durkheim and Max Weber that remain relevant for contemporary medical sociology. They were the first to be canonized and accomplished more than anyone else in establishing sociology as an academic discipline in the late nineteenth and early twentieth centuries. Their work will be examined here as it applies to medical sociology in the twenty-first century, beginning with Durkheim. The relevance of doing so is evident in the comment of Talcott Parsons (1981:183) as the leading sociologist of his time, who said:

> And here is a methodological or procedural point I want to leave with you. If the works in question really belong in the category of great human achievements—and this is certainly true of a great deal of Weber's and Durkheim's work—you can never exhaust their meaning and their influence for your work in a single reading. If you go back to them, you always find something new you did not understand before. Their texture is incredibly rich.

Durkheim

Émile Durkheim (1858–1917), as discussed in Chapter 3, had a particularly pivotal role in the founding of sociology and ranks as one of the greatest sociologists of all time because of his contributions to theory matched with his strong determination to establish sociology as a science (Fournier 2013; Heilbron 2015; Lukes 1973). In comparing what sociology initially was in Durkheim's time—namely philosophical speculation about the nature of society on the part of Auguste Comte and others—to what it is today, it is clear that Durkheim's prominence in sociology is well-deserved. As Durkheim ([1897] 1951:35) points out in *Suicide*, sociology was "still in the stage of system-building and philosophical syntheses" that preferred "brilliant generalities" in discourse to the "definite treatment of any one" particular question; noting, however, that "above all, such large and abrupt generalizations are not capable of any proof." In *Suicide*, he demonstrated a scientific methodology for sociology that provided the proof needed to allow the discipline to move beyond speculation and "grand" theorizing. His eventual stature is illustrated by Marcel Fournier's (2013:1) comment in his biography of Durkheim, where he says:

> The house on the boulevard de Talence in Bordeaux, where he [Durkheim] lived for several years, boasts a plaque bearing the legend: "Émile Durkheim, founder of sociology". Nothing more and nothing less!

Whereas another Frenchman, Comte, had given sociology its name, it was Durkheim more than any other individual who demonstrated that there was such a thing as a "sociology" that could explain society's influence on the social behavior of individuals with empirical evidence. His agenda was to promote the perspective that society has a reality of its own above and beyond the individual and that this reality could be studied scientifically. What Durkheim called attention to is the truism that people tend to act in particular and predictable ways because they know it is what society expects of them and, in doing so, society itself becomes a reality in their thinking. Durkheim ([1895] 1964:13, original emphasis) depicted this reality as a "social fact" and defined it as follows:

> *A social fact is every way of acting, fixed or not, capable of exercising on the individual an external constraint; or again, every way of acting which is general throughout a given society, while at the same time existing in its own right independent of its individual manifestations.*

Durkheim was therefore recognizing the importance of social structures, processes, norms, and values external to individuals that integrated them into the larger society and in doing so shaped their behavior along collective lines.

Box 4.1 Émile Durkheim

Durkheim was born on April 15, 1858 into a Jewish family in Épinal in the province of Lorraine in France. His mother was the daughter of a horse trader and his father was a rabbi, as was his grandfather and great-grandfather before him. Durkheim, however, a "studious and conscientious" student wanted to further his education and his father, who had wished more schooling for himself, did not object (Fournier 2013:23). He left home for a prep school in Paris and from there he gained admission on his third attempt in 1879 to one of France's most selective and prestigious schools of higher education, the Paris campus of the *École normale supérieure*. Durkheim's father wanted him excused from Saturday classes for religious reasons and to give him a clothing allowance. The administration said no. As Fournier (2013:28) describes it:

> He [Durkheim] had entered a small, closed world: the regime was austere, the discipline was strict and academic standards were both high and demanding. No exceptions were allowed.

As a student, Durkheim was rated as very serious, responsible, hardworking, well-informed, and exceptionally clever, with a rather cold

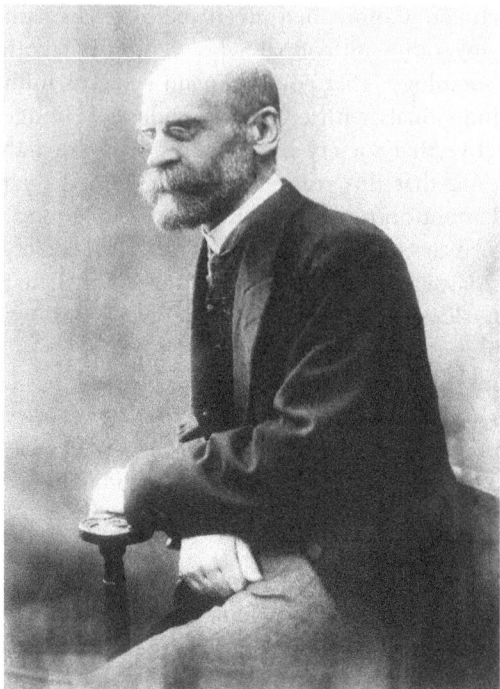

Image 4.1 Émile Durkheim

appearance, and a penetrating mind "more capable of assimilation than invention" (Lukes 1973:64–5). He completed his final examination (*agrégation*) in 1882, with an unexceptional but passing result. Of interest is that the person who became *the* major figure in the founding of sociology was not considered innovative, although it could well be said that this period was a time for the assimilation of knowledge providing a foundation for the innovation to come later. Durkheim was exposed to the works of Auguste Comte and Herbert Spencer and came to see that the topic he had chosen for his doctoral thesis (individual personality and social solidarity) was best addressed by way of the new but undeveloped science of "sociology" (Fournier 2013; Lukes 1973).

His thesis was published as *The Division of Labor in Society* in 1893, followed by *The Rules of Sociological Method* in 1895, and *Suicide* in 1897. He moved from teaching positions in schools (*lycées*) of secondary education to a newly created junior lectureship in social science at the University of Bordeaux (1897–1902). While there he founded a new and important sociological journal in 1898, the *L'Année Sociologique*

[The Annals of Sociology]. As his reputation grew, he was appointed to the faculty of the leading French university, the Sorbonne in Paris (1902–1917), first as a Professor of Science Education. Then in 1913, after the publication of another landmark study, *The Elementary Forms of Religious Life* in 1912, Durkheim was named Professor of Science Education and Sociology, marking the initial establishment of sociology as an academic subject in France. He had married Louise Dreyfus (1866–1926) in 1897, whose father had risen from a working-class origin to become a wealthy pipe manufacturer. In what was apparently a happy marriage, they had two children, a daughter Marie and a son André. André was killed in 1915 serving in the French Army in Serbia during World War I. Intense grief over the death of his son, associated with stress and weariness, is thought by many to have hastened Durkheim's own death on November 10, 1917 at the age of 59 (Fournier 2013; Lukes 1973).

Durkheim's Study of Suicide

As noted in Chapter 3, Durkheim's ([1897] 1951) only work having a direct application to medical sociology is his theory of suicide that linked the act of taking one's life to the strength of an individual's ties to his or her community or society. He approached this topic by studying Western European suicide rates between 1850 and 1891 and identifying social conditions external to the individual that he believed stimulated the taking of one's life. He suggested that suicide, despite its being a highly personal decision, is not entirely an act of free choice by the individual. He based this observation upon his analysis that the suicide rates for the various countries he studied were relatively constant or similar, year after year. Therefore, something more than individual motives appeared to be involved.

Durkheim also did not think that suicide was due to physiological causes or the physical environment, nor did he believe it could be explained solely in psychological terms or "individual peculiarities"; rather, there were decisive social forces at play (Fournier 2013). Suicide, in his view, was a social fact explainable in terms of social causes. As Durkheim ([1897] 1951:209) put it: "First of all, it can be said that, as collective force is one of the obstacles best calculated to restrain suicide, its weakening involves a development of suicide." Therefore, he regarded the social bonds that tie people to society as the key variable. His idea was that whether or not a person chooses to take his or her life depended on how strong a grip society has upon that person; that is, how well an individual is integrated into society. Durkheim reasoned that people were more likely to kill themselves when the social relationships that gave meaning to their lives were weak and less likely when they were strong. Steven Lukes (1973:217) summarized Durkheim's theory of suicide, as amounting to the following:

> under adverse social conditions, when … [the] social context fails to provide … [individuals] with the requisite sources of attachment and/or regulation, at the appropriate level of intensity, then their psychological or moral health is impaired, and a certain number of vulnerable, suicide-prone individuals respond by committing suicide.

Durkheim's data, for example, disclosed that unmarried people and people without children were more likely to commit suicide than married people and people with children, who presumably had stronger social attachments. Moreover, Protestants were more likely to commit suicide than Catholics, perhaps because Protestantism takes a more individualistic approach to religion. His results likewise supported the view that a supposedly uniform phenomenon like suicide is in fact a set of different phenomena, each with its own social causes. Within this conceptual framework, Durkheim identified three principal types of suicide and suggested a fourth—all grounded in the relationship of the individual to society. The types are:

(1) *egoistic* suicide, in which individuals become detached from society and, suddenly finding themselves left upon their own, are overwhelmed by the resulting stress;
(2) *anomic* suicide, in which individuals find their own norms and values are no longer relevant to them, so the controls of society no longer restrain them from taking their lives;
(3) *altruistic* suicide, in which individuals feel themselves so strongly integrated into a society that requires their suicide for failure or other reasons; and
(4) *fatalistic* suicide which is related to a sense of powerlessness that someone might feel when there is no viable future and life is controlled to an intolerable extent that occurs when people are subject to excessive social regulation. An example of fatalistic suicide would be that of a prisoner or slave who commits suicide because of the hopelessness of the situation. Durkheim did not discuss fatalistic suicide in any depth, because he thought the other three types of suicide were more common and, thus, more important.

Of the first three types of suicide described by Durkheim, egoistic suicide appears to be the most prevalent. It occurs when an individual has too few ties to the community. Egoistic suicide is characteristic of the "loner," who becomes isolated from society either by choice or by chance. It results from stress brought on by the separation of a once strongly integrated individual from his or her social group. Egoistic suicide is supposedly based upon the overstimulation of a person's intelligence by the realization that he or she has been deprived of collective activity and meaning. An illustration of egoistic suicide would be that of people who cannot cope with being apart from the activities and group relationships that once gave significant meaning to their lives. The suicides of people who lose someone important to them, or action-seeking individuals like soldiers and police officers who cannot adjust to inactivity after retirement sidelines them, are examples of egoistic suicide. The determining factor in egoistic suicide is the degree to which an individual is integrated into the social groups—religious, family, occupational, economic, and political—to which that person belongs.

Anomic suicide is described by Durkheim as an overstimulation of emotion and a corresponding freedom from society's rules. It is the result of a sudden change that brings on a breakdown of the values and norms by which an individual has lived his or her life. Sudden wealth or sudden poverty, for instance, could disturb the usual life patterns for a person and induce anomie, which is a state of normlessness or loss of established guidelines for social behavior. The person is not really lacking norms; rather, his or her norms no longer seem to apply anymore. In this situation, the person is likely to be restless, in crisis, and unable to see meaning in living. For example, there are instances of people killing themselves after suddenly losing vast sums of money in the stock market or their business, or finding out they have a terminal disease.

In altruistic suicide an individual kills himself or herself because society or some socially prescribed code of behavior demands it. Altruistic suicide represents the strong presence of a society mandating suicide because of the social situation. When a person takes his or her own life in this circumstance, states Durkheim ([1897] 1951:219), "it is not because he [or she] assumes the right to do so but, on the contrary, because it is his [or her] duty." One current example of altruistic suicide is that of terrorists who blow themselves up in order to kill enemies of their group or religion. Other examples are the practice of *harakiri* in feudal Japan, where certain social failure, wrongdoing, or loss of face by an individual, especially samurai, was expected to be redressed by the individual's suicide, or the traditional Hindu custom of the widow committing ritual suicide at her husband's funeral.

Durkheim's study of suicide, however, contains some shortcomings. His typologies, for example, cannot explain all suicides or be used to predict whether a particular individual is going to take his or her life. It is also not a complete theory of suicide in that it only attempts to explain its social causes, not its psychological ramifications. Overall, Durkheim's work reflects an emphasis on structure at the expense of agency and, by doing so, is an example of "downwards conflation" in which the causal power of structure is overstated (Archer 1995:3). Nevertheless, he was among the first to call attention to the reality of structural effects on individual behavior in relation to suicide. In doing so, he set the stage for sociology to become a science.

And, today, it is difficult, if not impossible, to publish a study of suicide in sociology without citing Durkheim, as his analysis remains the foundation for subsequent sociological investigations of this topic. What he accomplished was to identify the impact of society on the individual by noting that individuals commit egoistic or anomic suicide because the meaning and stability in their lives provided by the social order have been modified or weakened, or have disappeared. He contributes to our understanding of suicide by showing social factors can foster intolerable emotion or unbearable despair in individuals, which in turn leads to suicide. Or, conversely, that social solidarity offsets suicidal tendencies by providing support and a sense of stability. As for altruistic suicide, society is in control of requiring suicide and takes choice away from the individual. Yet the significance of Durkheim's work in this regard extends well beyond the issue of suicide. What is particularly insightful is Durkheim's recognition that societal processes can create stressful situations in which people are forced to respond to external conditions not of their own choosing.

Thus, Durkheim helps us not only to understand the social facets of suicide, but to recognize that social events can affect health in a variety of ways, both physical and mental, and that the effects of stress can be mitigated through social support or feelings of social solidarity. His depiction of social integration in relation to suicide anticipated concepts of social support in stress research in medical sociology (Pescosolido and Kronenfeld 1995). Jo Phelan and her colleagues (2004) credited Durkheim with providing a bold model for medical sociology to follow. The boldness in his work was his insistence that social forces outside of an individual's direct control can have a reality affecting people's health and in some situations curtailing their lives. This thesis can be extended to show that a person's health can be negatively affected through stressful conditions requiring responses to social situations not necessarily chosen by the individual. There is growing evidence, as seen in studies of poverty, social class, neighborhood effects and social capital, that social structures and conditions may ultimately be responsible for causing many health problems in ways that are consistent with Durkheim's perspective (Cockerham 2013a; Phelan et al. 2004).

Durkheim and Social Capital

While sociology has moved a considerable distance since Durkheim's pioneering efforts, one area in particular where we see his influence today in medical sociology is in the rapidly growing number of studies of social capital and health which will be discussed in more detail in Chapter 14. As Irish medical sociologist Orla McDonnell and her colleagues (McDonnell et al. 2009:17) point out:

> This body of work may be interpreted as neo-Durkheimian in the sense that social capital is understood as a property of social structures and social relationships whose function is to promote social support through norms and values of trust and reciprocity and that, at the same time, regulate deviant behavior.

Social capital is generally described in the research literature as a characteristic of social structures consisting of a network of cooperative relationships between residents of particular neighborhoods and communities. Networks providing social capital are distinguished by interpersonal trust, norms of reciprocity and mutual aid, and a supportive social atmosphere within which people look out for one another and interact positively with a sense of belonging. People embedded in such supportive networks have been consistently found to have better health and longevity than those who lack this resource (Song 2013). In locales where there are serious social problems (e.g., crime, stress, slums) and breakdowns in social networks, social capital is reduced or absent with the residents having poorer health and shorter lifespans (Scambler 2012).

Bryan Turner (2004) and others (De Maio 2010; McDonnell et al. 2009) suggest that the various theories of social capital, such as those by Robert Putnam, Nan Lin, and Pierre Bourdieu, are contemporary applications of Durkheim's theory of suicide in which individuals are protected by their close integration into society. Turner (2004) acknowledges that Durkheim never actually used the term "social capital," but maintains that his concepts of social solidarity and social facts are still valid in illustrating how social capital is protective of the health of the individual. Theories of social capital are of interest to medical sociologists because they can be a social mechanism linking inequality to health or, conversely, enhancing the health of people in neighborhoods and communities with high levels of it.

The message of social capital research, however, is not to claim individual-level characteristics are unimportant or are superseded by such capital, but that structural variables like communities can have a causal impact on health. This outcome is also seen in research in medical sociology on "neighborhood disadvantage" that investigates unhealthy urban living conditions. This research focuses on variables specific to neighborhoods, not individuals, such as the physical environment (e.g., quality of housing, water, air), availability of services (e.g., banks, police, fire, sanitation, health care), and social and cultural factors (e.g., social networks, single-parent families) that impair health through psychological distress or exposure to unhealthy living situations (Pearlin et al. 2005). While Durkheim studied other topics of importance, his analysis of suicide—an obviously unhealthy practice—and his influence underlying notions of social capital remain his most notable theoretical contributions to medical sociology.

Weber

Max Weber (1864–1920) was one of the leading intellectuals of his day and his insights place him in the front rank of sociological scholars. As his most recent biographer Joachim Radkau (2009:3) points out: "Weber is currently one of the thinkers through whom the social sciences have acquired a distinctive complexion and against whom one can often sharpen one's own thinking: he seems to grow and grow as you keep reading his texts." While Weber did not formulate theories on health, his work nevertheless has been influential in medical sociology as it is in much of sociology today.

According to his friend and colleague, the German psychiatrist and philosopher Karl Jaspers (1989), Weber was the greatest German of his time. "Max Weber's essence," states Jaspers (1989:113), "seemed to stand between a vanishing and a rising era." The vanishing era was the end of the last vestiges of Europe's old feudal social structures (i.e., landed aristocracy, serfdom) and the rising era was modernity as exemplified by industrialization and urbanization. Weber had noted this transition in his first study in 1890 of the social changes taking place in the agricultural areas east of the Elbe River in Germany as peasants were leaving the area's agricultural estates to seek employment in urban factories. He did not go on to formulate a general theory of society, but he did provide a wide range of lasting concepts for sociology and recognize many aspects of Europe's oncoming transition to modernity. He was also among the first major scholars to effectively criticize Karl Marx who had passed away in 1883. Much of his work was, in fact, characterized as "a debate with Marx's ghost."

Weber ([1919] 1946) also strongly believed that sociology should be value-free; that is, sociologists should not use their personal values and prejudices to shape their insights and conclusions about society. Sociologists, in his view, must *always* be objective in reporting their findings in order to portray social conditions as accurately as possible, namely, as they really are—without injecting their own personal agenda or desired outcomes into shaping the results of their research. This position strongly contrasts with that of Marx and his supporters, who argued that the social sciences should be used to actively change society in order to meet political and social goals.

Weber ([1922] 1978) further pointed out the limitations of Marx's analysis of social class. He explained that class (as determined by money and property) was only one dimension of socioeconomic status and that power (or political influence) and especially status (or prestige) also contribute to determining an individual's social ranking. Whereas a person's social-class membership is principally determined by wealth, an individual may have influence or status for reasons other than financial, as by holding an important political office or attaining a high level of education. Therefore, a person's position in relation to the means of economic production, as indicated by Marx, is not the only factor influencing which rung of a social ladder he or she may occupy.

Weber also analyzed aspects of the sociology of law, religion, art, politics, organizations and institutions, and economics. As the German social historian Wolfgang Mommsen (1989:195) pointed out, Weber's major focus was on determining the political and social conditions that, in the course of history, have promoted responsibility and creativity despite institutional forces—like bureaucracies or tradition—that tend to stifle individual initiative. In *Economy and Society* ([1922] 1978), Weber analyzed the manner in which modern bureaucracies impose rigid rules and regulations—an "iron cage"—on individuals in the name of efficiency. In *The Protestant Ethic and The Spirit of Capitalism* ([1905] 1958), he detailed how a lifestyle of entrepreneurship, investment, thrift, and hard work associated with the Protestant ethic in the sixteenth century gave rise to the development of modern capitalism.

Box 4.2 Max Weber

Max Weber was born in Erfurt in the German state of Thuringia on April 21, 1864. He was first of eight children, six of whom survived into adulthood. His father, Max Weber, Senior, was a lawyer from a family of industrialists who was active in politics and became an important figure in the National Liberal Party. He served in various municipal positions in Erfurt and Berlin before being elected to the Prussian Chamber of Deputies and later to the German Reichstag (1872–1884). His mother, Helene Fallenstein Weber, was a deeply religious and "morally rigorous" woman from a family of teachers (Ringer 2004). Her piety strongly contrasted with that of Weber's father who as a politician enjoyed socializing with friends and colleagues, often hosting gatherings of leading academics and political figures in the family's home in a Berlin suburb (Radkau 2009).

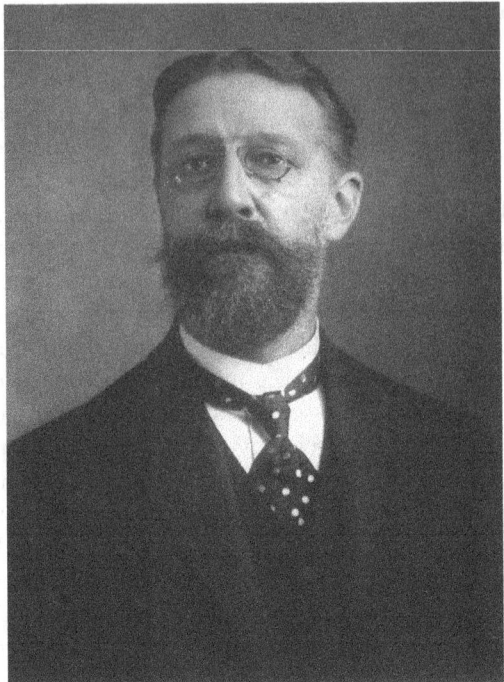

Image 4.2 Max Weber

The younger Max Weber left home in 1882 to study law, history, and economics at the University of Heidelberg where he enjoyed student life, joining a drinking and dueling fraternity, before spending a year in the German Army in 1883–1884 to qualify as a reserve officer (Ringer 2004). He returned home to continue his studies at the University of Berlin and lived in his parents' house until he married his cousin, Marianne Schnitger (1870–1954), the daughter of a physician, in 1893. Weber completed his doctoral dissertation (on the history of medieval trading companies) in 1889 and his *Habilitation*, a second dissertation (on Roman law), required for teaching in German universities in 1891. By 1897, he had held professorships at the Universities of Berlin, Freiburg, and Heidelberg and became increasingly interested in sociology. In July of that year, he had a serious argument with his autocratic father over his mother's right to visit him without his father accompanying her. His father died the next month without a reconciliation. Weber felt extreme guilt about this situation and became exceedingly distressed to the point that he suffered a nervous breakdown complicated by the conflicting values of his parents, a rigid and obsessive self-imposed work schedule, and perhaps a family tendency toward bipolar (manic-depressive) disorder (Radkau 2009; Ringer 2004).

Weber found it difficult to teach or keep up a heavy writing schedule. He finally resigned from his professorship at Heidelberg in 1903 at the age of 39. He became a private scholar, living off a comfortable inheritance from his wife's grandfather, traveled extensively, including to the United States where he ventured as far west as Oklahoma. He resumed writing for publication and other professional activities during periods of wellness. He also accepted a co-editorship of the journal *Archiv für Sozialwissenschaften und Sozialpolitik* [Archive of Social Science and Social Policy] in 1904, published his influential book on capitalism and the Protestant ethic in 1905, and helped found the *Deutsche Gesellschaft für Soziologie* [German Sociological Society] in 1910. When World War I broke out in 1914, he served for over a year as an Army captain establishing hospitals and acting as a staff disciplinary officer in the Heidelberg area. In 1918 he accepted a faculty position on a temporary basis at the University of Vienna and moved to the University of Munich in 1919 after service on the German peace delegation that ended World War I. He became ill with pneumonia and died on June 14, 1920 at the age of 56.

His wife, Marianne, collected and edited his writings that were published posthumously as *Economy and Society* in 1922, which became a seminal work in sociology. She also published his biography in 1926 and organized the "Weber Circle" that met regularly for tea on Sunday afternoons at her home in Heidelberg, overlooking the Neckar River, which began when Weber was still alive and continued after his death. Usually there was a presentation by a well-known academic figure, followed by discussion, which came to include Talcott Parsons. Weber's influence in Germany after his death was marginal and his publications were suppressed by the Nazis when they came to power in the 1930s. It remained for Parsons to *reintroduce* Weber to sociology by including Weber's work in his own theorizing, which initiated the pathway to Weber's canonization.

As for contemporary medical sociology, Weber's contributions generally fall into three areas, namely his conceptualization of (1) socioeconomic status, (2) lifestyles, and (3) formal rationality and bureaucracy (Cockerham 2013b, 2015). These concepts underlie many current studies in medical sociology on social class and health, health lifestyles, and hospital organization. Weber himself did not formulate theories unique to medical sociology or cause it to come into existence, but, as in the example of Durkheim, medical sociologists have found success in utilizing some of his theories.

Weber on Socioeconomic Status

The concept of socioeconomic status consisting of measures of income, occupational prestige, and level of education comes from Weber and is the standard determination of social stratification in American sociology that extends into medical sociology in the United States. Western European sociology, in turn, is not so Weberian. Europeans primarily focus on various dimensions of occupation, such as type of work, salary, supervisory status, level of responsibility, and the like as indicators of class position. For example, the European Socio-Economic Classification (ESC), a standardized measure intended for use throughout Europe, is based on the premise that occupation is the central indicator of class position since it is directly related to education and income (Kunst and Roskam 2010; Rose and Harrison 2010). However, American sociologists tend to think that more is involved in determining someone's class location than the characteristics of their job; consequently, they tend to take more of a Weberian approach in which occupation, income, and education are treated as distinct but interrelated variables.

Weber ([1922] 1978) had pointed out that the determinants of social stratification were more complex than a person's position in relation to the prevailing means of economic production as Marx had advocated. Instead, he advanced the idea of status groups (*Stände*) to account for the other factors involved. Weber defined status groups as communities of people linked together on the basis of wealth, status, and power. Wealth was viewed only as an indicator of money and property. Status, however, indicated a person's level of social prestige, which may or may not correspond to wealth. Whereas wealth is an *objective* dimension of a person's social standing based on how much money and material goods he or she possesses, status is a *subjective* dimension in that it consists of how much esteem someone is accorded by other people. Wealth and status were not considered the same thing, as a person could have wealth but not social status (a mob kingpin) or high status but not wealth (a ranking member of the clergy or a distinguished academic). As for power, Weber defined it as the ability to realize one's will even against the resistance of others. But he was otherwise vague about what power meant in relation to status, and while most sociologists today view its contemporary meaning as the amount of political influence a person has, power is more implied than operationalized in measures of SES in that higher SES persons are presumed to have it in comparison to lower SES individuals.

Weber's term "status groups," however, did not replace the concept of "social class" in sociology; rather, the term "class" in its popular usage came to incorporate notions of status within it. Weber had viewed classes more strictly as groups with similar income levels distinct from considerations of status. Yet, as the concept of social class evolved, it took on a more comprehensive meaning that included status and the term "status groups" has generally disappeared from sociological vocabularies. Nevertheless, Weber's influence on modern studies of social stratification is now seen in the widespread use of socioeconomic status to determine an individual's class position. SES not only reflects a person's economic situation, but also allows for differences in status that are not necessarily grounded in income or property. A large income, high occupational prestige, and an education from a notable college or university generally indicate upper- or upper-middle-class social standing, while low incomes or poverty, unemployment or a menial occupation, and a lack of education relegate an individual to the bottom of society. The three dimensions of SES—income, occupation, and education operate in combination to produce a person's social rank.

The advantage of using SES in quantitative studies is that income, occupation (through the use of scales ranking different jobs in terms of their respective levels of prestige), and number of years of education can all be assigned numerical values that sort people into social classes based on their scores. Each of these variables, although interrelated, reflects different dimensions of a person's position in the class structure of a society and when combined can pinpoint their overall location. SES is particularly useful in studies of health and illness because, as Marilyn Winkleby and her colleagues (Winkleby et al. 1992:816) determined:

- income reflects spending power, housing, diet, and quality of medical care;
- occupation signifies job status, responsibility at work, physical activity, and health risks associated with one's work; and
- education is indicative of a person's skills for acquiring positive social, psychological, and economic resources such as good jobs, nice homes, health insurance, access to quality health care, and knowledge about healthy lifestyles.

Although different models of class structure exist in medical sociology, including the basic three-class scheme of upper, middle, and lower, the model often followed in the U.S. by medical sociologists who desire greater precision in their analysis, evolved out of Weber's perspective. This is a five-class model consisting of (1) the upper class (extremely wealthy top corporate executives and professionals); (2) the upper-middle class (affluent well-educated professionals and high-level managers); (3) the lower-middle class (office and sales workers, small business owners, teachers, managers, etc.); (4) the working class (skilled workers, lower-level clerical workers, etc.); and (5) the lower class (semi-skilled and unskilled workers, the chronically unemployed, etc.).

Weber on Lifestyles

Weber's concept of lifestyles appears in his discussion of status groups in *Economy and Society* ([1922] 1978). His ideas form the basis for theorizing about lifestyles in sociology generally (Bourdieu 1984; Giddens 1991) and is the foundation for health lifestyle theory in medical sociology (Cockerham 2005, 2013a, 2013b). Weber ([1922] 1978:932) begins his analysis of lifestyles by pointing out that a distinguishing characteristic of status is what he called "status honor" (or prestige) which was normally expressed by the fact that a particular lifestyle is expected from all who wish to belong to a certain group (or social class). To be part of a group and share its status, then, means to live in the manner or style of that group.

However, Weber made the pertinent observation that lifestyles are based not on what a person produces, but on what the individual consumes. Thus, for him, the difference between status groups lay not in their relationship to the means of production as suggested by Marx, but in their relationship to the means of consumption as exemplified by their lifestyle. As Weber ([1922] 1978:933) explains, "status groups are stratified according to the principles of their *consumption* of goods as represented by special styles of life." The pattern and style of lifestyle consumption can therefore be regarded as a set of social and cultural practices that *establish* differences between social groups, not merely as a means of *expressing* differences that are already in place because of economic factors (Bourdieu 1984). That is, people of a similar station in society generally share the same or similar lifestyle that is seen in the way they live and differs from the lifestyles of those characteristic of other status groups or classes.

As shown in Figure 4.1, Weber used three distinct terms in German to express his concept of lifestyles: *Lebensstil* (lifestyle) and its two basic components, *Lebensführung* (life conduct), and *Lebenschancen* (life chances). *Lebensführung*, or life conduct, refers to self-direction in behavior and is the element of choice (or agency) that people have in the lifestyles they adopt, but the potential for realizing these choices is influenced by their *Lebenschancen*, or life chances.[1] Weber is ambiguous about what he really means by life chances, but the most accepted interpretation is that of British-German sociologist Ralf Dahrendorf (1979:73) who determined that life chances in Weberian terms can be defined as the "crystalized probability of finding satisfaction for interests, wants, and needs, thus the probability

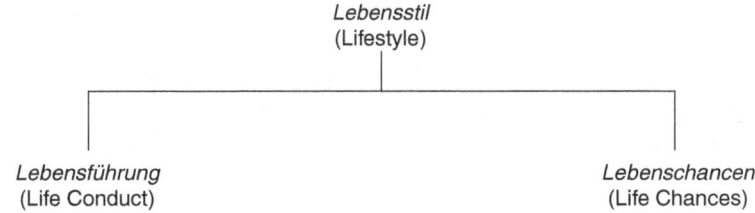

Lebensstil
(Lifestyle)

Lebensführung
(Life Conduct)

Lebenschancen
(Life Chances)

Figure 4.1 Weber's Lifestyle Components

of the occurrence of events which bring about satisfaction." For Weber, the notion of life chances therefore refers to the probability of acquiring satisfaction which is anchored in structural conditions that are predominately socioeconomic—consisting of income, property, the opportunity for profit, and the like—but also involving rights, norms, and social relationships (the probability that others will respond in a certain manner).

Weber's intent in conceptualizing lifestyles appears to be that of recognizing that people have choices (agency) in lifestyle selection, but the actualization of those choices is influenced by their life chances (structure). Life chances are socially determined, and class structure is an arrangement of those chances from top to bottom—all of which underscores the central role of social stratification in shaping lifestyle options as different classes reflect the lifestyles unique to them. When it comes to health, as will be discussed in Chapter 10, we will see how agency and structure operate in a dialectical fashion to mold lifestyle practices in particular ways that result in either healthy or unhealthy outcomes consistent with Weber's outlook.

Max Weber on Formal Rationality, Rational-Legal Authority, and Bureaucracy

Formal Rationality. Weber ([1922] 1978:85) defined formal rationality as the purposeful calculation of the most efficient means and procedures to realize goals. It is the type of thinking and process of logical deduction that people use to determine what is most important in particular situations and the most efficient method available for accomplishing what needs to be accomplished. Tradition, sentimentality, custom, piety, and various other types of potentially restraining ways of doing things innovatively or more efficiently are rejected in favor of calculating the most effective action that can be undertaken to achieve a desired outcome—what is sometimes called the "bottom line." In formal rationality all the past history, noise, and clutter on the margins is ignored and the focus is placed on what really matters.

Drawing upon his studies of Oriental societies, Weber found that traditional patterns of reasoning or rationality in Asian countries were different from the West, which he characterized as "substantive rationality." Substantive rationality is the realization of values and ideals based on custom, piety, or personal devotion. Weber ([1922] 1978) described how, in Western society, formal rationality became dominant over its substantive counterpart as people sought to achieve specific ends by employing the most efficient means and, in the process, tended to disregard substantive rationality because it was often cumbersome, time-consuming, inefficient, and stifled advancement on the basis of merit. This practical or formal type of rationality led to the rise of the West and the spread of capitalism.

The formal form of rationality that was most characteristic of Western society was by no means absent or insignificant in Asian civilizations (in fact, today it is especially prevalent in China, Japan, Singapore, and South Korea), but in the past "it operated from entirely different premises and accordingly it had a totally different impact upon the social fabric" (Mommsen 1989:161). The rationality prevalent in many Asian societies was strongly influenced by Confucianism and emphasized the abstract and the ideal, while advocating a lifestyle oriented toward harmony and an avoidance of embarrassment or loss of face. Conformity, deference to superiors, and obedience to traditional rules and customs were stressed. In the West, in contrast, the prevailing form of rationality was focused more on the practical than the abstract and strict codes of behavior, dogma, and tradition were disregarded if they impeded progress, creativity, or the achievement of practical goals.

Weber did not believe that formal rationality characterized Western society as a whole, but that it did become a more popular way of thinking than substantive rationality. In fact, it was a disregard of substantive ends and values in favor of calculated efficiency that made the West unique in his view. This form of rationality featured the freedom to inquire, experiment, and dispute, while it emphasized a concern for the practical over the abstract and a belief in the continued possibility of improvement unhindered by cultural, ideological, and political orthodoxy. Weber went on to link formal rationality to the origin and expansion of capitalism and connected it to modern institutions through bureaucratic forms of organization. He took the position that the most rational and efficient form of organization in managing complex human activity is the bureaucracy with its specialized tasks, hierarchy of formal offices with fixed channels of communication, emphasis on written and recorded orders, and so on. As Weber ([1905] 1958:25) points out, "modern rational capitalism has need, not only of the technical means of production, but of a calculable legal system and of administration in terms of formal rules."

A past example of how Weber's notion of formal rationality has been applied to the work of physicians is the concept of "deprofessionalization," which means a decline in a profession's autonomy and control over its clients. It does not mean a profession becomes less professional; rather, the profession is undergoing a decrease in power. Eliot Freidson's (1970a, 1970b) seminal work on the medical profession in the 1970s described American medicine's professional dominance over patients and its relations with external organizations, including the federal government. Medicine was *the* model of professionalism, with physicians having absolute authority and power over their work and ranked at or near the top of society in occupational status by sociologists. However, George Ritzer and David Walczak (1988) observed the loss of *absolute* authority by American physicians as their treatment decisions came under increasing scrutiny in the late twentieth century by patients, health care organizations, health insurance companies, and government agencies.

They found that government policies controlling health care costs and the rise of the profit motive in medicine identified a trend in medical practice away from substantive rationality (stressing ideals like serving the patient) toward greater formal rationality (stressing rules, regulations, and efficiency). Government and insurance company oversight in reviewing and approving patient care decisions, and the growth of private health care corporations hiring physicians as employees and controlling their work—joined with greater questioning and negotiation on the part of patients—to decrease the autonomy of medical doctors by reducing their professional power. Thus, the "golden age" of medical power and prestige that was prevalent in the mid-twentieth century ended, as medicine's efforts to avoid outside control left open an unregulated medical market in the U.S. that was quickly filled by fiscal controls over medical work, by corporate controls and government regulation.

Rational-Legal Authority. Before discussing Weber's concept of bureaucracy, it is useful to briefly review his insights on authority. Weber ([1922] 1978:215) identified three distinct types of authority: (1) traditional, (2) charismatic, and (3) rational-legal, with the latter providing the framework for bureaucratic decision-making. Traditional authority is the authority of a monarch based on the sanctity of past traditions that are handed down from one generation to another. People obey the monarch because they believe he or she has the right to rule. This right is not based on reason, but tradition. Charismatic authority rests on devotion to an exceptional individual whose personal qualities of heroism, personality, character, and/or perhaps wisdom inspire obedience. Such authority is often expressed dramatically and associated with radical change. However, as Weber points out, charismatic authority is not, by its nature, stable or lasting. Charisma can be maintained only for so long, and, once it becomes routine, it begins to have less effect on people. Therefore, Weber explains, it is the fate of charismatic leadership eventually to be transformed into traditional or rational-legal authority once it becomes routine. That is, the charismatic leader eventually adopts either a traditional or a rational-legal approach to leadership if he or she stays in power.

Rational-legal authority, in contrast, rests on a belief in the legality of enacted rules and the right of those occupying positions of authority under such rules to issue commands. Obedience is thus owed to legal orders and extends to persons whose office gives them the authority to issue those orders. People who obey orders issued from such authority do so because they are members of the organization or society that has recognized the authority's right to give these orders. In this situation, people are obeying impersonal rules, not the personal commands of a sovereign or charismatic individual. Rational-legal authority is the basis upon which bureaucracies operate and is intended to apply to all people over whom it has legal jurisdiction. It follows orderly procedures for appointments and dismissals from office, appeals, decision-making, allocations of areas of responsibility, and similar matters. Authority is attached to the office, not to the person holding the office. When the person is no longer the officeholder, he or she no longer has the authority that goes with it. Rational-legal authority is the dominant authority system in the world.

Bureaucracy. Weber's ([1922] 1978:809) concept of formal rationality at the macro level and his ([1922] 1978:24) notion of *zweckrztionalität* (calculation of purposeful goal-oriented action by individuals) at the micro level, along with his projection of the replacement of traditional and charismatic forms of authority by rational-legal systems, are all part of a general *process* of rationalization constructed on principles of efficiency and calculation. This process includes the emergence of the bureaucracy as the most efficient form of rational-legal organization in managing complex human affairs. In *Economy and Society* ([1922] 1978:956–8), Weber described bureaucracy as a rational and impersonal division of labor characterized by the principles of office hierarchy and levels of graded authority (lower offices are supervised by higher ones) and by fixed and official areas of jurisdiction governed by laws or administrative regulations. In bureaucracies, tasks are specialized; communication between the hierarchy of offices, with their designated channels of communication and authority, is based on written and recorded orders; there is a sharp separation of official from personal identity in the management of work; and rules and regulations are intended to be objective and logical in their application.

What makes Weber's theory of bureaucracy distinctive is that it sees bureaucracies evolving in business, government, religion, education, medicine, and elsewhere as an outcome of the process of formal rationalization. Although bureaucracies are an outgrowth of rationalism, Weber notes they also contain inherent tendencies toward dehumanization, since their procedures and decisions are generally impersonal. Weber ([1922] 1978:988) analyzed the manner in which modern bureaucracies impose rigid rules and regulations—an "iron cage"—on people in the name of efficiency and warns of the possibilities of bureaucracies becoming so rigid and inflexible that individuals find themselves trapped and their lives overregulated as "a small cog in a ceaselessly moving mechanism" traveling along a "fixed route of march."

However, Weber's warning can be seen as more of a possibility than a certainty, since his writings contain evidence that he also viewed rationality as an enhancement of freedom. This is seen in Weber's (1949:124–5) statement that:

> we associate the strongest empirical "feeling of freedom" with precisely those actions which we know ourselves to have accomplished rationally, i.e., in the absence of physical or psychic "compulsion"; actions in which we "pursue" a clear conscious "purpose" by what to our knowledge are the most adequate means.

Therefore, Weber also seems to have viewed formal rationality as means to achieve creative goals through the exercise of logic (Mommsen 1989). This is because rationality provides individuals with a basis for self-responsibility and allows them to chart their own goals and aspirations by assuming control over their circumstances and engaging in opportunities for creativity and self-expression. Even though bureaucratic procedures can be inflexible and tedious, the bureaucracy remains the most efficient type of organization yet devised to manage complex work and that includes health care delivery systems and hospitals.

Hospitals. Hospitals are not a perfect match for Weber's concept of bureaucracy because of their dual system of authority. One authority system is administrative and bureaucratic, and the other is clinical which can require a flexible, non-bureaucratic response, especially in critical or emergency situations. Weber's perspective on bureaucracy can nevertheless be applied to the general organization of hospital work (Cockerham 2015). The key to hospital efficiency and its effectiveness as an institution is its coordination of the work performed by various departments and individuals focused on the overall objective of patient care. Hospital work represents a complex and highly specialized division of labor whose elements are both interlocking and interdependent. In order to accomplish its tasks and coordinate its activities, the hospital's hierarchy of authority is well defined. The overall supervision of general and specialized hospitals comes under the auspices of its governing body, such as a board of trustees, a corporate headquarters, or government agency. Whereas the medical director and the hospital administrator are both directly responsible to the governing body, they are typically only indirectly responsible to each other. This system of dual authority is an outgrowth of the organizational division in hospitals between bureaucracy and professionalism. The basis of the division consists of the professional's (the physician's) insistence on exercising an autonomous judgment on patient care, while the bureaucrat (the hospital administrator) seeks to follow a rationally based management approach that favors the efficient coordination of the hospital's activities through formal rules and impersonal regulations applicable to all persons in all situations, including physicians.

Since the physician's professional practices can set specific limits on the hospital administrator's authority and vice versa, the result has been a system of dual authority. The occupational groups in the hospital most affected by its system of dual authority are the nurses and auxiliary nursing workers who perform health care tasks based on a physician's orders. Nurses are responsible to physicians for carrying out their orders, but they also are responsible to the hospital's administration for following its standardized procedures. Even though the communication and allegiance of ward personnel tend to be channeled along occupational lines within and toward the "administrative channel of command," medical authority can and does cut across these lines. Although this system may at times result in an overlapping of responsibility, it functions because all involved share a common goal of providing quality patient care.

While hospital services are oriented toward patient welfare, hospital rules and regulations are nevertheless designed for the benefit of hospital personnel, so that the work of treating large numbers of patients can be more systematic and efficient. Consequently, the sick and the injured are organized into various patient categories (such as maternity-obstetrics, orthopedics, surgery, pediatrics, psychiatry, and so on) that reflect the medical staff's diagnosis of their problem and are then subject to standardized, staff-approved medical treatment and administrative procedures. While it can be argued that standardizing patient care results in increased organizational efficiency—and ultimately serves the best interest of the patient—it is clear that hospital bureaucracy is organized to expedite the work of the staff and involves bureaucratic control over the patient's activities and options.

In order for the hospital to function effectively, it has therefore been necessary to construct a decentralized system of authority organized around a generally acceptable objective of service to the patient. While the administrator directs and supervises hospital policy, the medical staff has traditionally retained control over medical decisions. Hospitals, however, can be held legally responsible for what happens within their premises. This means hospitals have responsibility for patients separate from that of physicians. Liability for patient care results in the hospital imposing more of its rules and regulations on physicians, raising the standards of qualification required for staff privileges, and generally reducing the amount of professional discretion and autonomy physicians have traditionally been allowed to exercise. This is especially the case in corporate-owned profit-making hospitals, but also extends to nonprofit and government-owned facilities. Thus, control by hospital administrators may affect not only professional discretion, but also professional effectiveness, as the practitioners within the hospital are provided with better coordination of services and staff support. Enhanced coordination and control of services are already being provided for hospital administrators through the information systems made available by modern computer technology. In all probability, the hospital administration in nonprofit, profit-making, and government hospitals have increased control over the staff through computerization of information as a basis for decision-making.

Studies of hospital bureaucracies typically begin with Weber's concept, even though his model is not totally compatible with the norms of hospital authority. Nevertheless, the trend today is more toward his model than away from it. The essence of the conflict between bureaucracy and the professional (such as a physician) consists of the professional's insistence on exercising an autonomous individual judgment, while the bureaucrat (here, the hospital administrator) seeks to follow a rationalistic management approach that favors the efficient coordination of the hospital's activities through formal rules and impersonal regulations applicable to all persons in all situations. But in contemporary times, legal liability, computerization, government regulation, private and government insurance fee schedules, and organizational changes like managed care have eroded the professional status and autonomy of physicians in making independent decisions and, correspondingly, bureaucratic managers of hospitals have assumed greater control. Weber's concept of bureaucracy is therefore more applicable to hospitals today than ever before.

Summary

This chapter examines the contributions of Durkheim and Weber to medical sociology. Durkheim's work most directly applicable to the field is his study of suicide with its typology of egoistic, anomic, and altruistic forms of suicide, along with his influence on the concept of social capital. A particularly pertinent insight is his recognition that societal processes beyond the individual can create stressful situations in which people are forced to respond to external conditions not of their own choosing.

Weber noted the early dominance of formal rationality over its substantive counterpart in the West and its role in spreading capitalism, as well as promoting the rise of the bureaucracy for managing complex human activities.

While not a perfect fit for hospitals, such institutions have nevertheless adopted bureaucratic procedures as the basis for their managerial structure. As we move into the future, the hospital bureaucratic model appears to be coming closer to, not further from, Weber's concept. Consequently, when it comes to hospital bureaucracies and other areas of medical sociology, Weber's work still informs us about the effects of social conditions associated with the onset of modernity. Weber's ideas led to the development of socioeconomic status consisting of income, education, and occupational prestige as a major indicator of social-class position and provided a foundation for research on lifestyles generally and health lifestyles in particular.

Guide to Critical Thinking

1. What is a "social fact" according to Durkheim? How do social facts represent society's influence on the individual?
2. How do Durkheim's four types of suicide differ from one another? What is the key variable common to each type?
3. What are the major components of socioeconomic status according to Weber and how does each component relate to considerations of health?
4. Describe Weber's concept of formal rationality and its application to hospital bureaucracy.

Note

1 Weber did not regard lifestyles simply as a matter of choice or agency, nor did he ignore the effects of structure on lifestyle choices. Both agency (life choices or *Lebensführung*) and structure (life chances or *Lebenschancen*) are included in his lifestyle concept. However, in researching Weber's ([1922] 1978) work on lifestyles in the original German in his seminal chapter, "*Machtverteilung innerhalb der Germeinschaft: Klassen, Stände, Parteien*" ["The Distribution of Power within the Community: Class, Status, Party," in *Wirtschaft und Gesellschaft* [Economy and Society] ([1922] 1956:531–540), German medical sociologist Thomas Abel and the author (Abel and Cockerham 1993) found that the English-language translation of *Economy and Society* ([1922] 1978) by Guenther Roth and Claus Wittich contained a mistake in translation. The mistranslation occurred when "*Lebensstil*" (lifestyle) and "*Lebensführung*" (life conduct or self-direction) were both translated from German into English as "lifestyle," and this error was carried forward in other publications over time (i.e., Weber 1946, translated and edited by Hans Gerth and C. Wright Mills). Consequently, Weber's use of *Lebensführung*, referring to choice (agency) appears as "lifestyle" in English and does not have the distinctive meaning he intended in English translations of his work.

Suggested Reading

Fournier, Marcel. 2013. *Émile Durkheim*. Cambridge: Polity.
An account of the life and work of Émile Durkheim.
Radkau, Joachim. 2009. *Max Weber: A Biography*. Cambridge: Polity.
A thorough biography of Max Weber.

References

Abel, Thomas and William C. Cockerham. 1993. "Lifestyle or Lebensführung? Critical Remarks on the Mistranslation of Weber's 'Class, Status, Party.'" *Sociological Quarterly* 34(3):551–6.
Archer, Margaret S. 1995. *Realist Social Theory: The Morphogenetic Approach*. Cambridge: Cambridge University Press.
Baert, Patrick. 2007. "Conceptualizing Max Weber." *International Sociology* 22(2):119–28.
Bourdieu, Pierre. 1984. *Distinction*. Cambridge, MA: Harvard University Press.
Cockerham, William C. 2005. "Health Lifestyle Theory and the Convergence of Agency and Structure." *Journal of Health and Social Behavior* 46(1):51–67.
Cockerham, William C. 2013a. *Social Causes of Health and Disease*, 2nd ed. Cambridge: Polity.
Cockerham, William C. (ed.). 2013b. *Medical Sociology on the Move: New Directions in Theory*. Dordrecht: Springer.
Cockerham, William C. 2013c. "Sociological Theory in Medical Sociology in the Early Twenty-First Century." *Social Theory & Health* 11(3):241–55.
Cockerham, William C. 2015. "Max Weber: Formal Rationality and the Modern Hospital," in Fran Collyer (ed.), *Palgrave Handbook of Social Theory in Health, Illness and Medicine*. London: Palgrave Macmillan, pp. 124–38.
Connell, R.W. 1997. "Why is Classical Theory Classical?" *American Journal of Sociology* 102(6):1511–57.
Dahrendorf, Ralf. 1979. *Life Chances*. Chicago, IL: University of Chicago Press.
De Maio, Fernando. 2010. *Health and Social Theory*. Basingstoke: Palgrave Macmillan.
Durkheim, Émile. [1893] 1964. *The Division of Labor in Society*. New York: Free Press.
Durkheim, Émile. [1895] 1964. *The Rules of Sociological Method*. Glencoe, IL: Free Press.
Durkheim, Émile. [1897] 1951. *Suicide: A Study in Sociology*. New York: Free Press.
Durkheim, Émile. [1912] 1965. *The Elementary Forms of Religious Life*. New York: Free Press.
Fournier, Marcel. 2013. *Émile Durkheim*. Cambridge: Polity.
Freidson, Eliot. 1970a. *Profession of Medicine*. New York: Dodd, Mead.
Freidson, Eliot. 1970b. *Professional Dominance*. Chicago, IL: Aldine.
Giddens, Anthony. 1991. *Modernity and Self-Identity*. Stanford, CA: Stanford University Press.
Giddens, Anthony, Mitchell Duneier, Richard P. Applebaum, and Deborah Carr. 2018. *Introduction to Sociology*, 10th ed. New York: W.W. Norton.
Heilbron, Johan. 2015. *French Sociology*. Ithaca, NY: Cornell University Press.

Henslin, James M. 2019. *Essentials of Sociology: A Down to Earth Approach*, 14th ed. Boston, MA: Sage.

Jaspers, Karl. 1989. *On Max Weber*. New York: Paragon House.

Kunst, Anton E. and Albert-Jan Roskam. 2010. "Using the ESeC to Describe Socio-economic Inequalities in Health in Europe," in David Rose and Eric Harrison (eds.), *Social Class in Europe: An Introduction to the European Socio-economic Classification*. London: Routledge, pp. 216–34.

Lukes, Steven. 1973. *Émile Durkheim*. Harmondsworth: Penguin.

Macionis, John J. 2018. *Sociology*, 16th ed. Harlow: Pearson Education.

McDonnell, Orla, Maria Lohan, Abbey Hyde, and Sam Porter. 2009. *Social Theory, Health and Healthcare*. Basingstoke: Palgrave Macmillan.

Mommsen, Wolfgang. 1989. *The Political and Social Theory of Max Weber*. Cambridge: Polity.

Parsons, Talcott. 1981. "Revisiting the Classics throughout a Long Career," in Buford Rhea (ed.), *The Future of the Sociological Classics*. London: George Allen & Unwin, pp. 183–94.

Pearlin, Leonard I., Scott Schieman, Elena M. Fazio, and Stephen C. Meersman. 2005. "Stress, Health, and the Life Course: Some Conceptual Perspectives." *Journal of Health and Social Behavior* 46(2):205–19.

Pescosolido, Bernice A. and Jennie J. Kronenfeld. 1995. "Health, Illness, and Healing in an Uncertain Era: Challenges from and for Medical Sociology." *Journal of Health and Social Behavior* 35(extra issue):5–35.

Phelan, Jo C., Bruce G. Link, Ana Diez-Roux, Ichiro Kawachi, and Bruce Levin. 2004. "Fundamental Causes of Social Inequalities in Mortality: A Test of the Theory." *Journal of Health and Social Behavior* 45(3):265–85.

Radkau, Joachim. 2009. *Max Weber: A Biography*. Cambridge: Polity.

Ringer, Fritz. 2004. *Max Weber: An Intellectual Biography*. Chicago, IL: University of Chicago Press.

Ritzer, George and Jeffrey Stepnisky. 2018. *Sociological Theory*, 10th ed. Los Angeles, CA: Sage.

Ritzer, George and David Walczak. 1988. "Rationalization and the Deprofessionalization of Physicians." *Social Forces* 67(1):1–22.

Ritzer, George and Wendy A. Wiedenhoft Murphy. 2019. *Essentials of Sociology*, 3rd ed. Thousand Oaks, CA: Sage.

Rose, David and Eric Harrison (eds.). 2010. *Social Class in Europe: An Introduction to the European Socio-economic Classification*. London: Routledge.

Royce, Edward. 2015. *Classical Social Theory and Modern Society: Marx, Durkheim, Weber*. Lanham, MD: Rowman and Littlefield.

Scambler, Graham. 2012. "Health-related Stigma." *Sociology of Health & Illness* 31(3):441–55.

Song, Lijun. 2013. "Social Capital and Health," in William Cockerham (ed.), *Medical Sociology on the Move: New Directions in Theory*. Dordrecht: Springer, pp. 233–58.

Turner, Bryan S. 2004. *The New Medical Sociology*. New York: W. W. Norton.

Weber, M. [1905] 1958. *The Protestant Ethic and the Spirit of Capitalism*. Talcott Parsons (trans.) New York: Scribner's.

Weber, Max. [1919] 1946. "Science as a Vocation," in Hans Gerth and C. Wright Mills (eds. and trans.), *From Max Weber: Essays in Sociology*. New York: Oxford University Press, pp. 129–56.

Weber, Max. [1922] 1956. *Wirtschaft und Gesellschaft [Economy and Society]*. Tübingen: J. C. B. Mohr.

Weber, Max. [1922] 1978. *Economy and Society*, 2 vols, Guenther Roth and Claus Wittich (trans. and eds.). Berkeley, CA: University of California Press.

Weber, Max. 1946. *From Max Weber: Essays in Sociology*. Hans Gerth and C. Wright Mills (trans. and eds.). New York: Oxford University Press.

Weber, Max. 1949. *The Methodology of the Social Sciences*. Edward Shils and H. Finch (eds.). New York: Free Press.

Winkleby, Marilyn A., Darius E. Jatulis, Erica Frank, and Stephen P. Fortmann. 1992. "Socioeconomic Status and Health: How Education, Income, and Occupation Contribute to Risk Factors for Cardiovascular Disease." *American Journal of Public Health* 82:816–20.

Chapter 5

Classical Theory

Marx

This chapter reviews the theoretical formulations of Karl Marx that remain relevant for medical sociology. He has a controversial history with sociology, was the last of the Durkheim–Weber–Marx trio to be canonized, and did not establish sociology as an academic discipline. Nonetheless, some of his ideas have persisted as lasting influences on sociological theory and, by extension, on medical sociology. The chapter also examines how Marxist theory affected sociological theory under communism in order to provide a more complete account of its historical impact on sociology and medical sociology.

Marx

Karl Marx (1818–1883), born in present-day Germany and spending most of his life in exile because of his political views, was a distinct latecomer to canonization (Connell 1997). He was a socialist theorist and revolutionary, not a sociologist. His approach to theory is evident in *The German Ideology* (Marx and Engels [1888] 1976:620), originally published in 1845, where Marx and his colleague Friedrich Engels famously declared: "Philosophers have only *interpreted* the world in various ways; the point, however, is to *change* it." And while social change, namely the overthrow of capitalism and the establishment of a classless society, was the clear intent of Marx's activist theoretical philosophy, his views nonetheless became influential in sociology because of his analysis of the economic basis of social stratification.

However, Marx's theorizing was not particularly visible in mainstream sociology for a lengthy period, other than Weber's critiques of his ideas. Talcott Parsons, for example, in his seminal book, *The Structure of Social Action* (1937), does not treat Marx as an equal to Durkheim and Weber or even Alfred Marshall and Vilfredo Pareto. Parsons (1937:110) does at least recognize Marx as an important bridge between the positivist and idealist traditions in sociology, but otherwise Marx is treated as a background figure in sociology.[1] Moreover, Marx is absent in a mid-twentieth-century review of sociology's major theorists in *An Introduction to the History of Sociology* (Barnes 1948) and scarcely mentioned in Robert Merton's influential theory book *Social Theory and Social Structure* (1957).

During the Cold War between the United States and other Western democracies and the Marxist-inspired former Soviet Union and its allies, there was both rejection of, and hostility toward, Marx (Ritzer and Stepnisky 2018). As Fran Collyer (2015:35) points out: "In the West, their [Marx and Engels] works have always been contentious and controversial, and there have been, and continue to be, profound disagreements over interpretation and even disputes about the authors' intentions." Following the collapse of the communist version of socialism in the former Soviet Union and Eastern Europe, Marx's influence in sociology went into an observable decline.

As Alex Callinicos (2007) described it, Marxism began losing influence from the late 1970s onward, with political events sinking Marxist theory in Western universities. First, French scholars turned their back on Marxism as a "theory of domination" in response to Soviet labor camps, the Cold War, and the crackdown on the Solidarity labor union in Poland in 1981, followed by similar reactions elsewhere in Europe and Latin America. "The process of retreat was slower in the English-speaking world," states Callinicos (2007:261), "but by the beginning of the 1990s, under the impact of postmodernism and the collapse of 'existing socialism' in Eastern Europe and the Soviet Union, Marx was a dead dog for most intellectuals there as well."

Yet despite being pronounced dead many times, Marxist theory has seen somewhat of a revival in sociology as it is no longer burdened so completely by its association with communism (Antonio 2011). As the gap in income between the rich and poor in many countries has grown larger, renewed interest on the part of some scholars in what Marx had to say has taken place. This situation has relevance for medical sociology as differences in health and life expectancy have correspondingly widened along with the income gap, thereby revitalizing pro-Marxist scholarship (Garnham 2014; Scambler 2012; Scambler and Scambler 2014). Much of this work is termed "neo-Marxist" because it extends Marxist thought beyond the boundaries of its classical stage (Muntaner et al. 2014; Scambler 2018). Neo-Marxism has taken many forms, some no longer relevant, including structural (social developmental) Marxism, analytical (rigorous) Marxism, cultural (race, gender, and the arts) Marxism, Western (philosophical) Marxism, libertarian (less authoritarian) Marxism, and Marxist feminism (blaming capitalism for the oppression of women)—resulting in a multiplicity of perspectives.

However, to claim in a clear straightforward manner that Marxism is "back" (or noticeably "still here") is not entirely accurate; instead, "it is *Marx*, rather than *Marxism*, whose strengths are being appreciated" (McLennan

2001:52). What this means in relation to medical sociology is that while Marx's political ideology about revolution, historical materialism, and a class-less society have lost influence, his ideas about the causes of social inequality in relation to health and sickness still resonate. Although Marxist theory failed to produce a sustainable political and economic system when it was put into practice in the former socialist countries of Europe, it did illustrate the division of society along economic lines. According to Robert Antonio (2011:115), perhaps no other social theorist has provoked more intense and contradictory responses from more globally dispersed audiences than Marx—whose name is associated with some of the last century's greatest emancipatory struggles and worst repression. Nevertheless, as Antonio (2011:116) summarizes: Marx's "work is as analytical and sociological as it is political; it has generated diverse lines of social research and social theory," and he remains important because the issues of class, exploitation, poverty, ideology, and capitalism are still alive and subjects of contemporary debate.

Box 5.1 Karl Marx

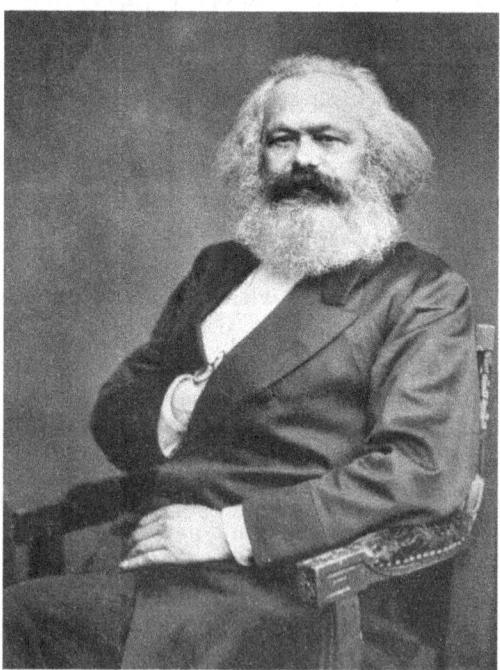

Image 5.1 Karl Marx

Karl Marx was born on May 5, 1818 in Trier in the province of Rhineland of what was then Prussia and now Germany. Marx's family was originally Jewish, but his father converted to Christianity (Lutheranism) and adopted the name of Heinrich Marx (previously it had been Herschel Levi) as he pursued a secular career in law. His mother, Henrietta Philips, was from a family of Hungarian Jews who emigrated to Holland and whose descendants founded Philips Electronics. She was a housewife who had eight children of whom Karl Marx was the second. In 1835, at age 17, Marx attended the University of Bonn, but his father had him transfer to the University of Berlin because of arrests for drunkenness and disturbing the peace, running up debts, and dueling. In Berlin, Marx studied law and philosophy and joined the politically left-wing group, the "Young Hegelians," whose outlook was based on the dialectical philosophy of Georg Hegel (1770–1831). In 1836, he became secretly engaged to Jenny von Westphalen (1814–1881), whom he had known since childhood. She was four years older and from a wealthier family.

Marx received his doctorate in 1841 at the age of 23, but was unable to obtain an academic position because of his politics. Instead, he became a journalist and then editor of a Cologne newspaper, the *Rheinische Zeitung*, until the paper was closed down by the Prussian government in 1843 for its leftist opinions. He married Westphalen in 1843 and they moved to Paris where he edited a journal, was active in revolutionary politics, and became friends with Friedrich Engels (1820–1895), his long-time colleague and supporter. The two collaborated on several writing projects, including *The German Ideology* in 1845 and *Manifesto of the Communist Party* in 1848.

In 1849, Marx moved to London since he had been declared unwelcome by governments in Prussia, France, and Belgium. He lived there the rest of his life, living off a small salary he received as a correspondent for European affairs for the *New York Daily Tribune* and money provided by friends, especially Engels. He resided in poverty in one of the worst sections of the city until his financial situation improved later in life. Much of Marx's time was spent in London's British Museum, where he produced his most notable work, *Das Kapital* [Capital], the first volume of which was published in 1867 and two others posthumously from notes found by Engels after his death. Marx was apparently a loving father, but his family life was tragic. Of his seven children, three died in infancy, one in childhood, and two adult daughters, both socialist activists, committed suicide at ages 43 and 66, respectively, after his death. A year after his wife died in 1881, his much beloved first-born daughter, also named Jenny, died of cancer at age 38 in 1882, and Marx himself passed away on March 14, 1883 at the age of 64 sitting in a chair in his study. Marx was never personally popular or even widely read in his lifetime, and much of his life was spent in obscurity; only 11 mourners attended his funeral in London and his death was mostly unnoticed by the general public (Ritzer and Stepnisky 2018).

Why was Marx eventually canonized as one of the three most important classical theorists in sociology? According to Australian sociologist Raewyn Connell (1997): (1) he was the founding father of social science for socialists; (2) his writings were readily available in translation because of his importance to socialism; (3) his work was prominent because of opposition to many of his ideas by other theorists (notably Weber); and (4) there was strong interest in his ideas by the radical left in Western societies and universities in the 1960s. More recently, Marx's ideas resurfaced in response to the global economic crisis of 2008 that fit his analysis of capitalism's cyclic swings disadvantaging workers.

It should also be said that Marx developed an influential science of society some 40 years before Durkheim. His concepts turned out to be the leading explanation of revolutionary social change in the twentieth century. They served as the foundation for communism that continues as the dominant political and social ideology of present-day China, North Korea, Vietnam, and Cuba, as well as in the former Soviet Union and Eastern Europe before imploding in those locales in 1989–1991. For some historians (e.g., Lukacs 1993), the momentous peacetime collapse of socialism in communist Europe could be said to be a defining event of the twentieth century—which underscores the magnitude of Marx's once prominent influence.

Wendell Bell (1990:161) noted long ago that despite the eventual failure of his economic ideas when put into practice or the oppression that accompanied the social systems developed by his followers, Marx nevertheless "incorporated and gave life to the idea that humans can, through action, change their own circumstances and thus change themselves as well as society." The oppression that Bell refers to is that as Marxist groups achieved power, they invariably either executed, imprisoned, or exiled to labor camps or other countries, those who did not agree with them and even some who did in the case of Joseph Stalin's "show trials" in the former Soviet Union in the 1930s. The exact number of people who perished or were sent to labor camps is unknown, but it is estimated to be in the millions (Brown 2009). By 1939, the Gulag—the Soviet system of labor camps—was the largest employer in

Europe (Davies 1996). While socialism under Stalin may not have been what Marx intended and considered a perversion of his theories, it was nevertheless based on an authoritarian version of his ideas (Brown 2009; Pipes 2001).

Because of such circumstances, it could be considered unlikely that Marxist theory persists and Marx himself is canonized in sociology. Yet as Bell (1990) explains, as a *theory*, Marx's perspective emphasizes values that have a universal appeal—an end to alienation, inequality, and conflict between social classes, along with goals of social justice and opportunities for self-fulfillment. What is not mentioned by Bell is that in order to realize these values, a revolution and destruction of the existing social order under capitalism was required, thereby highlighting conflict as a fundamental feature of Marx's view of society. This is seen in Marx's concept of historical materialism and class struggle that are of particular significance in understanding how his thinking has been applied to medical sociology.

Historical Materialism and Class Struggle

Historical materialism is the view that social, cultural, and political phenomena are historically determined by a society's mode of producing its material goods. Control over the means of production is the critical variable because it is the basis upon which an individual is assigned to a social class. Those who own or control the means of production sit at the top of society and in a position to monopolize whatever surpluses (or profits) are produced by labor at the bottom. Exploitation in capitalist economies results when business owners use the labor of workers to increase their wealth, which is based on paying workers far less than the full value of what they produce when it is sold in the marketplace. This situation is inherently unequal and inevitably leads to class conflict between the owners, who try to protect the economic system on which their wealth, privilege, and power depend, and the workers, who seek a larger share of the profits and a better life. As Russian Marxist theorist V. D. Zotov (1985:116) once explained, "the underlying reason for the struggle between antagonistic classes is very simple indeed: exploiters oppress the exploited, while the exploited act to rid themselves of exploitation and the exploiters."

Briefly stated, Marx's theory is that class inequality leads to conflict that causes social change. This view is based on Hegel's theory of dialectics, which holds that any idea or event (a thesis) generates its opposite (an antithesis) and the resulting interaction eventually leads to a reconciliation or change (a synthesis) that is new and more advanced. The new synthesis then becomes the new thesis, which is subjected to its own antithesis that results in yet another synthesis and so on through history until the ultimate synthesis (what Hegel called the "absolute idea") is reached.

In this context, Marx maintained that societies follow a set path of universal laws in which two social classes struggle against one another for social and economic domination throughout history. His analysis begins with primitive communism in which tribes of early humans shared their resources, but over time some people accumulated more things of value than other people leading to the rise of aristocracies who developed the power to enslave others. Whatever was produced by slaves was owned solely by their masters. Slavery was replaced by feudalism, yet the economic mode of production remained largely agricultural and was controlled by a land-owning aristocracy. Labor was provided by serfs, who were not slaves and had some rights, but still were not entirely free to move elsewhere. Serfs agreed to work specific parcels of land and to turn over part of their crops to the landowner, and often to work without pay a certain number of days each year on the landowner's estate. This system gave way to industrialization and the rise of capitalism. Those at the bottom of society now had to sell their labor to factory owners in exchange for wages in order to live. Thus, capitalism joins slavery and feudalism as forms of exploitation. Class struggle continues until capitalism is overturned and socialism is achieved in which the state assumes ownership of private property (factories, buildings, railroads, etc.) and no one's labor is exploited for someone else's financial gain. Socialism then transforms into communism as "the state withers away" and consists of a society in which there are no social classes and total equality.

In Marx's view, the history of class relationships is therefore one of constant struggle between the "haves" and the "have-nots." In fact, Marx argues that individuals form a class only as they become engaged in a common struggle against another class. Struggle leads to social change as new classes and class relationships emerge over time and continues to the end state of communism. The transfer of economic and political power from one class to another underlies the process by which society evolves from one phase to the next. Marx believed that two historical periods were particularly important. One was the transition from feudalism to capitalism, in which the struggle between lords and serfs was replaced by conflict between two new classes, the bourgeoisie (capitalist owners and managers) and the proletariat (industrial workers). The second important period would begin when the workers destroyed capitalism through revolution and established a classless (communist) society after a period of socialism in which wealth was shared equally. Writing in the *Manifesto of the Communist Party*, Marx and Engels (1848:473) summarized class struggle as follows:

> The history of all hitherto existing society is the history of class struggles. Freeman and slave, patrician and plebeian, lord and serf, guildmaster and journeyman, in a word, oppressor and oppressed stood in constant

opposition to one another, carried on an uninterrupted, now hidden, now open fight, a fight that each time ended either in a revolutionary reconstitution of society at large, or in the common ruin of the contending classes.

Workers do not become revolutionaries, claims Marx, until they recognize (develop a class consciousness of) the shared nature of their exploitation and the need for collective action against the system that gave them their class identity. This process is assisted by the inherent instability of the capitalist system, whose contradictory periodic swings from prosperity into economic recessions or depressions cause workers to lose their jobs and become even more desperate. After a revolution and the end of capitalist society, a new social order evolves in which private ownership of property is abolished and replaced with state ownership, and all persons are equal in a genuinely classless society with equal shares in what is produced. Just how this classless utopia was to be ultimately achieved, however, was never fully articulated. There is no hint in Marx's writing about how state ownership of property under socialism was to transition to the highest stage of full communism, marking the establishment of a classless social system. As French economist Thomas Piketty (2014:10) describes it:

> Marx ... devoted little thought to the question of how a society in which private property had been totally abolished would be organized politically and economically—a complex issue if ever there was one, as shown by the tragic totalitarian experiments undertaken in states where private capital was abolished.

It also needs to be pointed out that social conflict in capitalist societies has not been reduced to antagonism between capitalists and workers that drive history; rather, power struggles oriented toward some type of hegemony have mostly involved a variety of interest groups and their political allies. Furthermore, the notion that there are only two social classes is obviously flawed, as existing class models are exceedingly more complex, beginning even with the basic three-class configuration (lower, middle, and upper) and extending to as many as ten social classes in the current European Socio-Economic Classification (ESeC) model (Rose and Harrison 2010) and 12 class positions in Erik Olin Wright's (1997) reformulated neo-Marxist class scheme.

There has also been the emergence of a relatively large middle class of managerial, technical, and administrative specialists who interpose themselves between owners and workers. This middle group, consisting of both upper- and lower-middle-class individuals, was generally ignored by Marx, yet has grown substantially since Marx's time and represents a large and highly diverse array of middle-level occupations. Wright (1997) addressed this anomaly in his attempt to reconstruct Marxist class analysis by adding in what he called "contradictory class locations" that included middle-class groupings, but his class scheme is not generally used in sociological research because other models of class position more readily lend themselves to statistical analysis (Atkinson 2015:38–9).

Moreover, some sociologists, as British sociologist Will Atkinson (2015) points out, question whether "class" as conceptualized by Marx and others in the past is even relevant today; that is, is it still useful? This is because the class structure of advanced societies has moved on from its industrial form into a postindustrial era profile in which manufacturing jobs have increasingly disappeared into developing economies (especially in Asia) where labor costs are cheaper. Expansion has come instead in technology and the service sector (health care, banking, finance, hospitality, tourism, personal services, etc.). The predicted proliferation of various forms of artificial intelligence in manufacturing and other areas of the economy is likely to produce even more changes from the world known by Marx. Postindustrialism is, in reality, deindustrialization—all of which makes Marx's basic view of a two-class system in which the industrial working class eventually becomes all-powerful no longer pertinent as a model of social stratification.

While it could easily be surmised from the critiques of historical materialism and class struggle discussed above that Marxism has run its course in sociology and is now out of date, this chapter is obviously here because there are Marxist concepts applicable to medical sociology that persist. First, we will see how sociological theory and medical sociology fared under Marxist regimes before examining how Marxist-oriented theories currently perform in medical sociology.

Sociological Theory and Medical Sociology

Soviet Union/Russia

Marx was not only *the* central social theorist in communist countries, he was the *only* theorist of consequence other than Vladimir Lenin (1870–1924) who led the Bolshevik (communist) takeover in Russia and contributed his own political ideas to Marxism. However, instead of Marx's theories promoting the establishment of sociology under communism, his prominence stunted the field's growth. Marxism was a theory of society and no other science of society, namely sociology, was considered needed nor allowed to develop by those in power. Past work in sociology was ignored and efforts to continue it curtailed, since only Marxism-Leninism was considered the "true" social science (Zotov 1985:326). Sociology was, in fact, labeled in the Soviet Union by Lenin's successor Stalin as a "bourgeois pseudoscience" which resulted in it being banned until after Stalin's death in 1953. As Russian sociologist Vladimir Shlapentokh (1987:14) stated:

> under Stalin sociology in the USSR was effectively destroyed. Its very mention instilled fear. The term "sociology" was declared bourgeois; it appeared exclusively in quotations and then only in a pejorative sense. It was ironic that the only person to use the term in a positive way was Stalin himself, in his last speech to a party congress, when he suddenly spoke about "general sociological laws" (1952). Yet the fear born of habit was deeply rooted and even after Stalin himself had employed the term "sociology," no one else risked its public use.

Sociology was not organized in the former Soviet Union as a formal discipline until 1958 when a small group of Soviet intellectuals and academics convinced the government that the work of Marx, Engels, and Lenin was associated with sociological principles and, moreover, that sociology could further socialism by providing scientific studies of the social processes justifying socialism and leading to communism (Titarenko and Zdravomyslova 2017). Yet allegiance to Marxism-Leninism was not enough when government officials were uncomfortable with a sociology that sometimes investigated social problems (i.e., prostitution, crime, inadequate housing) that were officially nonexistent under communism. As Raisa Gorbachev (1991:94), holder of a Ph.D. in sociology from Moscow State University and wife of the Soviet Union's last leader, Mikhail Gorbachev, pointed out, "sociology told us rather unpleasant things that don't fit in with official doctrine." Patterns of social stratification were a particularly sensitive issue in societies that were supposedly headed toward being "classless." Consequently, sociology experienced advances and retreats, along with supervision and control by the Communist Party, and was largely reduced to public opinion polling *within* the boundaries of Marxist-Leninist doctrine.

Since communism ended, sociology in Russia has seen a division emerge between sociologists who are international in outlook (Western) and others who are regionally oriented (Slavophiles), with the split most visible in theory (Titarenko and Zdravomyslova 2017). Still unresolved is the debate over whether to construct their own nation-based theories or assimilate theories that originated in the West. The result is that Russia has "—as of yet— failed to produce any comprehensive theories or at least partial hypotheses to explain the Russian 'scenario'" (Dmitriev 2006:162; see also Titarenko and Zdravomyslova 2017).

If sociology wasn't much under communism, neither was medical sociology. The subdiscipline was not institutionalized in the Soviet Union's university system prior to 1991, nor did it emerge in strength in Russia after the fall of communism. In the post-Soviet era, there have been studies on health-related topics by a few sociologists, so the field exists and a few university courses are available on the subject. However, as for sociological theory, Russian medical sociologist Elena Dmitrieva (2005:330) pointed out some years ago in an assessment that remains current, that the "theoretical foundation of medical sociology in Russia is fairly poor as the result of the dominance of Marxist-Leninism theory."

Moreover, Russian medical sociology lacked visibility when an extraordinary health crisis dating back to the 1960s under communism was revealed in its entirety in the 1990s. It was not until 2012 that male longevity consistently returned to mid-1960s levels. In 1965, for example, male life expectancy in the Russian part of the former Soviet Union was 64.0 years compared to 64.6 years in 2012. Female life expectancy had been 71.1 years in 1965 but eventually normalized with a gain of nearly five years to 75.9 years by 2012. The most recent figures for Russian life expectancy as this book goes to press are for 2016 showing that men lived an average of 66.5 years and women 77.1 years—that still remains among the largest gender gaps in longevity in the world.

The principal causes of the downturn in life expectancy included a dramatic increase (some called it an "epidemic") in mortality from heart disease, but also from accidents, alcohol poisonings, homicide, and suicide that were associated with an extraordinary level of alcohol consumption and binge drinking. The high mortality was most prevalent among middle-aged, working-class men brought on by unhealthy lifestyles (not only heavy alcohol consumption and binge drinking, but smoking, poor diets, lack of leisure-time exercise, and a general lack of attention to personal health), neglect in Soviet times of social and material needs, stress associated with the transition out of socialism to state capitalism, and the poor performance of the health care system—particularly in reducing cardiovascular mortality (Cockerham 1997, 1999, 2009, 2012; Grigoriev et al. 2014:107; Gugushvili et al. 2018; Manning and Tikhonova 2009; Parsons 2014; Rose 2009; Scheiring, Irdam, and King 2019).[2]

The Soviet Union had deliberately stopped publishing data on life expectancy in 1972 and infant mortality after 1974. These data and other statistics on homicide, suicide, plague, cholera, and work-related accidents were considered "politically dangerous" and ordered to be kept away from observers both in and outside of the Soviet Union (Shkolnikov, Meslé, and Vallin 1996:133). It was not until 1988 and Mikhail Gorbachev's policies of *perestroika* (restructuring) and *glasnost* (openness) that state statistics were opened to Russian and French demographers who took the lead in verifying and initially analyzing the trends shown in the data (Shkolnikov et al. 1996). Although the Center for Sociological Studies at Moscow State University and the Institute of Sociology of the Russian Academy of Sciences were subsequently involved in collecting survey data on health problems in post-Soviet Russia, the majority of sociologists participating in the various research projects were foreign (American, British, Finnish, and Swedish).

Eastern Europe

In the Soviet-dominated communist countries of Eastern Europe, sociology's experiences generally paralleled those in the Soviet Union. For example, in Hungary, sociology was reinstated in the 1960s as its advocates argued that the discipline was not anti-Marxist; rather, it was a special field of research that could investigate "concrete social reality" from a Marxist viewpoint (Kolosi and Szelényi 1993). Sociology was also reinstated in the former Czechoslovakia in the 1960s with the mission of helping to build state socialism within the confines of Marxist-Leninist theory (Skovjsa and Balon 2017). Sociology in Poland resurfaced in 1956 when the communist government allowed it to return to universities with a focus on applied studies. Theory was generally avoided (Buchole 2016; Kwasniewicz 1993).

In East Germany, sociology was firmly grounded in Marxism-Leninism (Assmann and Stollberg 1979; Meyer 1994). The extent of official dogma was so pervasive that its universities had Departments of Marxism-Leninism reviewing literally all scientific papers before dissemination, even those in the physical sciences, to insure they were consistent with socialist ideology as laid down by Marx and Lenin. East German sociologist Hansgünter Meyer (1994:34) observed the following:

> East German sociology was … permeated by the Soviet Russian understanding of the social sciences, a heritage of the Stalin period, subjugated by the dogmas of so-called Marxism-Leninism, which, when looked at in the light of day, was no scientific synthesis of Marx and Lenin but a collection of extremely simplified postulates on a historical finalism that, one believed, was precisely now well on the way to realization.

Sociology was decidedly not sociology in a Western sense in Europe's communist countries, but a sociology locked into a Marxist-Leninist model. What this meant for sociological theory was a lack of innovation and discourse about competing theories, along with theoretical regimentation. After communism collapsed, Poland, like the other countries of Eastern Europe, has been largely dependent on imported theories and concepts; in fact, academic sociology in Poland has been described as a "foreign import" from its beginning (Buchole 2016). Eastern Europe as a whole has been depicted as "hardly even present on the map of contemporary social theory" (Szakolczai and Wydra 2006:138).

Not surprisingly, medical sociology experienced varying stages of underdevelopment in Eastern Europe. This was the case even though these countries experienced differing levels of the same crisis in life expectancy that had occurred in the Soviet Union between the mid-1960s and 1990s—leading to the comment that "communism was bad for your health" (Cockerham 1999). In Bulgaria, sociology was in a Marxism-Leninism orbit, while in Romania it was used to glorify the achievements of the government (Ostrowska 1996). Medical sociology did not have a realistic presence in either country. Medical sociologists in Czechoslovakia, East Germany, and Hungary were generally affiliated with Institutes of Social Hygiene that focused on social medicine not medical sociology. In the former Czechoslovakia (the present-day Czech Republic and Slovakia), nearly all of the sociologists active in the study of medicine left the field after the peaceful revolution in 1989 that ended communism and closed the institutes (Janečková 2005). The subdiscipline has been slow to recover because of a lack of institutionalization in Czech universities and sociologists with an interest in health care.

East Germany, like the Soviet Union, rigidly followed Marxist-Leninist dogma in sociology, but at least had a medical sociology textbook in the German language during the latter stage of communism with contributions from East German, Czech, and Hungarian medical sociologists that included sociological theory, even Parsons' concept of the sick role (Hüttner 1987). Polish medical sociologist Nina Ostrowska (1996, 2005) clarified the attraction of Parsons and structural-functionalism in Eastern European sociology by pointing out that a general sociological theory like structural-functionalism could more readily be adapted to their social conditions than other theoretical concepts common in Western medical sociology. As Ostrowska (2005:344) explained:

> The structural functionalist theory was most popular among researchers. This theory was especially attractive for eastern European societies. The Marxist emphasis on conflict could not be applied to the analysis of a socialist society, which was expected to be conflictless. Parsons's vision of cooperation, goodwill, and the mutually complementary components of a system met the ideological pattern of a socialist society in many respects. Paradoxically, in Poland there were very few medical sociology studies that could be directly derived from the traditions of Marxist sociological theory.

Consequently, structural-functionalism was adopted as the leading theoretical perspective outside of Marxism in Eastern European sociology in the 1960s. "The wave of criticism of functionalism that developed in the Western sociology" observed Ostrowska (1996:101), "was perceived in Eastern Europe mostly as a theoretical oddity." Many East European medical sociologists were in favor of structural-functionalism, which was ironic given that a major weakness of the functionalist approach was an inability to adequately account for revolutionary social change. In an oncoming classless utopia, consensus and social solidarity was an inherent feature of society, not conflict, and structural-functionalism fit this model.

Polish medical sociology was the most advanced and independent in Eastern Europe. It was initiated by Magdalena Sokolowska (1922–1989), a physician and sociologist, who had studied at Columbia University in New York City. While maintaining international contacts and a prominent role in the International Sociological Association, she had institutionalized medical sociology in Poland by establishing the Polish Academy of Science Institute of Philosophy and Sociology in Warsaw in 1965 and then steered the subdiscipline in that country toward a strictly sociological, rather than biomedical, orientation toward health and illness (Piątkowski and Skrzypek 2012, 2013). In doing so, Sokolowska (1986) wrote the first Polish medical sociology textbook that was the first published anywhere under communism.

Sokolowska also fostered a critical approach to health problems and medical practice as seen in her 1980 book, *Granice medycyny* [*Limits to Medicine*] that disparaged the Polish medical profession for its "engineering orientation" toward health care, driving up costs with poor results, and failing to appreciate the role of lifestyles and behavior as possible causes of disease (Piątkowski and Skrzypek 2013:617). This influence is seen in the work of Polish medical sociologist Wlodzimierz Piątkowski (2012:46), in his book, *Beyond Medicine*, in which he utilizes symbolic interaction, phenomenology, and ethnomethodology to analyze alternative methods of health care in Poland and argue that "daily life," along with "everyday ideas of health and illness, value hierarchies, patterns of health behaviors, and health awareness have a stronger effect on mortality and incidences of most diseases than the influence of institutional medicine." While Polish medical sociology has moved beyond traditional Marxism, the development and use of sociological theory is not strong—as is the case throughout the former communist world or in those countries where communism survives.

China

In China, sociology was not formally established until 1979 when the communist leader Deng Xiaoping decided that studies of Chinese society were needed as the country underwent a transition to a market capitalist economy while maintaining its communist political system (Bian and Zhang 2008; Chen 2018; Rocca 2015; Wilson 2007). Unlike other communist countries, including those that still exist, China readily accepted the influence of American sociology and numerous Chinese students with government funding attended universities in the U.S. for sociology degrees, including studies in medical sociology. Chinese post-graduates also trained in American institutions. In the meantime, sociology programs, both undergraduate and graduate, were established in Chinese universities. In 1998, nine Western (eight American, one French) sociology textbooks were selected and translated into Chinese to meet student needs and published by Huaxia Publishing House in Beijing. These books were mostly on theory and research methods, but also included the author's medical sociology textbook.[3] This translation and those of subsequent editions made an American textbook on medical sociology available to Chinese-speaking students.

While Chinese sociology has increasingly been modeled on the American version, its research orientation is applied in order to justify government support (Bian and Zhang 2008; Chen 2018). As Hon Chen (2018:133) notes, the institutionalization of Chinese sociology has been "Janus-faced" (two-sided) in that while the state has resourced sociological research, it has reduced sociology's autonomy at the same time. In a continuing era of one-party (communist) rule, sociology is expected to be constructive and supportive of public policy, not critical. The concept of the sick role, for example, was expanded from a dyad (doctor–patient relationship) to a triad (doctor–patient–Party/state relationship) after the government established official sick role expectations and norms (the "cooperative patient" model) for sick persons who were supposed to behave along Party–state guidelines (Yang 2019).

Marxist-Based Views in Medical Sociology

As for Marx, he was literally written off as finished in sociology over a decade ago (Callinicos 2007), or at best characterized as being at a low ebb (Atkinson 2015), while critiqued by this author (Cockerham 2013) for the failure of Marxist-Leninist doctrine to produce healthy societies in Europe's former communist states. Yet work in the political economy of health and conflict theory nevertheless shows something of a Marxist revival. Marxist theory clearly emphasizes structure over agency, which may still be useful for medical sociologists seeking to explain the top-down effects of capitalism on disadvantaged populations. This perspective is seen in Marx's ([1852] 1954:10) oft-cited statement that:

Men make their own history, but they do not make it as they please, they do not make it under circumstances chosen by themselves, but under circumstances directly found, given, and transmitted from the past.

So while individuals have choices, their choices are constrained by already existing social structures, primarily the economic system in which they work and the class system in which they live. This perspective is especially reflected in Marxist-based concepts seen in political economy theory, conflict theory, and the income inequality hypothesis.

Political Economy Theory

The political economy approach in medical sociology seeks to explain how differences in class relations in economic markets cause differences in health outcomes along class lines. It centers on examining inequalities in the health marketplace when health care is treated as a "commodity" under capitalism to be sold to those who have the means to pay for it and beyond the reach or with lessened availability on the part of those who cannot. In *Das Kapital*, Marx ([1867] 1949:1) defines a commodity as an "object outside us, a thing that by its properties satisfies human wants of some sort or another." He says that the value of a commodity does not depend on how much labor has gone into producing it, but upon how useful it is in the process of consumption— namely, what it will bring (can be sold for) in the marketplace.

The commodification of health is central to understanding health inequalities in cases where the poor lack health care because they cannot pay for it directly or for the insurance to cover it. When the provision of health care is a commodified product, it becomes a privilege to be purchased, not a right of citizenship or a public good. In this context, socioeconomic disadvantage in society is further converted into a health disparity as reduced opportunities to obtain quality health care combine with the greater likelihood of having an unhealthy lifestyle and increased exposure to unhealthy living conditions, disease, and injury. Both Marxists and non-Marxists would likely agree this circumstance (commodification) is key to explaining health inequality in the world at large.

Health care, of course, is not the only health-related commodity, as the health market is substantial on a global scale. The high costs of drugs and profit-seeking on the part of pharmaceutical companies and the advertising of unhealthy products like cigarettes, alcohol, and unhealthy foods high in sugar and fat are all related to the market and consumer demand. In addition to the extensive advertising of medicinal drugs and procedures (e.g., laser surgery to remove fat or improve vision) in the media, there is also the marketing of health foods, vitamins, fitness equipment, weight-loss programs, eyeglasses, and a vast array of other health-related products and services constituting a virtual flood of products to help the individual "manufacture" his or her own health. Commercial products associated with health not only produce profits, but also reinforce the idea that health and fitness constitute a practical goal to be achieved through the use of these products.

In order to offset commodity-related health disparities, most welfare state capitalist countries, with the major exception of the U.S., provide some form of universal health insurance. The U.S. only subsidizes the health needs of the poor (Medicaid) and the elderly (Medicare). Universal benefits, however, are usually awarded on the basis of citizenship or legal residency to make sure some level of health care is generally available, regardless of income. Some 130 nations provide a right to health in their constitutions (Gostin 2014); yet, they vary considerably in their implementation since a universal health care system is at odds with the dynamics of the marketplace (G. Cockerham 2018:214). This is because health care is a commodity in a free-market economy, not a right, which results in inequality.

The market can be a hegemonic presence in health care because health care delivery systems do not evolve randomly. They are deliberate creations that reflect the social and political philosophies of the societies that create them. These philosophies underlie the policies made, institutions formed, and levels of funding provided for health care. One can therefore argue that health care delivery systems are themselves social constructions in that they reflect the cultural orientation of the countries that establish them.

From a neo-Marxist perspective, it is the dominance of the free market (neo-liberalism) in international trade and politics that prevents or constrains the establishment of health as a human right (Coburn 2000, 2004, 2015). Neo-liberalism is an economic theory and political philosophy that favors an enhanced role for free-market economies and a minimized role for state control and intervention. Marxists maintain that neo-liberalism needs to be curtailed and markets subjected to much greater regulation by the state since it cannot be assumed that the dynamics of the marketplace on its own will ever favor humanitarian aims over economic interests. It is therefore necessary for the state to intervene and impose health-promoting measures. Yet as neo-Marxists acknowledge, ideological support for capitalism and free-market neo-liberalism is deeply entrenched globally and the competition to replace it with communism was a spectacular failure (Hudis 2013). Consequently, as political scientist Geoffrey Cockerham (2018:271) concludes, the dominance of the market in global governance makes the transformation of health as a human right from a principle to a fully implemented practical right very problematic.

However, a neo-Marxist political economy perspective has not disappeared. The global economic crisis of 2008 stimulated a resurgence in interest. A review of the causes of that crisis shows an ideology of wealth appropriation and profit-maximizing strategies on the part of individuals and major financial corporations, along with a disregard for risk that led to the global sub-prime mortgage debacle. Some financial institutions failed, massive government loans and grants were required for others, and there was a sharp rise in unemployment, loss of investments, a weakened economy, a few criminal indictments, and the dispossession of assets, particularly homes, from vulnerable people. The effects of that crisis and other economic problems lingered for years afterwards in some cases.

Even though safety nets are provided by the state in capitalist economies in the form of welfare benefits, such benefits can be insufficient in a major fiscal crisis thereby accelerating the vulnerability of the disadvantaged in a number of ways—including their health (Scambler 2012). The basic message of political economy theory for medical sociology is that the concept of health as a commodity remains very relevant in the real world and health itself can be harmed from macro-level economic conditions over which individuals have no control.

Conflict Theory

As British medical sociologist Graham Scambler (2018:45) points out, any account of conflict theory begins with Marx. Other sociological theorists, such as Weber, Georg Simmel, Ralf Dahrendorf, and Lewis Coser made important contributions over the years, but conflict theory evolved out of Marx's perspective on class relations. He initiated the view that conflict is the basis of social change. It is an alternative to consensus theories, like structural-functionalism, that maintain social order is based on mutual consent and social change is a process that weaves slowly through society as its component parts adjust to new developments over time. Marx's perspective in conflict theory is seen in the rejection of the observation put forth by structural-functionalism that society is held together by shared norms and values. Conflict theory claims instead that true consensus does not exist; rather, society's norms and values are those of the dominant group and are imposed by them on the less privileged in order to maintain their advantage. Social processes are therefore essentially struggles over resources. All social systems contain inequality, which causes conflict, which, in turn, causes reorganization of the social system.

In Marx's view, people usually act in accordance with the interests of the class in which they find themselves—as typically the upper end of the social scale functions to protect its privileged position through political and economic means, and the lower segments try to improve their situation as best they can. Marx's analysis also helps us to understand the economic roots of racial and ethnic exploitation, in which minorities are exploited for their cheap labor—whether it is the slave trade of past centuries or migrant workers today. For example, in advanced technological societies, migrants or "guest workers" in particular, are generally employed in low-wage occupations, have little career opportunity, and lack job security. Illegal migrants, in particular, reside not just at the bottom of their host societies but on its margins, without effective control over their work.

Whereas Marxist-based versions of conflict theory have emphasized class struggle, other conflict theorists have instead concentrated on analyzing the competition that takes place among interest groups such as labor and management, geographical regions, political parties, business corporations, professional groups such as the American Medical Association, and agencies within governments. In this instance, as Dahrendorf (1988) argued long ago, inequality stems from the unequal distribution of political power, rather than economic factors being the prime source of inequality. Power and authority are scarce resources and, in Dahrendorf's view, those who have them are interested in maintaining the status quo, while those who lack them are interested in acquiring them and changing the status quo.

Another view of conflict theory comes from Bryan Turner (1988) who says modern societies are best understood as having a conflict between the principles of democratic politics emphasizing equality and universal rights and the organization of their economic systems involving the production, exchange, and consumption of goods and services, about which there is considerable inequality. This unresolved contradiction is relatively permanent and a major source of conflict and tension in democracies as they try to resolve this situation through the provision of government welfare benefits that are either universal (as in Europe) or based on income or age (as in the U.S.).

Conflict theory can therefore explain the maneuvers of various groups or social entities, like the medical profession, insurance companies, pharmaceutical companies, the business community, and the public, as they struggle politically to acquire, protect, or expand their interests against existing government regulations and programs, and those under consideration. This situation represents one of conflict theory's most important assets for medical sociology; namely, the capacity to explain the politics associated with health inequalities.

There is also a side of neo-Marxism that remains more connected to a classical Marxist version of conflict theory by continuing to emphasize class competition to explain health policy outcomes and the disadvantages of the lower and working classes in obtaining health care in capitalist medical systems where health is a commodity (De Maio 2010; Muntaner et al. 2014; Scambler 2018; Waitzkin 2001). This view does not consider political struggles between interest groups as a sufficient strategy for understanding health inequalities and instead continues to strongly emphasize class conflict and exploitation as the most complete explanation for the poor health of disadvantaged groups. In essence, there is what can be called a "soft" (interest group competition) and "hard" (class exploitation) approach to conflict theory in medical sociology that has yet to be unified or resolved one way or the other. Nonetheless, Fernando De Maio (2010:49) maintains that conflict theory has made profound contributions to understanding global health issues, health inequalities, the power of pharmaceutical corporations, and the politics of health reform.

However, conflict theory, despite its supporters and status as a major twentieth-century sociological theory, joins structural-functionalism in the category of what George Ritzer and William Yagatich (2012:105) describe as "zombie theories." Zombie theories, as mentioned in Chapter 3 in relation to structural-functionalism, are theories that may seem alive to some devotees, but they are actually either dead or "at least in the process of dying while moving toward a zombie-like state" (Ritzer and Yagatich 2012:105). Conflict, of course, is ongoing in the social world and the topic remains significant, yet finding conflict in social situations does not automatically verify the relevance of conflict theory in their view. The theory sparked opposition because, like structural-functionalism, it accorded the individual little opportunity for innovation and creativity—as conflict was predetermined by class struggle. Additionally, conflict theory was not extensively developed and was severely criticized for ignoring social order and stability, just as it had earlier attacked structural-functionalism's failure to account for conflict and change (Ritzer and Stepnisky 2018). Once structural-functionalism disappeared, conflict theory's value as an alternative faded, leading Ritzer and Yagatich (2012) to assign it to the zombie category. As they (Ritzer and Yagatich 2012:105) put it: "This is the case even though many still see society as defined by conflict …, but merely seeing society in that way does not mean that one is a conflict theorist."

Moreover, conflict theory never became a *dominant* theory in medical sociology and arguably gained even less of a foothold than structural-functionalism which could at least point to the seminal contribution of Parsons' (1951) concept of the sick role. A particular problem with conflict theory, in the author's opinion, is that conflict is not common in most health situations. Cooperation is typically the norm in care-giving environments. Other than Howard Waitzkin (1971), few medical sociologists in the U.S. utilized conflict theory and the number has since diminished. While conflict theory has relevance for explaining the political competition between interest groups with respect to health policy and reform, along with situations in which class warfare harms health, there nevertheless are inherent limitations in the use of the theory for medical sociologists. This is because while some health situations are affected by conflict-laden conditions, others are not. People may either maintain their health or become sick, seek medical care, and even die, but these outcomes can have little or nothing to do with conflict, politics, interest group competition, and class struggle, and mostly or everything to do with ailments caused by aging and physical deterioration, smoking for pleasure, poor dietary habits, the onset of viruses and cancerous cells in the body, the genetic inheritance (family history) of certain diseases, and other conditions that do not involve conflict at all.

The Income Inequality Hypothesis

British health economist Richard Wilkinson (1996) introduced the "income inequality hypothesis" that fostered considerable interest among neo-Marxists (De Maio 2010), although Wilkinson himself did not cite any of Marx's work nor frame his argument in Marxist terms. Wilkinson (1996:15), instead, modeled his research after Durkheim's ([1897] 1951) study of suicide. However, De Maio (2010) finds that Wilkinson's thesis on income inequality is similar to that of Engels' [1845] 1969) nineteenth-century examination of the effects of class exploitation on the health of British factory workers, and additionally has links to social theory beyond Durkheim that extend to conflict theory. Based on a review of several international studies, Wilkinson had hypothesized that when countries make the transition to high living standards and achieve a positive level of health, they can continue to increase their wealth but not be any healthier if class differences do not diminish. "What this means," says Wilkinson (1996:5), "is that the quality of the social life of a society is one of the most important social determinants of health and that this, in turn, is very closely related to the degree of income equality."

The key variable is the degree of social and economic equality *within* a population. If there is a significant income gap between the rich and the poor, then substantial health inequalities will exist inside a society, even though the overall level of health is generally good. Yet if the gap in income is small, inequalities in health will also be small. Wilkinson's basic thesis was that among advanced countries, it is not the richest nations that have the highest overall levels of health, but the ones who are most egalitarian. He called attention to the positive level of population health in relation to the relatively smaller gaps in income in Norway and Sweden as examples of his argument. In his view, it is the degree of inequality within a country, not between countries, that determines a population's health.

On the surface, this looked like a promising hypothesis. But over time it was subjected to widespread and intense criticism. The hypothesis was politically provocative because it implied income needed to be redistributed by taking money away from the wealthy, likely through increased taxation, and giving it to the poor as welfare benefits to raise their standard of living and by extension their health. But it did not get to a policy level debate because it became academically contentious rather quickly, even among some neo-Marxist scholars who might have been expected to be sympathetic toward it. Canadian public health researchers Carles Muntaner (2003) and David Coburn (2000, 2004) were among those finding fault with the hypothesis. Muntaner argued that Wilkinson's focus on income inequality neglected the effects of class, gender, and racial influences on health disparities, while Coburn contended that Wilkinson did not pay enough attention to the social context of income inequality, particularly what *causes* income inequality to occur in the first place. Coburn believed the ultimate cause was the neo-liberal doctrines of advanced capitalist societies that have spread through globalization. The greater the degree to which neo-liberal policies were in effect in a particular country, Coburn insists, the more it promoted wealth accumulation on the part of big business, lessened the power of the working class to obtain health benefits, fostered poverty in the lower class who were deprived of good-paying jobs and welfare subsidies, and caused unequal access to health-relevant resources.

Wilkinson and Kate Pickett (2009; Pickett and Wilkinson 2015) countered that most studies support the hypothesis as originally stated and further highlighted the importance of a psychosocial sense of relative deprivation in fostering poor health. That is, being stressed and depressed about one's deprived socioeconomic situation was considered a critical factor in promoting an unhealthy state in an individual. It was not just having a low income that was damaging to a person's health, but the perception of one's income relative to the income of others. The notion of relative deprivation, however, is controversial in itself. As British medical sociologist Mel Bartley (2017) observed, this suggests that poor health is triggered by a person's perception of his or her status in a social hierarchy. Therefore it is not just what someone possesses, but what that person possesses relative to other people that affects their health. According to Bartley (2004:125):

> There is something rather depressing about this idea that not being a "top dog" in some kind of fixed hierarchy could be so psychologically catastrophic as to have an effect on life expectancy itself. Do people really care so much about not having a bigger car than their neighbours that their immune defense systems collapse in protest? ... Do people really die of envy?

It is far from clear that this is the case. The relative deprivation thesis lacks convincing evidence on this point, although Bartley finds there is some support for feelings of isolation and loneliness being harmful to health.

She also maintains that while people who feel inferior may be motivated to not take care of themselves or their stresses may induce unhealthy forms of consumption (i.e., alcohol, drugs, sweets), a sense of relative deprivation would likely have to be part of a larger negative phenomenon to significantly affect one's health.

As for income inequality, Coburn (2015) insists that it is only *one* indicator of health differences. He maintains that compensating factors also needed to be taken into consideration, such as the extent of health insurance programs for the poor, subsidies for prescription drugs, housing, and utilities, unemployment insurance, and additional variables beyond income that can offset income differences and are also relevant for determining the health situation of the disadvantaged. While recognizing there is data linking income inequality with poorer health, Coburn nevertheless points out that the relationship between income inequality and other social factors is more complex than presented and it has not yet been proven that income inequality is the main cause of the health effects they describe. Other research, for example, shows that poverty is a more important overall determinant of poor health than income inequality (Rambotti 2015).

However, what especially damaged the income inequality hypothesis in the author's opinion was when several researchers failed to replicate Wilkinson's findings and/or found his statistical analysis flawed (Bakkeli 2016; Blázquez-Fernández, Cantarero-Prieto, and Pascula-Saez 2018; Eberstadt and Satel 2004; Jen, Jones, and Johnston 2009; McLeod, Nonnemaker, and Call 2004). Jason Beckfield (2004), for example, in an award-winning paper, replicated previous work in a carefully designed study using a large sample from 115 countries and found no evidence to support the income inequality thesis. Nicholas Eberstadt and Sally Satel (2004) identified a persuasive body of scholarship showing that by controlling for household income, living conditions, education, and race, the relationship between income inequality and health either diminishes significantly or disappears completely. Eberstadt and Satel (2004:36) concluded that instead of being a scientific hypothesis, a better way to describe the income inequality hypothesis is to call it "a doctrine in search of data" because of a lack of verifiable supporting evidence. A problem in using the income inequality hypothesis in one's research is the challenge it brings to responding to criticism.

Summary and Conclusion

This chapter has reviewed the contributions of Marx to medical sociology and, as discussed, his influence in sociology generally has been both profound and contentious. His notion of historical materialism and class struggle as the driver of human history has been severely critiqued. One effect of Marxist theory in communist countries was that of suppressing sociology and medical sociology by extension, since Marxism was the only theory of society deemed acceptable by the ruling authorities. Consequently, contributions to sociological theory have yet to emerge from former or current communist countries. While there are also several criticisms of neo-Marxist theory and it occupies more of a niche area in contemporary medical sociology rather than dominating it, the perspective survives in a diminished state of influence. Nevertheless, it can be useful in selected areas of research, namely (1) political economy studies in which health is viewed as a commodity, (2) conflict theory that deals with the effects of class division on health and interest group differences in health policy disputes, and (3) the beleaguered income inequality hypothesis that has been subjected to extensive criticism.

Guide to Critical Thinking

1. Describe Marx's concepts of historical materialism and class struggle. Are they relevant concepts for medical sociology today?
2. What has been the effect of Marxism on sociology and medical sociology in communist countries?
3. What does the political economy approach in medical sociology explain and how does the concept of health as a commodity enter into this discussion?
4. Is conflict theory a zombie theory when it comes to explaining health? Explain.
5. What are the strengths and weaknesses of the income inequality hypothesis?

Notes

1 The positivist approach in sociology maintains that social reality needs to be determined by scientific evidence, which means that theories needed to be tested by the facts or data. Idealists, in contrast, see such social reality determined by how people subjectively define it. Marx presented his theory of historical materialism as a scientific law although it was grounded in idealism.
2 Whereas Soviet-style health care delivery systems could be effective in treating collective health problems with large-scale inoculations and public hygiene programs, it was ineffective in coping with heart ailments requiring individual and personalized attention. This mortality crisis lasted nearly 50 years in Russia from its beginning in the mid-1960s to what appears to be an eventual end around 2012 under a non-Marxist political and economic system. As a political doctrine, Marxism–Leninism had failed to construct healthy living conditions, along with an adequate health care delivery system, in the countries that adopted it.

3 William C. Cockerham, 2000. *Medical Sociology*, 7th edition, Yang Hui and Zhang Tuohong (trans.). Beijing, China: Huaxia Publishing House. Subsequent Chinese editions were published in Beijing in English by Peking University Press, translated into Chinese by the People's University Press (Yuoping Guo and Baoyen Yang) and in Chinese simplified by Pearson Education Asia (Yiliao yu Shehui), and also in Taiwan by Wu-Nan Book Company (Chou-yen Cho and Jia-hwa Xiao) and Yeh Yeh Book Gallery (Rosa Ho). Other Asian language translations are Korean (Hojin Park) and Mongolian (S. Munkhbaatar). There is also a Spanish language translation (Lourdes Lostao and Enrique Regidor).

Suggested Reading

Atkinson, Will. 2015. *Class*. Cambridge: Polity.
An excellent analysis of class concepts, including Marx, with a chapter on health, life, and death.
Antonio, Robert J. 2011. "Karl Marx," in George Ritzer and Jeffrey Stepnisky (eds.), *The Wiley-Blackwell Companion to Major Social Theorists*, Vol. 1. Oxford: Wiley-Blackwell, pp. 115–64.
A review of Marx's theories and a realistic assessment of their applicability to contemporary social conditions.

References

Antonio, Robert J. 2011. "Karl Marx," in George Ritzer and Jeffrey Stepnisky (eds.), *The Wiley-Blackwell Companion to Major Social Theorists*, Vol. 1. Oxford: Wiley-Blackwell, pp. 115–64.
Assmann, Georg and Rudhard Stollberg (eds.). 1979. *Grundlagen der marxistisch-leninistischen Soziologie* [*Foundations of Marxist-Leninist Sociology*]. Berlin: Dietz Verlag.
Atkinson, Will. 2015. *Class*. Cambridge: Polity.
Bakkeli, Nan Zou. 2016. "Income Inequality and Health in China: A Panel Data Analysis Study." *Social Science & Medicine* 157:39–47.
Barnes, Harry Elmer. 1948. *An Introduction to the History of Sociology*. Chicago, IL: University of Chicago Press.
Bartley, Mel. 2004. *Health Inequality*. Cambridge: Polity.
Bartley, Mel. 2017. *Health Inequality*, 2nd ed. Cambridge: Polity.
Beckfield, Jason. 2004. "Does Income Inequality Harm Health? New Cross-National Evidence." *Journal of Health and Social Behavior* 45(3):231–48.
Bell, Wendell. 1990. "Values and the Future in Marx and Marxism." *Futures* (March):146–62.
Bian, Yanjie and Lei Zhang. 2008. "Sociology in China." *Contexts* 7(3):20–5.
Blázquez-Fernández, Carla, David Cantarero-Prieto, and Marta Pascula-Saez. 2018. "Does Rising Income Inequality Reduce Life Expectancy? New Evidence for 26 European Countries (1995–2014)." *Global Economic Review* 47(2):1–16.

Brown, Archie. 2009. *The Rise and Fall of Communism*. New York: Ecco.

Buchole, Marta. 2016. *Sociology in Poland*. Basingstoke: Palgrave Macmillan.

Callinicos, Alex. 2007. *Social Theory: An Historical Introduction*, 2nd ed. Cambridge: Polity.

Chen, Hon Fai. 2018. *Chinese Sociology*. Basingstoke: Palgrave Macmillan.

Coburn, David. 2000. "Income Inequality, Social Cohesion and the Health Status of Populations: The Role of Neo-Liberalism." *Social Science & Medicine* 51:135–46.

Coburn, David. 2004. "Beyond the Income Inequality Hypothesis: Class, Neo-Liberalism, and Health." *Social Science & Medicine* 58:41–56.

Coburn, David. 2015. "Income Inequality, Welfare, Class, and Health: A Comment on Pickett and Wilkinson, 2015." *Social Science & Medicine* 146:228–32.

Cockerham, Geoffrey B. 2018. *Global Governance and Public Health*. London: Rowman and Littlefield.

Cockerham, William C. 1997. "The Social Determinants of the Decline of Life Expectancy in Russia and Eastern Europe: A Lifestyle Explanation." *Journal of Health and Social Behavior* 38(2):131–48.

Cockerham, William C. 1999. *Health and Social Change in Russia and Eastern Europe*. London: Routledge.

Cockerham, William C. 2009. "Understanding the Russian Health Crisis: A Sociological Perspective." *Sociology Compass* 3:327–40.

Cockerham, William C. 2012. "The Intersection of Health and Gender in a Transitional State: The Case of Russia." *Sociology of Health & Illness* 34(6):943–57.

Cockerham, William C. 2013. "Sociological Theory in Medical Sociology in the Early Twenty-First Century." *Social Theory & Health* 11(3):241–55.

Collyer, Fran. 2015. "Karl Marx and Frederich Engels: Capitalism, Health and the Healthcare Industry," in Fran Collyer (ed.), *The Palgrave Handbook of Social Theory in Health, Illness and Medicine*. Basingstoke: Palgrave Macmillan, pp. 35–58.

Connell, R.W. 1997. "Why is Classical Theory Classical?" *American Journal of Sociology* 102(6):1511–57.

Dahrendorf, Ralf. 1988. *The Modern Social Conflict*. Berkeley, CA: University of California Press.

Davies, Norman. 1996. *Europe: A History*. New York: Oxford University Press.

De Maio, Fernando. 2010. *Health & Social Theory*. Basingstoke: Palgrave Macmillan.

Dmitriev, Alexander. 2006. "Contemporary Russian Social Theory," in Gerhard Delanty (ed.), *Handbook of Contemporary European Social Theory*. London: Routledge, pp. 153–67.

Dmitrieva, Elena. 2005. "The Russian Health Care Experiment: Transition of the Health Care System and Rethinking Medical Sociology," in William C. Cockerham (ed.), *The Blackwell Companion to Medical Sociology*. Oxford: Blackwell, pp. 320–33.

Durkheim, Émile. [1897] 1951. *Suicide: A Study in Sociology*. New York: Free Press.

Eberstadt, Nicholas, and Sally Satel. 2004. *Health and the Income Inequality Hypothesis*. Washington, DC: AEI Press.

Engels, Friedrich. ([1845] 1969). *The Condition of the Working Class in England in 1844*. Oxford: Oxford University Press.

Garnham, Lisa M. 2014. "Understanding the Impacts of Industrial Change and Area-Based Deprivation on Health Inequalities, Using Swidler's Concepts of *Cultured Capacities* and *Strategies of Action.*" *Social Theory & Health* 13(3/4):308–39.

Gorbachev, Raisa M. 1991. *I Hope.* New York: HarperCollins.

Gostin, Lawrence O. 2014. *Global Health Law.* Cambridge, MA: Harvard University Press.

Grigoriev, Pavel, France Meslé, Vladimir M. Shkolnikov, Evgeny Andreev, Agnieszka Fihel, Marketa Pecholdova, and Jacques Vallin. 2014. "The Recent Mortality Decline in Russia: Beginning of the Cardiovascular Revolution?" *Population and Development Review* 40(1):107–29.

Gugushvili, Alexi, Aytalina Azarova, Darja Irdan, Whitney Crenna-Jennings, Michael Murphy, Martin McKee, and Lawrence King. 2018. "Correlates of Frequent Alcohol Consumption Among Middle-Aged and Older Men and Women in Russia: A Multilevel Analysis of the PrivMort Retrospective Cohort Study." *Drug and Alcohol Dependence* 186:39–44.

Hudis, Peter. 2013. *Marx's Concept of the Alternative to Capitalism.* Chicago, IL: Haymarket.

Hüttner, Hannes (ed.). 1987. *Medizin Soziologie [Medical Sociology].* Berlin: Verlag Volk und Gesundheit.

Janečková, Hana. 2005. "Transformation of the Health Care System in the Czech Republic—A Sociological Perspective," in William C. Cockerham (ed.), *The Blackwell Companion to Medical Sociology.* Oxford: Blackwell, pp. 347–63.

Jen, Min Hua, Kelvyn Jones, and Ron Johnston. 2009. "Global Variations in Health: Evaluating Wilkinson's Income Inequality Hypothesis using the World Values Survey." *Social Science & Medicine* 68:643–53.

Kolosi, Tomás and Ivan Szelényi. 1993. "Social Change and Research on Social Structure in Hungary," in Birgitta Nedelmann and Piotr Sztompka (eds.), *Sociology in Europe.* Berlin: de Gruyter, pp. 141–64.

Kwasniewicz, Waldyslaw. 1993. "Between Universal and Native: The Case of Polish Sociology," in Birgitta Nedelmann and Piotr Sztompka (eds.), *Sociology in Europe.* Berlin: de Gruyter, pp. 165–87.

Lukacs, John. 1993. *The End of the Twentieth Century and the End of the Modern Age.* London: Ticknor and Fields.

Manning, Nick and Nataliya Tikhonova (eds.). 2009. *Health and Health Care in the New Russia.* Farnham: Ashgate.

Marx, Karl. [1852] 1954. *The Eighteenth Brumaire of Louis Bonaparte.* Moscow: Progress Publishers.

Marx, Karl. [1867] 1949. *Capital.* London: Allen & Unwin.

Marx, Karl and Friedrich Engels. 1848. *Manifesto of the Communist Party.* New York: International Publishers.

Marx, Karl and Friedrich Engels. [1888] 1976. *The German Ideology.* Moscow: Progress Publishers.

McLennan, Gregor. 2001. "Maintaining Marx," in George Ritzer and Barry Smart (eds.), *Handbook of Social Theory.* London: Sage, pp. 443–53.

McLeod, Jane D., James M. Nonnemaker, and Kathleen Thiede Call. 2004. "Income Inequality, Race, and Child Well-being: An Aggregate Analysis in the 50 United States." *Journal of Health and Social Behavior* 45(3):249–64.

Merton, Robert K. 1957. *Social Theory and Social Structure*. Glencoe, IL: Free Press.

Meyer, Hansgünter. 1994. "Sociological Research in the GDR (DDR)." *Soziologie*, Special Edition (3):33–51.

Muntaner, Carles. 2003. "Social Epidemiology and Class: A Critique of Richard Wilkinson's Income Inequality and Social Capital Hypothesis." *Rethinking Marxism* 15(4):551–64.

Muntaner, Carles, Edwin Ng, Haejoo Chung, and Seth J. Prins. 2014. "Two Decades of Neo-Marxist Class Analysis and Health Inequalities: A Critical Reconstruction." *Social Theory & Health* 13(3/4):267–87.

Ostrowska, Antonina. 1996. "The Development of Medical Sociology in Eastern Europe, 1965–1990." *European Journal of Sociology* 6(2):100–4.

Ostrowska, Nina. 2005. "In and Out of Communism: The Macrosocial Context of Health in Poland," in William C. Cockerham (ed.), *The Blackwell Companion to Medical Sociology*. Oxford: Blackwell, pp. 334–46.

Parsons, Michelle A. 2014. *Dying Unneeded: The Cultural Context of the Russian Mortality Crisis*. Nashville, TN: Vanderbilt University Press.

Parsons, Talcott. 1937. *The Structure of Social Action*. New York: McGraw-Hill.

Parsons, Talcott. 1951. *The Social System*. New York: Free Press.

Piątkowski, Wlodzimierz. 2012. *Beyond Medicine: Non-Medical Treatments in Poland*. Frankfurt am Main: Peter Lang.

Piątkowski, Wlodzimierz and Michal Skrzypek. 2012. "The Social Nature of Health and Illness—Evolution of Research Approaches in Polish Classical Medical Sociology." *Annals of Agricultural and Environmental Medicine* 19(4):821–35.

Piątkowski, Wlodzimierz amd Michal Skrzypek. 2013. "To Tell the Truth: A Critical Trend in Medical Sociology—An Introduction to the Problems." *Annals of Agricultural and Environmental Medicine* 20(3):613–23.

Pickett, Kate E. and Richard G. Wilkinson. 2015. "Income Inequality and Health: A Causal Review." *Social Science & Medicine* 128:316–28.

Piketty, Thomas. 2014. *Capital in the Twenty-First Century*. Cambridge, MA: Belknap Press.

Pipes, Richard. 2001. *Communism*. New York: Modern Library.

Rambotti, Simone. 2015. "Recalibrating the Spirit Level: An Analysis of the Interaction of Income Inequality and Poverty and its Effect on Health." *Social Science & Medicine* 139:123–31.

Ritzer, George and Jeffrey Stepnisky. 2018. *Sociological Theory*, 10th ed. Los Angeles, CA: Sage.

Ritzer, George and William Yagatich. 2012. "Contemporary Sociological Theory," in George Ritzer (ed.), *The Wiley-Blackwell Companion to Sociology*. Oxford: Wiley-Blackwell, pp. 98–118.

Rocca, Jean-Louis. 2015. *A Sociology of Modern China*. New York: Oxford University Press.

Rose, David, and Eric Harrison (ed.). 2010. *Social Class in Europe*. London: Routledge.

Rose, Richard. 2009. *Understanding Post-Communist Transformation*. London: Routledge.

Scambler, Graham. 2012. "Health Inequalities." *Sociology of Health & Illness* 34(1):130–46.

Scambler, Graham. 2018. *Sociology, Health and the Fractured Society*. London: Routledge.

Scambler, Graham and Sasha Scambler. 2014. "Theorizing Health Inequalities: The Untapped Potential of Dialectical Critical Realism." *Social Theory & Health* 13(3/4):340–54.

Scheiring, Gabor, Darja Irdam, and Lawrence P. King. 2019. "Cross-country Evidence on the Social Determinants of the Post-socialist Mortality Crisis in Europe: A Review and Performance-based Hierarchy of Variables." *Sociology of Health & Illness* 41:673–91.

Shkolnikov, Vladimir, France Meslé, and Jacques Vallin. 1996. "Health Crisis in Russia I. Recent Trends in Life Expectancy and Causes of Death from 1970 to 1993." *Population* 8:123–54.

Shlapentokh, Vladimir. 1987. *The Politics of Sociology in the Soviet Union.* Boulder, CO: Westview Press.

Skovjsa, Marek and Jan Balon. 2017. *Sociology in the Czech Republic.* Basingstoke: Palgrave Macmillan.

Sokolowska, Magdalena. 1980. *Granice medycyny* [*Limits to Medicine*]. Warsaw: Wiedza Powszechna.

Sokolowska, Magdalena. 1986. *Socjologia medycyny* [*The Sociology of Medicine*]. Warsaw: PZWI.

Szakolczai, Arpad and Harold Wydra. 2006. "Contemporary East Central European Social Theory," in Gerard Delanty (ed.), *Handbook of Contemporary European Theory.* London: Routledge, pp. 138–52.

Titarenko, Larisa and Elena Zdravomyslova. 2017. *Sociology in Russia.* Basingstoke: Palgrave Macmillan.

Turner, Bryan S. 1988. *Status.* Milton Keynes: Open University Press.

Waitzkin, Howard. 1971. "Latent Functions of the Sick Role in Various Settings." *Social Science & Medicine* 5:45–75.

Waitzkin, Howard. 2001. *At the Front Lines of Medicine.* Lanham, MD: Rowman and Littlefield.

Wilkinson, Richard D. 1996. *Unhealthy Societies: The Afflictions of Inequality.* New York: Routledge.

Wilkinson, Richard and Kate Pickett. 2009. *The Spirit Level: Why Greater Equality Makes Societies Stronger.* New York: Bloomsbury Press.

Wilson, Jeanne. 2007. "China's Transformation towards Capitalism," in David Lane and Martin Myant (eds.), *Varieties of Capitalism in Post-Communist Countries.* London: Palgrave Macmillan, pp. 239–53.

Wright, Erik Olin. 1997. *Class Counts: Comparative Studies in Class Analysis.* Cambridge: Cambridge University Press.

Yang, Jingqing. 2019. "State and the Sick Role: A Study of Sick Models in the Pre-reform China." *Social Theory & Health* 17(4), https://doi.org/10.1057/s41285-019-00114-z.

Zotov, V. D. 1985. *The Marxist-Leninist Theory of Society.* Moscow: Progress Publishers.

Chapter 6

Symbolic Interaction and Labeling Theory

This chapter reviews two of the three leading micro-level theories in medical sociology, namely symbolic interaction and its variant labeling theory. The other micro theory is social constructionism, which is examined in Chapter 9. Micro-level theories focus on explaining patterns of face-to-face social interaction occurring between individuals and within small groups. These theories emphasize "agency" or the capacity of the individual to select his or her behavior and orient it in the direction chosen. When individuals engage in making choices, they become the "agent" of their own behavior which is the origin of the term "agency." According to this perspective, society is created from the bottom up by people who construct the structures in their lives through patterned forms of social interaction. This is obviously a different mode of theorizing than the structurally oriented perspectives of Durkheim and Marx discussed earlier and takes into account the micro-level features of social life they did not consider.

Typically, micro-level theories are based on the use of qualitative methods, such as participant observation, in-depth face-to-face interviews, focus groups, life histories, conversation analysis, situational analysis, and similar non-quantitative approaches to collecting data (Clarke, Friese, and Washburn 2018; Denzin 2017a, 2017b; Denzin and Lincoln 2018). The social behavior theoretically explained by the use of these methods has in some cases been directly observed, and in others recorded or reported by an informant or interviewee. The intent is to capture reality from the standpoint of those being studied or come as close to it as possible. Qualitative methods in medical sociology show how people perceive, evaluate, and experience health and illness, health care, disability, and health disparities in their own voices, attitudes, perspectives, and behaviors (Barker 2005; Charmaz and Belgrave 2013; Timmermans 2013). As David Karp and Lara Birk (2013:23) point out: "One of the most important missions and mandates of sociology has been to 'give voice' to those who have been forgotten, made socially invisible, or otherwise marginalized." Qualitative methodologies are typically utilized for this type of research.

The primacy of agency is strongly embedded in the core of the symbolic interactionist perspective whose popularity in the 1960s and 1970s signaled the beginning of the end of the dominance of structural-functionalism in sociological theorizing. Symbolic interaction theory had been utilized extensively in medical sociology to explain illness behavior, doctor–patient interaction, death and dying, disability and identity, and mental illness. At that time, a case could have been made that symbolic interaction was the leading theoretical perspective in medical sociology in the United States, as the field was a major battleground in the successful theoretical assault on structural-functionalism. This is no longer the situation.

However, among the so-called "big three" sociological theories—structural-functionalism, conflict theory, and symbolic interaction—that once dominated all of sociology, including medical sociology, symbolic interaction survived the best. It is still featured as a leading school of sociological thought in introductory textbooks. As George Ritzer and William Yagatich (2012:105) observed, symbolic interaction theory is indeed "clearly still alive and kept that way by a number of supporters, especially in the US." Yet they also characterize the theory as being on life support and headed toward a zombie-like state—so there are grounds for saying it is in decline although surviving.

Of course, one might ask if the theory is in decline, why consider it? The answer is that symbolic interaction has an exceptionally rich tradition in medical sociology, as seen in the seminal contributions of Anselm Strauss and Erving Goffman. The theory still persists, and has extended its influence with some interactionists moving into the study of aging, emotions, and social constructionism (Charmaz and Belgrave 2013). Labeling theory, that evolved out of symbolic interaction and was a central concept in several studies of mental illness, had also faltered but been buoyed by modified labeling theory (Link et al. 1989; Link and Phelan 2010). This chapter, accordingly, will assess the strengths and weaknesses of these micro-level theories and their use in medical sociology, beginning with symbolic interaction.

Symbolic Interaction

The general orientation of symbolic interaction will be discussed by way of George Herbert Mead and Herbert Blumer, which is its dominant perspective, followed by the work of Strauss on the negotiated order, awareness contexts, and other topics, Goffman on impression management, the mental hospital, and stigma, Edwin Lemert and Howard Becker on labeling theory, and Thomas Scheff on mental illness, and other approaches to the study of health and illness.

Early Influences

Symbolic interaction is a distinctly American perspective whose roots in sociology can be initially traced to the ideas of William James, John Dewey, Charles Cooley, and William I. Thomas at the beginning of the twentieth century. Some sources credit Max Weber's notion of "*Verstehen*," translated literally as "understanding" and sometimes held to mean "interpretive understanding," as a basis for the origin of symbolic interaction because it advocated a subjective approach to the analysis of social action. However, as footnoted in Guenther Roth's and Claus Wittich's translation of Weber's *Economy and Society* ([1922] 1978:57), a rigorous use of the English term for "*Verstehen*" is inadvisable because Weber assigned different meanings to it in different contexts in German. However, Weber's concept does not appear to have a direct connection to symbolic interaction or other micro approaches. It seems to apply not to individual behavior but to patterned (that is, collective) forms of behavior in order "to assist macro sociologists in quite practical ways ... to take cognizance of the importance of subjective meaning" (Kalberg 1994:48; Ritzer and Stepnisky 2018). Mead, for example, in his seminal book, *Mind, Self, and Society* (1934), the foundation of symbolic interaction, does not refer to Weber at all.

Instead, the origin of symbolic interaction rests solidly in American pragmatism which is an approach to philosophical discourse that maintains "truth" or "meaning" is determined by its practical consequences or how it affects the real world. Therefore, the function of human thought is not simply to describe something, but to apply it to explaining situations, predicting outcomes, and solving problems empirically. William James (1842–1910), for example, a philosopher and psychologist, and an early pioneer in pragmatism, strongly supported the notion of free will, which he defined as a person's ability to choose his or her behavior and take action to achieve that choice. James' ([1892] 1977) influence on symbolic interaction is also seen in his claim that the relatively less important and simple things people do regularly in life (e.g., go to a store and buy something) become habitual forms of behavior that do not require concentrated thought while doing them, yet provide stability in daily activities as people know what to expect from one another in advance and can themselves act accordingly. Additionally, James ([1909] 1977) advocated what he called "radical empiricism," which was a view that theoretical propositions should not be developed prematurely and based on speculation, but formulated on the basis of the evidence that has been acquired.

This outlook is seen in Barney Glaser and Strauss's book, *The Discovery of Grounded Theory* (1967), a fundamental research methodology in symbolic interaction, recommending that theory be "grounded" in data through the process of discovery. In this context, theorizing does not begin with a set of preformulated and precisely defined hypotheses to be tested; instead, its direction is toward generating and testing hypotheses that are discovered or deduced as they emerge from the data being analyzed. Grounded theory methods thus begin with data that the researcher codes, analyzes, verifies, and utilizes to construct abstract hypotheses or theoretical propositions (Charmaz 2006). A researcher's deductions or theories are developed, extended or modified through ongoing data analysis rather than existing as a finalized product awaiting either verification or negation before data are analyzed. This approach also allows the researcher to discover social phenomena whose existence was not apparent at the beginning of an investigation, but is discovered during the research process. It ensures that a theory is representative of the data in which it originates.

When it comes to theory construction, however, a shortcoming of grounded theory is that it has not generated much theory (Timmermans and Tavory 2012). Instead, it has become a useful *method* for conducting exploratory research and grounding findings in the data collected. So the utilization of grounded theory not only continues, but has even been extended, as seen in Adele Clarke's (Clarke et al. 2018) addition of situational analysis that includes "mapping" the various elements present in particular situations to determine the respective positions and behavioral agendas of the participants.

John Dewey (1859–1952), another pragmatic American philosopher and psychologist, focused on education. Dewey ([1896] 1981) advanced the idea that the meaning of an object depends on what people decide its use is and they communicate its meaning through social interaction with other people. He also noted that people do not always respond automatically to a stimulus, but can delay or even modify their response through the exercise of judgment and choice.

Also important is the work of Charles Horton Cooley (1864–1929), a sociologist at the University of Michigan, who studied social organizations and formulated the theory of the "Looking-Glass Self." According to Cooley ([1902] 1962), our self-concepts emerge from social interaction in which we see ourselves reflected in other people. Cooley compares this reflection of ourselves in others to reflections in a mirror or "looking glass." His concept has three basic components: (1) We see ourselves in our imagination as we think we appear to the other person; (2) we see in our imagination the other person's judgment of ourselves; and (3) as a result of what we see in our imagination about how we are viewed by the other person, we experience some sort of self-feeling, such as satisfaction, pride, or humiliation. The contribution of this concept to symbolic interaction theory is that an individual's perception of himself or herself as a social object is based on the reaction of other people. The failure of the other person (the subject) to reflect a self-image consistent with that intended by the onlooker (the observer) can be stressful, while a successful reflection can not only generate positive feelings but confirm the person's sense of self.

This view is apparent in Cooley's concept of the primary group, which has been influential in the study of small groups, such as families and military units at the platoon, squad, or team level. Cooley ([1902] 1962:23) maintains that a primary group is "characterized by intimate face-to-face association and cooperation" and is primary in the sense that it is "fundamental in forming the social nature and ideals of the individual." The fusion of individuals into a common whole involves a mutual identification, a "we-feeling" between members of that group. Primary groups have an emotional character that binds them together and a functional character that is expressed in its activities as it functions collectively to achieve a common end.

The work of William I. Thomas (1863–1947), a University of Chicago sociologist, and part of the "Chicago School of Sociology" that dominated American sociology from the early twentieth century until World War II, also made a relevant contribution to symbolic interaction through his notion of the "definition of the situation." Thomas (Thomas and Thomas 1928:572) pointed out that situations defined as real are real in their consequences. That is, people define the situations they find themselves in and the consequences of the definitions they apply are "real" (even if mistaken) as individuals act upon them. As long as definitions of a social situation remain relatively constant, behavior is generally orderly. However, when rival definitions appear and habitual behavior becomes disrupted, a sense of disorganization and uncertainty may appear. The ability of an individual to cope with an intrusive situation will be based upon socialization experiences that have taught the person how to define and adjust to it.

This is seen in Thomas's view of a crisis. First, he notes that the same crisis *will not produce the same effect uniformly in all people.* This is because reactions depend upon how the situation has been defined by the individual. Second, he explains that adjustment to, and control of, a crisis result from an individual's ability to compare a present situation with similar ones in the past and to revise judgment and action upon the basis of past experience. Therefore, the outcome of a particular situation depends upon an individual's definition of that situation and how that individual comes to terms with it.

When the ideas of these various scholars are considered as a whole, they illustrate a theoretical foundation for understanding social behavior from the standpoint of the individual according to that person's assessment of the nature of the interaction that he or she has with other people.

George Herbert Mead

George Herbert Mead (1863–1931) is considered the originator of symbolic interaction theory. He was an American philosopher, who, like James and Dewey, favored pragmatism. He taught social psychology at the University of Chicago between 1894 and 1931, and his book *Mind, Self, and Society* (1934), based upon student notes from his courses and unpublished manuscripts, is a sociological classic. Mead posited that the individual is a creative, thinking organism able to choose his or her behavior instead of reacting more or less mechanically to the influence of large-scale social forces, as implied by structural-functionalism. Basic to the symbolic interactionist's conception of human behavior is the assumption that all behavior is self-directed on the basis of symbolic meanings that are shared, communicated, and manipulated by interacting human beings in social situations (Denzin 2017a). The process of social interaction between people forms behavior in a creative fashion, rather than being merely a means by which behavior is expressed. Therefore, society is seen as a human product and people as a social product, since both are formed in a continuing dialectical process in which human beings and their social environment act and react toward each other (Berger and Luckmann 1967; Denzin 2017a).

As a theory, symbolic interaction is expressly focused on understanding the individual's stream of consciousness, internal self-conversations, the development of the individual's self-concept in relation to social experiences with other people, self-definitions of social situations, and the merging of individual behavior into collective expressions of joint or group activities (Blumer 1969; Dennis, Philburn, and Smith, 2013; Denzin 2017a; Mead 1934; Rohall 2020; Strauss 1964). Although the emphasis is on agency and the thesis is that reality is socially constructed, symbolic interactionists nevertheless acknowledge that society and its institutions precede and constrain individuals—leaving them to respond as they will to external constraints on their behavior (Charmaz and Belgrave 2013).

Box 6.1 George Herbert Mead

Mead was born in South Hadley, Massachusetts on February 27, 1863 during the American Civil War. His father, Hiram Mead, was a Congregationalist minister, who went to Oberlin College in Ohio in 1870 to preside over courses on the art of preaching. His mother, Elizabeth Storrs Billings Mead, taught English composition and went on to serve as president of Mount Holyoke College in Massachusetts between 1890 and 1900. Mead earned a BA in history and literature

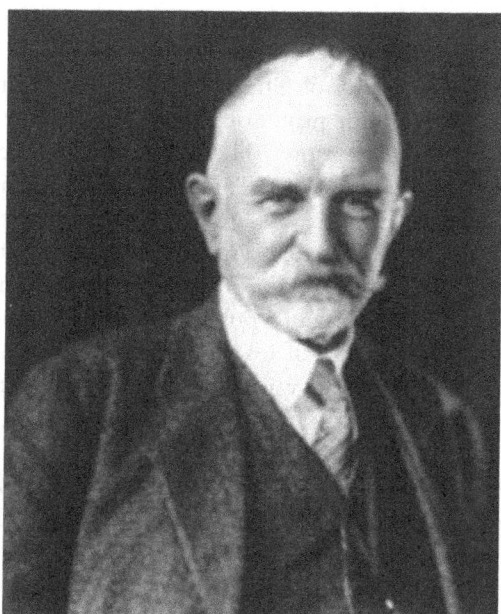

Image 6.1 George Herbert Mead

from Oberlin in 1883 and worked at various jobs the next four years, such as teaching grade school, tutoring, and working as a surveyor for a railroad, before enrolling at Harvard College. At Harvard, he obtained an MA in philosophy in 1888 and came to know William James, tutoring his children. James advised Mead, who had become interested in psychology, to go to Germany for his doctoral training, which was not uncommon for American academics in that era.

Mead spent the fall semester of 1888 in a Ph.D. program in philosophy and physiological psychology at the University of Leipzig under the noted psychologist Wilhelm Wundt. He also was able to reunite with his close friend and former Oberlin roommate Henry Castle, a wealthy scion of a prominent family in Hawaii, who was in Leipzig at the time with his sister Helen who was studying languages. Mead transferred to the University of Berlin in the spring of 1889 and married Helen Castle (1860–1929) in Berlin on October 1, 1891. He left Berlin shortly thereafter to accept a faculty position in philosophy and psychology at the University of Michigan. He never completed his Ph.D.

His only child, Henry Castle Albert Mead, who became a physician, was born in Ann Arbor in 1892. While on the Michigan faculty,

Mead became closely acquainted with Charles Horton Cooley and especially John Dewey. When Dewey became chair of the philosophy department at the University of Chicago in 1894, he insisted on bringing along Mead as a junior professor, considering him "the most original thinker of his generation" (Huebner 2014:2). Mead spent some 37 years on the University of Chicago faculty teaching philosophy and social psychology. He was a popular instructor who lectured without notes and attracted large numbers of graduate students, especially from sociology, to his classes. He may not have been at ease with writing, however, even though he published over 125 papers in various disciplines. Apparently, few of his papers were considered major contributions for someone who was recognized as one of the most brilliant pragmatists and he did not publish any books (Strauss 1964). An exception was a book manuscript, *Essays on Social Psychology*, that existed in printed galley proofs in 1910 and later found in family archives, but it went unpublished in Mead's lifetime for reasons that remain a mystery (Deegan 2010). Hospitalized in early 1931, Mead resigned from his university position and died the day after he went home on April 26, 1931 at the age of 68.

Nevertheless, his ideas formed the basis for symbolic interaction and his book, *Mind, Self, and Society* (1934), as noted earlier in this chapter, was published from the class notes of his students after his death. It became a landmark work in sociology. In fact, Mead's work became more prominent in sociology than either philosophy or psychology. As Daniel Huebner (2014:3) ironically points out: "Put in admittedly oversimplified terms, Mead is known in a discipline [sociology] in which he did not teach for a book he did not write."

The starting point for the symbolic interactionist perspective is how self-awareness and agency emerge in the individual through social experience. Mead (1934) maintains that a child's concept of self originates in his or her capacity to view themselves as a social object through the process of social interaction in which the individual experiences him or herself from the standpoints of other individuals in his or her social group and the generalized standpoint of the group as a whole to which he or she belongs. First is primary socialization consisting of childhood experiences with significant others (significant because they provide the child with his or her basic identity and self-concept) which is normally the family. For older children, significant others can also be teachers, peers, or other people—provided that they impart a sense of self to the child.

As the child becomes older and takes as his or her own the values and opinions of the immediate family, or those of the wider society as presented by the family, the child is considered to be on the way toward becoming properly socialized to the extent that he or she behaves in accordance with these same values and opinions. Ultimately the child can either accept or reject the social perspective put forth by the family, but the choices offered are set by older persons who determine what information is provided and in what context it is presented. As Peter Berger and German sociologist Thomas Luckmann point out in their seminal work, *The Social Construction of Reality* (1967), children have no choice in the selection of parents, so identification with parents and internalization of their values is virtually automatic. This outcome is seen in contemporary studies of health lifestyles involving adult practices of smoking, alcohol use, dietary habits, and exercise. These studies provide consistent findings showing that health lifestyles learned and adopted in childhood continue into adulthood although they may be modified over time (Lee et al. 2018; Mize 2017; Mollborn et al. 2014; Mollborn and Lawrence 2018).

Primary socialization is followed by secondary socialization that inducts an already socialized individual into a new role or position in society, usually as an adult. Symbolic interaction, for example, provided the theoretical framework for the most extensive (but seriously outdated) study of secondary socialization among medical students by Becker, Strauss, and their colleagues (1961) at the University of Kansas Medical School in the late 1950s. A goal of their research was to determine what the students learned in the culture of the medical school other than the mastery of medical knowledge. It was found that they developed a strong appreciation of clinical experience (actually working with patients rather than reading about disease and studying it in the laboratory) and acquired a sense of responsibility toward patients. They additionally learned to view disease and death as medical problems and to be emotionally detached in treating them. This study not only remains the foundational study on medical school socialization, but its methodological procedures later proved important in formulating the principles of grounded theory.

Mead (1934) goes on to say that a person is not socialized until he or she is able to comprehend a situation from the standpoint of someone else. Mead explains this in his analysis of play, the game, and the generalized other. Play is the first step in learning to understand roles. When children play at being parents, superheroes, and the like, they are imitating what they perceive are the roles of these types of people. When children become older, they begin to play organized games with formal rules. To do so, each child must understand his or her role in relation to the roles of the other participants.

For example, when playing baseball, a player must know how each participant is supposed to play a position. "They do not have to be present in consciousness at the same time," states Mead (Strauss 1964:215–16), "but at the same moment he or she has to have three or four individuals present in his or her own attitude, such as the one who is going to throw the ball, the one who is going to catch it, and so on." To achieve this, the player must be able to take the others' roles and anticipate how each of the others will attempt to play out the situation. When a player comes to know and anticipate how each teammate will play a position, he or she will be able to react more quickly and collectively to situations that develop during the game. When the child is able to understand the roles of others, and then fit his or her own actions into a common effort to reach a goal, the child is well on the way to becoming a member of society.

This sequence of socialization from the stage of play to that of games gives the child a progressive realization about the roles and attitudes of specific people to an understanding of roles and attitudes in general. Berger and Luckmann (1967:132–3) illustrate this process with an example of soup-spilling in which the child first learns that his or her mother will become angry at the child if he or she spills soup, which is followed by the realization that additional significant others will also get angry at soup-spilling, and on to the decisive step "when the child recognizes that *everybody* is against soup-spilling and the norm is generalized to '*One* does not spill soup'—'one' being himself [or herself] as part of a generality that includes in principle, *all* of society."

At this point the child can identify not only with significant others (specific people), but also with a generalized other, which Mead defines as the attitudes of a society, community, or group as a whole. The generalized other is not a person; rather, it is a person's conscious awareness of the society, community, or social group that he or she is part of. Mead's example of a generalized other is a sports team on which a child may play. Even though there are individuals on the team, the team itself has a name and an identity, and it represents an organized effort to achieve collective goals. The team is a generalized other for each player because it enters into the experience of all the individual members and acts to influence their behavior. One plays well so that "the team" can win; but "the team" is an abstract social concept consisting of the collective attitudes and roles of all the players brought together in a single identity for a particular goal.

Mead (1934:155) states that it is in the form of the generalized other that a social group or society exercises control over the conduct of its members. An awareness of the generalized other enters into a person's thinking, influencing how that person will act in certain situations. A person may have many generalized others, including family, friends, religion, work group, political party, community, nation, and society in general. Some of these generalized others are more important than others but nevertheless are taken into account when a person decides they are relevant in choosing what form of behavior to adopt.

Mead goes on to explain that socialization is never perfect or complete. He makes a distinction between what he calls the "I" (the unsocialized self) and the "me" (the socialized self). Both are part of a person's self-concept in his view. The "me" is that part of the self that is conscious of the norms, values, and traditions of the community; it governs the "I" in such a way that the person's expression of self reflects the attitudes of the generalized other. At times, however, the "I," which is that part of the self that is selfish, impulsive, and oriented toward self-fulfillment, takes over and directs behavior toward purely individual ends. Consequently, people do not always do what society expects, since someone more under the influence of the "I" may break rules or fail to conform to the expectations of others.

Mead's notion of the "I" and the "me" is mentioned here because its omission would be noticed by symbolic interaction purists, but its research value is logically questionable and exceedingly difficult to measure with any scientific precision. The "I" and "me" dichotomy, in fact, seems similar to Austrian psychoanalyst Sigmund Freud's concept of the personality in which the id (the "I") follows the pleasure principle and the superego (the "me") strives for what is ideal, which is likewise an untestable concept. Margaret Archer (2003) rejects Mead's notion of the "I" and the "me" altogether by pointing out that one cannot simultaneously be both subject and object in thinking about one's self and that the "me" as a reflection of the "generalized other" means the individual is actually conversing with society in one's mind, not one's self.

Herbert Blumer

The most influential interpretation of Mead's work is found in the writings of Herbert Blumer (1900–1987), one of Mead's students at the University of Chicago, who drew together and explained much of the material that is the basis of symbolic interactionist thought. Blumer (1969) pointed out that a central feature of symbolic interaction is the assumption that all behavior is socially directed and the key to understanding human conduct is the symbolic meanings shared, communicated, and manipulated by people interacting in social situations. Interaction is symbolic in the sense that actors respond to the behavior of others not for some inherent quality in what they say and do, but for the significance imputed to their actions by those present. Social reality does not exist unless we make it so. Blumer maintains that Mead's analysis of social action has five central features: the self, the act, social interaction, objects, and joint action.

1. First, Mead believed that the *self* of a person is formed through social interaction and experience with other people; thus, the self is a social product developed from a person's relationships with others. In this context, the human being is able to perceive, have conceptions of, communicate with, and act toward himself or herself as a social object in relation to other people.

2. Second is Mead's concept of the *act*. Mead insisted that human beings do not just respond more or less automatically to a given social influence but are able to interpret and define their own particular situation and organize their behavior to meet their circumstances. Blumer (1969:64) says: "In order to act the individual has to identify what he [or she] wants, establish an objective or goal, map out a prospective line of behavior, note and interpret the actions of others, figure out what to do at other points, and frequently spur himself [or herself] on in the face of dragging dispositions or discouraging settings."

3. Third is the concept of *social interaction*, which consists of two forms, the non-symbolic and the symbolic. Non-symbolic interaction is essentially the stimulus–response paradigm in which a person makes a non-thinking response to a certain stimulus, such as stepping back from a growling dog or raising a hand to catch a ball. Symbolic interaction, in contrast, is a situation in which human beings interpret and define actions and objects based upon symbolic meanings (notably language) shared with other people.

4. Fourth is the notion of the *object*, which maintains that objects do not possess inherent meanings but become what they are defined as by human beings interacting with each other. Thus, human beings act toward an object on the basis of the meaning that object has for them. Humans, for instance, define gold as valuable and act toward it accordingly. Yet there is nothing intrinsic to gold that makes it valuable; the social meaning of gold or anything else depends upon how humans define it. If gold was not defined as valuable, it would not be valuable.

5. Fifth is the *joint act*, which is the focal point of group behavior. Each participant in a social gathering brings his or her own individual social act or line of behavior to a situation. By fitting together all of those separate acts or lines of behavior into a single collective or joint act involving each person present, it is possible to ascertain the overall direction of group behavior. The result is that group activities are socially constructed by individual people coming together and interacting with one another in respect to the overall group enterprise. Joint actions may be open to many outcomes; once started they may be interrupted, abandoned, modified, or continued as expected. What happens depends

upon what those involved decide to do and how they act upon their decisions. The joint act, not the individual, is the focus for symbolic interactionist analyses of social behavior.

Joint acts contribute a sense of stability to social situations because they require a participant to identify that activity and orient himself or herself in that direction when engaging in behavior suitable to the scene. Blumer (1969:71) states, "Thus, to act appropriately, the participant has to identify a marriage ceremony as a marriage ceremony, a holdup as a holdup, a debate as a debate, a war as a war, and so forth." However, as pointed out by Norman Denzin (2017b), it is necessary for the study of behavior to go beyond the surface of social situations and taken-for-granted meanings and extend analysis of the joint act to the more subtle nuances of social relationships between people, including verbal and nonverbal acts and gestures. Symbolic interaction therefore regards human social behavior as an ongoing process of definition, interpretation of, and calculated response to the actions of others and the conditions of the social environment. The interactionist view is that: *Reality is socially constructed as it emanates from the perceptions and actions of those involved.*

Symbolic Interaction: Assessment

Symbolic interactionism proved itself to be an insightful and creative theoretical approach to explaining how self-concepts are shaped by social interaction and small group behavior can be analyzed through the joint acts of its participants. It put a human face on data collected through its methodologies that emphasize explaining social behavior directly from the comments, viewpoints, and actions of those engaging in that behavior—rather than relying on statistical tests showing various numerical values illustrating the significance or lack thereof of behavioral outcomes. Moreover, the concept of the generalized other provided a bridge linking micro to macro-levels of social behavior as it represents the presence of society (that is, the influence of structure) in the thinking and decision-making of individuals.

Additionally, its early studies in medical sociology were highly informative, with the Becker et al. (1961) study of medical school socialization from the standpoint of the students themselves just one of many. Anselm Strauss (1916–1986), in particular, who studied under Blumer at the University of Chicago and was arguably the leading medical sociologist in the 1960s and 1970s, was a symbolic interactionist. In one of many projects, Strauss and his colleagues (1963) examined how a mental hospital operated as a bureaucracy with its standard procedures, rules, and regulations for its staff, but was not rigid about those rules when patient care required maximum "innovation and improvisation." Thus rules were flexible, and the social organization of the hospital's work resulted from negotiation about what rules did or did not apply in particular situations.

What glued this social order together and kept it cohesive, making it possible for the staff to function effectively, was the sharing of a common goal to return their patients to the outside world in a better condition than when they entered the hospital. Physicians were able to establish relatively stable understandings with nurses and others involved in patient care, which resulted in efficient behaviors that were not dependent upon special bureaucratic instructions for each and every contingency. Consequently, the work of the hospital was carried out through a set of relationships that produced the structure influencing the staff's interaction and establishing the "trajectory" of patient outcomes within its walls. Strauss et al. used this observation to introduce the concept of the "negotiated order" to the literature on social organizations generally and it is still used today to study the organization of hospital services (Nugus 2019).

Glaser and Strauss (1965) studied death and dying and used their research to introduce the notion of "awareness contexts" based upon participant observation in several hospitals in the San Francisco Bay area. These awareness contexts were all associated with the control of information about dying in a hospital in which the patient was either unaware he or she was in a terminal state (closed awareness), suspected it was such (suspected awareness), pretended along with the staff not to know even though they all did (mutual pretense awareness), or all were openly aware (open awareness). This research, along with the findings of others studying the self-protective strategies of coroners (Charmaz 1975) to avoid the emotion of the death scene and maintain the routine character of their work and those of medical examiners (Timmermans 2006) who define how individuals have died, contributed to an understanding of the social psychology of those persons whose occupations and professions require routine exposure to death.

Kathy Charmaz (1991) studied chronically ill patients and found that such persons frequently experience an impaired self-image because they live restricted lives, are socially isolated, perhaps stigmatized, and feel devalued and a burden to others due to their illness or disability. All of these factors combined to reduce their sense of self-worth, unless some alternative means of pride and satisfaction can be obtained. According to Strauss (1975), the chief business of a chronically ill person is not just to stay alive or keep symptoms under control but also to live as normally as possible. A lifelong illness, in Strauss's view, requires lifelong work to control its course, manage its symptoms, and live with it. In this context, the sick role that the person assumes is a permanent condition, not temporary.

Along with British medical sociologist Michael Bury (1997), Charmaz (1991) finds that most disabled and many chronically ill individuals are obliged by their physical condition to reconstruct their sense of self and personal biography. They do this because of what Bury (2000:177) calls a "biographical disruption" in their lives. At one point they were "normal" and then because of a health-related event their normality is disrupted, and they are "different" in a negative way—"marking a 'then' and 'now' divide between life before and after illness" (Saunders 2017:727).

Box 6.2 The Looking-Glass Self and Disability

Using Cooley's "looking-glass" (seeing one's sense of self reflected in others) approach, Charmaz and Dana Rosenfeld (2006) found people with disabilities can be extremely self-conscious about their handicap. This concern is seen, for example, in Alexandra Nowakowski's (2016:902) account of a chronic illness where it is stated that: "Even now, I hesitate to draw attention to myself because people might think that I am 'sick', and I know what that role brings." Charmaz and Rosenfeld (2006:35) reported another woman's observation about how other people respond to her difficulty in walking:

> I just feel real self-conscious when I'm downtown and people look at me, you know, … or they notice the way I'm not walking correctly or whatever. And it really bothers me. It's almost like it brings me up short or something … I don't know what they're thinking or anything, but I can see that they perceive something different about me because they're looking, and I get annoyed.

In other research about the "meaning" of being able to drive despite having a neurological disease, one woman (Stepney et al. 2018:1192) says that people must "freak out" when they see her park her car and hobble from it:

> … they must think "Jesus, is she allowed on the road?" But when I'm behind the wheel of my car, I'm the same as anybody else. Sudden, suddenly I've got nothing wrong with me. Nobody can tell. It's only when I park and get out or walk.

Biographical disruptions and their effects on the social lives of individuals have attracted attention from medical sociologists because they illustrate how sick and disabled people suffer, experience stigma, and are socially marginalized, as seen in qualitative studies of disabilities (Grue 2016), incapacitation (Garthwaite 2015), HIV (Wouters and De Wet 2016), mucositis

(Nowakowski 2016), and inflammatory bowel disease (Saunders 2017). Taken together, the concepts of loss of self and biographical disruption provide important insight into how people experience chronic illness and disability (Charmaz and Belgrave 2013).

Symbolic interaction's greatest strengths are in explaining the evolution of a person's self-concept through the process of social experience and coming to understand the viewpoints of others and society as a whole as imparted by significant others and through the awareness of the generalized other. By the 1980s, however, symbolic interaction entered a period of decline that extended to medical sociology. Seldom do medical sociologists study the concepts of self originating in childhood during primary socialization, while research on the secondary socialization of medical and nursing students has not been conducted for years. Furthermore, despite its merits in capturing the behaviors of people in natural social settings, the use of qualitative methods that depend on the subjective assessments of researchers places symbolic interactionists at somewhat of a disadvantage as most research in American sociology generally is quantitative and based on statistical analyses of survey data. The reverse is true in Britain, however, where qualitative research in medical sociology is dominant and there are medical sociology journals such as the UK-based *Sociology of Health & Illness* and *Social Science & Medicine* that feature qualitative work.

Yet an important point made by Denzin (1992) is that the larger body of theory represented by symbolic interaction generally appeared to have reached its limits and taken on the image of a "fixed doctrine." That is, the theory seemed to have hit a wall. Symbolic interaction explained primary and secondary socialization rather well, was able to account for the concept of self, and could interpret various features of small-group interaction. But having accomplished this, it seems to have said what it had to say, and thereafter simply got old—what Denzin (1992:13) calls "the greying of interactionism," thereby leaving more recent qualitative perspectives like social constructionism to take center stage. Nevertheless, in those areas of research in medical sociology where symbolic interaction excels, such as studies of the self in health and sickness, physical disability, and aging, the perspective remains theoretically relevant. Additionally, as Charmaz and Linda Belgrave (2013:31) note, symbolic interaction can be linked to the investigative procedures of grounded theory and "form a useful theory-methods package" in conducting research. So symbolic interaction has not quite reached a zombie status and its influence continues.

Erving Goffman

Erving Goffman (1922–1982) developed the dramaturgical or "life as theatre" approach in sociology, which is linked to symbolic interaction. In this context, people typically act out their roles in certain ways in public ("front stage") but are especially likely to reveal their true selves in more private settings ("backstage"). Goffman (1959) observed that in order for social interaction to be possible, people need information about the other participants in a joint act. This information is communicated through: (1) one's appearance; (2) previous experience with similar individuals; (3) the social setting; and, of most importance, (4) the information a person chooses to express about himself or herself through words and actions. This fourth category of information is decisive, says Goffman, because it is subject to control by the individual and represents the impression that person is projecting—which others may or may not come to accept. This information enables others to know in advance what a person expects of them and what they may expect of him or her. Goffman calls this process "impression management." In large social organizations, individuals with a particular social status may cooperate as "performance teams" to maintain a definition of a situation for those above and below them; in essence, they are staging a show.

Goffman maintains that people live in worlds of social encounters in which they act out a line of behavior that consists of verbal and nonverbal acts by which individuals express their view of a situation and their evaluation of the participants, including themselves. The social value that individuals claim for themselves by the line of behavior that others assume they have taken is termed a "face." This face is an image of self that is projected by the individual to other people. One's face is one's most personal possession, but Goffman points out that a person's face is only on loan from society and can be withdrawn or modified if the person conducts himself or herself inappropriately. A person may be in the "wrong face" when information about that person's social worth cannot be integrated into his or her line of behavior or a person may be "out of face" when he or she acts out a line of behavior that people in a particular situation would not be expected to take. Goffman further explains that the maintenance of face is a condition of interaction, not its objective. That is, when people engage in "face-work," they are taking action to make their activities consistent with the face they are projecting. This is important because every member of a social group is expected to have some knowledge of face-work and some experience in its use, such as the exercise of social skills like tact.

Goffman sees almost all acts involving other people as being influenced by considerations of face. People are aware of the interpretations that others have placed upon their behavior and that they themselves also have done the same. The face that a person adopts to project his or her self-image is important because it represents who he or she is and is always present in social interaction. Consequently, Goffman sees the self as a sacred object to be protected from embarrassment and for someone to challenge its integrity can be stressful. Otherwise, people might not take such great care in acting in ways considered appropriate to their situation. The self is viewed as a player in a ritual game who copes judgmentally with their social environment. This aspect of Goffman's work identifies the calculative element in dealings between people and presents them as information managers and strategists maneuvering for gain in social situations. It also implies a degree of superficiality and insincerity as the *appearance* of performing a role is more important than the role itself, in Goffman's opinion, but people can nonetheless sometimes act as superficially as he describes and play "games" to manage impressions. Goffman suggests that we can never really know other people; that is, we can never actually penetrate their "true" being. We can only construct an image of what we think they are like.

This framework of how people manage impressions of themselves is seen in *Asylums* (1961), Goffman's ground-breaking study of life in a mental institution and the rationales patients used for explaining how they got there. Goffman (1961:xiii) described the mental hospital as a "total institution," which he defined "as a place of residence and work where a large number of like-situated individuals, cut off from the wider society for an appreciable period of time, together lead an enclosed, formally administered round of life." The central feature of the total institution, which also includes prisons, monasteries, homes for the blind, and military bases, is uniformity. All aspects of life are conducted in the same place under the same authority and in the immediate company of others who are treated alike and who do the same thing together. All phases of activities are scheduled to fulfill the aims of a rational plan supposedly designed to meet the official goals of the institution, which in the case of the mental hospital is therapy, custodial care, or both.

The goals of the total institution are *the* determining factors in shaping the social life that takes place within its confines. In the case of mental patients, regardless of whether or not they have a positive or negative view of their situation, Goffman observes that such patients actually have very little choice but to adapt to the social environment of the hospital. He identifies four types of adjustment to the total institution: (1) situational withdrawal; (2) intransigence (rebellion); (3) colonization (using negative experiences of the life in the outside world to demonstrate the desirability of life on the inside); and (4) conversion (living up to the staff-sponsored ideal model). Goffman tells us that typically the inmates will not follow completely any one particular mode of adaptation but will most likely adopt a somewhat opportunistic combination of conversion, colonization, and loyalty to the inmate group. Instead of making what Goffman calls a primary adjustment of "giving in" to the system, the patient will make a secondary adjustment, which is to appear to conform to the system while gaining hidden satisfactions whenever possible.

Perhaps Goffman's most important contribution to medical sociology is his concept of stigma. Goffman (1963:3) defines stigma as "an attribute that is deeply discrediting." He reminds us that the term *stigma* apparently originated with the ancient Greeks, who used it to refer to marks on the body. These marks were intended to represent something unusual and morally bad about the people having them. Usually, the marks were brands cut or burned into the body to identify the bearer as a criminal, a slave, or a traitor. Thus, any citizen encountering the stigmatized person was entitled to treat him or her badly or, once aware of the mark, was expected to avoid contact altogether with that person.

In contemporary society, Goffman finds there are three main forms of stigma: (1) abominations of the body, such as various types of physical deformities; (2) blemishes of individual character—that is, mental disorder, sexual deviance, dishonesty, criminality, addiction to drugs, alcoholism, suicidal tendency, and so forth; and (3) the stigma of race, religion, and nationality. The person with such attributes is someone who is different from most other people, but in a negative (supposedly less human or socially unacceptable) way. "On this assumption," says Goffman (1963:5), "we exercise varieties of discrimination, through which we effectively, if often unthinkingly, reduce his [or her] life chances." When it comes to health, Graham Scambler (2012:441) describes stigma this way:

> Stigma is typically a social process, experienced or anticipated, characterized by the exclusion, rejection, blame or devaluation that results from experience, perception or reasonable anticipation of an adverse social judgement about a person or group. This judgement is based on an enduring feature of identity conferred by a health problem or health-related condition, and the judgement is in some essential way medically unwarranted.

Therefore, as Bruce Link et al. (1989) and others (Kroska et al. 2014) point out, one of the negative consequences of being diagnosed ("labeled") with a mental disorder is that cultural ideas about the mentally ill (such as incompetence and dangerousness) become relevant for that person and transformed into expectations that others will devalue, discriminate, stigmatize, and avoid that individual. Even the potential for being stigmatized can influence an individual's behavior and act as a barrier to seeking help, since awareness of being treated for mental symptoms can affect judgments of family, friends, coworkers, and others about the person. For example, persons submitting job resumes or applications may not want to mention that they were ever under psychiatric care even if that was the case. This same situation can apply to persons with stigmatizing physical illnesses who avoid or hide the fact they are receiving medical care, for example, by not parking their car near an AIDS clinic where passers-by might recognize it.

Link and Jo Phelan (2010, 2013:532) studied why people stigmatize others and determined that three basic goals are achieved by doing so: (1) exploitation/domination (keeping people down), (2) enforcement of social norms (keeping people in line), and (3) avoidance (keeping people away). When it comes to mental disorder, Link and Phelan favor "keeping people in line" as the major reason for stigmatizing them as violating norms is socially disruptive, although avoidance or "keeping people away" also happens frequently. They likewise note that stigmatization is an exercise of *power* in that it takes power to stigmatize and also confirms power on those able to do the stigmatizing. The effects of stigma on the person or group being stigmatized are a loss of status and subjugation to discrimination. To avert these social penalties, the stigmatized person is forced to behave differently, re-educate or confront others to change their mind, or engage in some form of activism to counter the stigma (Thoits 2011, 2016). Otherwise, the stigma can "stick" as an adverse social label carrying rejection, devaluation, and discrimination along with it. As Jason Schnittker (2013) explains, the stigma attached to mental illness is both severe and common. "Relative to other sources of stigma," states Schnittker (2013:81), "the stigma of mental illness may be unusually strong."

Consequently, we see in Goffman's scheme that a current or former mental patient or a person infected with a socially controversial disease such as HIV/AIDS, is someone who may be discredited because of a blemish of character, that blemish being, of course, past or present history of a socially discrediting affliction (Payton and Thoits 2011). Stigma can also be applied to an individual with a dread disease (i.e., Ebola, COVID-19) because of fear of contagion. Their stigma can cause others to keep their social distance from the stigmatized person (Martin et al. 2007; Perry 2011). Goffman's notion of stigma and how it operates in health-related situations is important not only because of how people are mistreated by others because of it, but also because of how they see themselves.

Labeling Theory

Labeling theory evolved out of symbolic interactionism, but is not really a theory at all; it is a view of deviance that qualifies as what Blumer (1969) calls a sensitizing concept. It is sensitizing in that it is intended to provide a *general* orientation and suggest directions for further inquiry; it is not intended as a definitive theoretical statement. Nevertheless, labeling theory emerged as a major sociological approach to understanding mental disorder. The foundations for labeling theory result principally from the work of Edwin Lemert (1912–1996) and Howard Becker.

Lemert (1972) argued that studies of deviant behavior needed to confront two problems: (1) how deviant behavior originates, and (2) how deviant acts become symbolically attached to certain persons and what the consequences of such attachment are for those individuals. Therefore, Lemert (1951) came up with the concept of *primary* and *secondary deviance*. Primary deviance is a situation in which a person who is "normal" temporarily acts differently or strangely, but the behavior is rationalized as atypical by others because it is perceived as not characteristic of the person's usual self. Secondary deviance, on the other hand, is more serious because it refers to a situation in which a person is regarded as a deviant; that is, being deviant is thought to be a typical characteristic of that individual. As Eliot Freidson (1970:218) explains: "Significant deviance is *secondary*—that is, it becomes socially recognized as *deviance* rather than as mere difference."

Secondary deviance occurs when a person continues over time to violate norms and is subsequently labeled by the reactions of other people as a deviant. Freidson notes that what is important is the imputation of deviance to an individual by others. Whether or not that person is actually deviant, in his view, is beside the point. What is the point is the power of society to organize and apply labels that affect how someone themselves and others classify that person, and how others treat that person because of the classification or "label." Heavy drinking, for example, can be regarded initially as being a case of primary deviance, but if such drinking is consistent over time, that person moves into a position of secondary deviance by the reactions of others who come to define that person as an alcoholic. A person labeled by others as an "alcoholic" may find it difficult to associate with "normals" (moderate drinkers or abstainers). The result may be that the person is forced (if he or she desires companionship) to develop associations with other people who drink heavily or accept alcoholism as normative behavior. Thus, we have the stereotypical situation of the once socially acceptable person whose heavy drinking leads to a disruption of normal relationships and downward social mobility into a world of alcoholics and "skid row" living conditions in which heavy drinking and drunkenness is the norm. Drug addicts can easily find themselves on the same path. Lemert's analysis thus implies an identity for deviants that is more or less lasting once the label has been applied.

Becker made further contributions to labeling theory in his book *Outsiders* (1973) in which he argues that social groups create deviance by making rules whose infraction constitutes deviance. *Deviance is therefore not a quality of the act a person commits but rather is a consequence of the definition applied to the act by others.* Whether an act is deviant therefore depends on how other people react to it. The responses of other people are problematic because their interpretation of the situation is the deciding factor, and not all people see things the same way. The focus of *Outsiders* is upon marijuana smokers who view marijuana use as normal behavior in their own subculture but who were criminals in the eyes of the wider society at the time. Other factors may also be important to how people respond to deviance, such as the timing of the deviance and it may depend upon *who* commits the act and *who* feels harmed by it as rules tend to be applied more to some people than to others.

Becker's (1973:20) model of deviant behavior is depicted in Table 6.1 as follows:

Table 6.1 Types of Deviant Behavior

	Obedient Behavior	Rule-Breaking Behavior
Perceived as deviant	Falsely accused	Pure deviant
Not perceived as deviant	Conforming	Secret deviant

In his typology, Becker notes that some behavior can be classified as obedient to rules and other behavior as rule breaking, yet whether a particular individual is defined as deviant depends upon the perceptions of others. Therefore, in the category of obedient behavior is the "conformist," who is not perceived as deviant and is not deviant in fact; then there is the "falsely accused," who is perceived as deviant but is in fact innocent. Under rule-breaking behavior, we have the "pure" deviant, who is both deviant and perceived as such, and the "secret" deviant, who is deviant but not perceived as such because they act deviantly only in secrecy. Thus, the labeling approach stresses that judgments of what is deviance are relative, depending upon the perceptions of others. The critical variable in understanding deviant behavior is the social audience that has knowledge of the act in question because the audience determines what is and what is not deviant.

Mental Illness

The labeling theory perspective was particularly viable in studies of mental patients. For example, in David Rosenhan's (1973) long ago research on voluntary mental hospital admissions, a group of eight supposedly normal persons—a psychiatrist, a pediatrician, a painter, a housewife, a psychology graduate student, and three psychology professors—presented themselves for admission as schizophrenics at 12 different mental hospitals located in five states on both the East and the West coasts. All were admitted, and once in the hospital they immediately reverted to their usual normal behavior.

Yet, despite their show of sanity after some initial nervousness over actually being in a mental hospital, the pseudo-patients were never detected by the hospital staffs as being "fakes." Rather, it was the "real" patients who correctly identified the pseudo-patients as imposters. Rosenhan believed that the failure of the hospital staff to discover the pseudo-patients (length of hospitalization ranged from seven to 52 days, with an average of 19 days) illustrates the power of labeling in psychiatric assessment. Once labeled as schizophrenics, there was *nothing* the pseudo-patients could do to overcome an identification that profoundly affected the perceptions of other people about them and their behavior. Their release from the mental hospital was contingent upon the staff's accepting the idea that the nonexistent schizophrenia was "in remission." Rosenhan (1973:251) noted that despite their public "show" of sanity, the pseudo-patients were never detected, were admitted with a diagnosis of schizophrenia, and were discharged with a diagnosis of schizophrenia "in remission." The evidence showed that once labeled a schizophrenic, the pseudo-patient was stuck with that label.

The sociologist best known for linking labeling theory and mental disorder is Thomas Scheff (1974, 1999) who claimed that mere rule breaking is not enough in itself to cause others to respond to a rule breaker as mentally ill. So he added the concept of *residual rule breaking* to the labeling view of mental illness. Residual rule breaking is based upon the idea that most social norms are fairly clear and widely understood, yet there is a residual area of social convention that is assumed to be so natural that it is part of "human nature," such as looking at the person you are talking to or responding to someone who calls your name. To violate these residual conventions goes beyond just violating norms; it involves acting contrary to human nature. Such "unnatural" behavior may come to be regarded by others as mental illness.

Scheff further suggested that social stereotypes shape symptoms of mental disorder. He claimed that people as young as elementary school children have grasped the literal meaning of "crazy." Such meanings are part of our culture, he says, as illustrated by the general understanding of phrases such as "The boogey man will get you!" He goes on to point out that the cultural stereotype of insanity stays with us into adulthood and is continually reinforced through social interaction; in fact, it is often the basis for our manner of reacting to people who have already been labeled insane. Furthermore, this stereotype is available to the patient and becomes part of the patient's orientation for guiding his or her own "crazy" behavior. Thus, in brief, Scheff considers mental disorder a social role whose behavior conforms to society's expectations of people who are "crazy."

Depending upon the identity of the rule breaker, the rule broken, the amount of tolerance available, any alternative explanation that might clarify or rationalize the behavior, and the social context in which the rule-breaking behavior takes place, the residual rule breaker may be labeled by others as "mentally ill." In Scheff's view, when this happens and people respond to that person in accordance with that label, a deviant has been created by society. He points out that, at some time, virtually everyone acts crazy. But if a person is labeled mentally ill and comes to the attention of a community's formal system of control for mental illness, that person will be launched on a career of chronic mental illness and is thus irreparably stigmatized as a mental patient.

Labeling Theory: Critique

Walter Gove (1970, 1975:48–51) was a leading critic of Scheff and he suggested, in contrast, that studies providing evidence of genetic inheritance, stress from critical life events, and the expression of symptoms by mental patients indicate there is much more to mental illness than simply labeling. Gove's criticism had three central themes. First, he rejects the notion that lower-class people are more readily labeled as mentally ill than the affluent because he feels there is quicker recognition of it and less tolerance for it among members of the upper social strata. Second, being labeled mentally ill does not, in his view, result in lasting stigma for former mental patients. And third, he believes that those people who are mentally ill have an inherent mental condition quite apart from how they are labeled. This last criticism is especially important because it recognizes that mentally ill people have something wrong with them, regardless of how they are labeled. Inferences of mental disorder are made from verbal and nonverbal behaviors that indicate a person's mental state and, therefore, what seems apparent is that before the onset of labeling, there likely exists a troubled mind independent of the labeling process. Once the individual who possesses that disturbed mind expresses his or her internal state to others, various factors then intervene to influence the responses to, and decisions made about, the individual in question, including the application of any labels.

This situation represents the most important weakness in the application of labeling theory to mental disorder. Labeling theory does not explain what actually causes mental disorder, other than societal reaction to residual rule breaking, nor does it explain why certain people become mentally ill and why others in the same social circumstances do not. Gove was justified in questioning the efficacy of labeling theory in this regard. His other major criticisms—who is most readily labeled mentally ill (the affluent), and the duration of that label's stigma—are not as strong. Past research, for example, has shown a powerful relationship between lower-class social position and mental disorder and that the stigma of being a mental patient either can be shed if the person concerned acts relatively normal over time or can endure for those persons with long-term mental disorders (Cockerham 2017).

This criticism is in line with the critique of Lemert's notion of primary and secondary deviance that neglects the issue of what caused the deviance in the first place. This criticism can be applied to labeling theory as a whole because societal reaction alone does not explain why certain people commit deviant acts and why others in the same circumstances do not. A label in itself does not cause deviance. Some situations (e.g., crime, alcoholism, drug addiction, suicide, mental disorder) are defined by many people as being deviant—yet people do these things regardless of how they are labeled, and their reasons for doing so may have nothing to do with the label that is attached to them. Another problem is Becker's notion of the secret deviant. If a deviant status is applied by a social audience, how does a secret deviant become labeled "deviant" if no one knows about it? Becker (1973) attempts to refute this criticism by claiming that secret deviance consists of being vulnerable to discovery, that is, of being in a position in which it would be easy to make a deviant label stick. In this circumstance, the secret deviant *knows* he or she will be labeled deviant if discovered. But here again, this does not tell us how or why the deviance began in the first place.

Another deficiency of labeling theory rests in its attempts to explain the characteristics of deviants and deviant acts. If deviant actors share characteristics (e.g., poverty, stress, childhood abuse, age, family background, or perhaps a desire for thrills or personal gain) other than societal reaction, the characteristics are not defined or explained. Such characteristics may be as important as, if not more important than, the reaction of the social audience. In fact, the reaction of the social audience may not be especially relevant in accounting for the social characteristics of the person exhibiting deviant behavior and cannot stand alone as the explanation for deviant conduct.

Another issue is that in line with their symbolic interactionist heritage, labeling theorists maintain that individual behavior is not automatically determined by social situations and structures; it is derived from how people define what they and others do based upon free choice. Yet once a person is labeled "deviant," labeling theorists seem to place the labeled individual in circumstances in which that person has little or no choice about what happens. In other words, once labeled, the deviant person is forced to assume a deviant status in society because that is how he or she is perceived and treated by others. Thus it seems a contradiction to assert that initially people have a choice about being deviant and later they do not (when they are labeled).

Although labeling theory has flaws, it nevertheless has merits. Its most important contribution is that it calls attention to the potentially powerful effects of labeling on individuals. People labeled "mentally ill" by others are likely to be stigmatized and find it difficult to rid themselves of the label. As Eric Wright and his associates (Wright, Gronfein, and Owens 2000) pointed out several years ago, social rejection is an enduring force in the lives of people with mental illness. Being shunned, avoided, socially devalued, and discriminated against by those who have applied the label is often a common experience. People, in turn, may not only expect and experience rejection but also come to think less of themselves because of the severity of their symptoms and the limited social opportunities that accompany their label. Therefore, Bruce Link and his colleagues (Link et al. 1989; Link and Phelan 2010) suggested a "modified labeling theory" that has given labeling theory new life. Modified labeling theory avoids the idea that labeling *causes* mental disorder and changes the theory's emphasis away from the defining role of the social audience to the illness's effects on the individuals being labeled. Those individuals whose symptoms are mild or moderate, or do not have a history of mental illness, are more likely to resist the stigma of being labeled mentally ill and deflect that identity to prevent self-stigmatization (Thoits 2016; Thoits and Link 2016).

Summary

This chapter reviewed symbolic interaction and labeling theory that focus on explaining patterns of face-to-face social interaction occurring between individuals and within small groups. These theories emphasize "agency" which, as previously noted, refers to the capacity of the individual to select his or her behavior and orient it in the direction chosen as he or she interacts socially with other people. When individuals engage in making choices, they become the "agent" of their own behavior, which is the origin of the term "agency." Society is therefore created from the bottom up by people who use agency to create the structures in their lives through patterned forms of social interaction. Symbolic interaction was introduced through the work of Mead who presented the theory to sociology which included his concept of socialization consisting of significant others, play, the game, and the generalized other. Blumer, the major interpreter of the interactionist perspective, identified the five central features of symbolic interaction as (1) the concept of self, (2) the act, (3) social interaction, (4) definitions of objects, and (5) the joint act. Next discussed was the work of Strauss on the negotiated order of the hospital, awareness contexts with respect to death and dying, and other topics, followed by Goffman's theories of impression management, the mental hospital as a total institution, and stigma, Lemert and Becker on labeling theory, and Scheff on mental illness.

Guide to Critical Thinking

1.   What are micro-level theories? Why does sociology have such theories?
2.   What makes "grounded theory" different from quantitative methodologies?

3. Describe how the "Looking-Glass" theory reflects a sense of self.
4. Explain Mead's concept of play, the game, and the generalized other.
5. What is the difference between significant others and the generalized other?
6. Explain what Goffman means by "face-work" and "impression management."
7. How can stigma be an important concept in studies of illness and disability? What are the effects of a biographical disruption?
8. Is labeling theory still useful in studies of mental illness? Explain why.

Suggested Reading

Dennis, Alex, Rob Philburn, and Greg Smith. 2013. *Sociologies of Interaction*. Cambridge: Polity.
A review of various micro-level approaches in sociology that includes a chapter on the body, health, and illness.
Denzin, Norman K. and Yvonna S. Lincoln (eds.). 2018. *The Sage Handbook of Qualitative Research*, 5th ed. Thousand Oaks, CA: Sage.
An authoritative compendium of qualitative research methods.
Aneshensel, Carol, Jo C. Phelan, and Alex Bierman (eds.). 2013. *Handbook of the Sociology of Mental Health*, 2nd ed. Dordrecht: Springer.
Several chapters include discussions of symbolic interaction, labeling theory, and social constructionism in relation to mental disorder.

References

Barker, Kristin K. 2005. *The Fibromyalgia Story: Medical Authority and Women's Worlds of Pain*. Philadelphia, PA: Temple University Press.
Becker, Howard. 1973. *Outsiders: Studies in the Sociology of Deviance*. New York: Free Press.
Becker, Howard S., Blanche Greer, Everett C. Hughes, and Anselm Strauss. 1961. *Boys in White: Student Culture in Medical School*. Chicago, IL: University of Chicago Press.
Berger, Peter L. and Thomas Luckmann. 1967. *The Social Construction of Reality: A Treatise in the Sociology of Knowledge*. Garden City, NY: Doubleday.
Blumer, Herbert. 1969. *Symbolic Interactionism: Perspective and Method*. Englewood Cliffs, NJ: Prentice-Hall.
Bury, Michael. 1997. *Health and Illness in a Changing Society*. London: Routledge.
Bury, Michael. 2000. "On Chronic Illness and Disability," in Chloe Bird, Peter Conrad, and Allen Fremont (eds.), *Handbook of Medical Sociology*, 5th ed. Englewood Cliffs, NJ: Prentice-Hall, pp. 173–83.
Charmaz, Kathy C. 1975. "The Coroner's Strategies for Announcing Death." *Urban Life* 4:296–316.
Charmaz, Kathy. 1991. *Good Days, Bad Days: The Self in Chronic Illness and Time*. New Brunswick, NJ: Rutgers University Press.

Charmaz, Kathy. 2006. *Constructing Grounded Theory: A Practical Guide through Qualitative Analysis*. London: Sage.

Charmaz, Kathy and Linda Liska Belgrave. 2013. "Symbolic Interaction Theory and Health," in William Cockerham (ed.), *Medical Sociology on the Move: New Directions in Theory*. Dordrecht: Springer, pp. 11–40.

Charmaz, Kathy and Dana Rosenfeld. 2006. "Reflections of the Body, Images of Self: Visibility and Invisibility in Chronic Illness and Disability," in D. Waskul and P. Vannini (eds.), *Body/Embodiment: Symbolic Interaction and the Sociology of the Body*. London: Ashgate, pp. 35–50.

Clarke, Adele E., Carrie Friese, and Rachel Washburn. 2018. *Situational Analysis: Grounded Theory after the Postmodern Turn*, 2nd ed. Thousand Oaks, CA: Sage.

Cockerham, William C. 2017. *Sociology of Mental Disorder*, 10th ed. New York: Routledge.

Cooley, Charles H. [1902] 1962. *Social Organization*. New York: Schocken.

Deegan, Mary Jo (ed.). 2010. *George Herbert Mead: Essays in Social Psychology*. New Brunswick, NJ: Transaction.

Dennis, Alex, Rob Philburn, and Greg Smith. 2013. *Sociologies of Interaction*. Cambridge: Polity.

Denzin, Norman K. 1992. *Symbolic Interactionism and Cultural Studies*. Cambridge, MA: Blackwell.

Denzin, Norman K. 2017a. *The Research Act*. New York: Routledge.

Denzin, Norman K. 2017b. *Sociological Methods*. New York: Routledge.

Denzin, Norman K. and Yvonna S. Lincoln (eds.). 2018. *The Sage Handbook of Qualitative Research*, 5th ed. Thousand Oaks, CA: Sage.

Dewey, John. [1896] 1981. "The Reflex Arc in Psychology," in John McDermott (ed.), *The Philosophy of John Dewey*. Chicago, IL: University of Chicago Press, pp. 136–48.

Freidson, Eliot. 1970. *Profession of Medicine: A Study of the Sociology of Applied Knowledge*. New York: Harper & Row.

Garthwaite, Kayleigh. 2015. "Becoming Incapacitated? Long-Term Sickness Benefit Recipients and the Construction of Stigma and Identity Narratives." *Sociology of Health & Illness* 37(1):1–13.

Glaser, Barney G. and Anselm L. Strauss. 1965. *Awareness of Dying*. Chicago, IL: Aldine.

Glaser, Barney G. and Anselm L. Strauss. 1967. *The Discovery of Grounded Theory: Strategies for Qualitative Research*. Chicago, IL: Aldine.

Goffman, Erving. 1959. *The Presentation of Self in Everyday Life*. Garden City, NY: Doubleday.

Goffman, Erving. 1961. *Asylums*. Garden City, NY: Doubleday.

Goffman, Erving. 1963. *Stigma: Notes on the Management of Spoiled Identity*. Englewood Cliffs, NJ: Prentice-Hall.

Gove, Walter R. 1970. "Societal Reactions as an Explanation of Mental Illness: An Evaluation." *American Sociological Review* 35:873–84.

Gove, Walter R. 1975. "Labeling and Mental Illness," in W. Gove (ed.), *The Labeling of Deviance: Evaluating a Perspective*. New York: Halsted, pp. 35–81.

Grue, Jan. 2016. "The Social Meaning of Disability: A Reflection on Categorisation, Stigma, and Identity." *Sociology of Health & Illness* 38(6):957–64.

Huebner, Daniel R. 2014. *Becoming Mead: The Social Process of Academic Knowledge.* Chicago, IL: University of Chicago Press.

James, William. [1892] 1977. "Habit," in John McDermott (ed.), *The Writings of William James: A Comprehensive Edition.* New York: Random House, pp. 9–21.

James, William. [1909] 1977. "Radical Empiricism," in John McDermott (ed.), *The Writings of William James: A Comprehensive Edition.* New York: Random House, p. 136.

Kalberg, Stephen. 1994. *Max Weber's Comparative Historical Sociology.* Chicago, IL: University of Chicago Press.

Karp, David A. and Laura B. Birk. 2013. "Listening to Voices: Patient Experience and the Meanings of Mental Illness," in Carol Aneshensel, Jo Phelan, and Alex Bierman (eds.), *Handbook of the Sociology of Mental Health*, 2nd ed. Dordrecht: Springer, pp. 23–40.

Kroska, Amy, Sarah K. Harkness, Lauron S. Thomas, and Ryan P. Brown. 2014. "Illness Labels and Social Distance." *Society and Mental Health* 4(3):215–34.

Lee, Chioun, Vera K. Tsenkova, Jennifer M. Boylan, and Carol D. Ryff. 2018. "Gender Differences in the Pathways from Childhood Disadvantage to Metabolic Syndrome in Adulthood: An Examination of Health Lifestyles." *SSM-Population Health* 4:216–24.

Lemert, Edwin M. 1951. *Social Pathology.* New York: McGraw-Hill.

Lemert, Edwin M. 1972. *Human Deviance, Social Problems, and Social Control*, 2nd ed. Englewood Cliffs, NJ: Prentice-Hall.

Link, Bruce G. and Jo C. Phelan. 2010. "Labeling and Stigma," in Teresa Scheid and Tim Brown (eds.), *A Handbook for the Study of Mental Disorder: Social Contexts, Theories, and Systems*, 2nd ed. Cambridge: Cambridge University Press, pp. 571–87.

Link, Bruce G. and Jo V. Phelan. 2013. "Labeling and Stigma," in Carol Aneshensel, Jo Phelan, and Alex Bierman (eds.), *Handbook of the Sociology of Mental Health*, 2nd ed. Dordrecht: Springer, pp. 525–41.

Link, Bruce G., Francis T. Cullen, Elmer Struening, Patrick E. Shrout, and Bruce P. Dohrenwend. 1989. "A Modified Labeling Theory Approach to Mental Disorders: An Empirical Assessment." *American Journal of Sociology* 92(6):1461–500.

Martin, Jack K., Bernice A. Pescosolido, Sigrun Olafsdottir, and Jane D. McLeod. 2007. "The Construction of Fear: Americans' Preferences for Social Distance from Children and Adolescents with Mental Health Problems." *Journal of Health and Social Behavior* 48(1):50–67.

Mead, George H. 1934. *Mind, Self and Society.* Chicago, IL: University of Chicago Press.

Mize, Trenton D. 2017. "Profiles in Health: Multiple Roles and Health Lifestyles in Early Childhood." *Social Science & Medicine* 178:196–205.

Mollborn, Stefanie and Elizabeth Lawrence. 2018. "Family, Peer, and School Influences in Children's Developing Health Lifestyles." *Journal of Health and Social Behavior* 59(1):133–50.

Mollborn, Stefanie, Laurie James-Hawkins, Elizabeth Lawrence, and Paula Fomby. 2014. "Health Lifestyles in Early Childhood." *Journal of Health and Social Behavior* 55(4):386–402.

Nowakowski, Alexandra C. H. 2016. "Hope is a Four-Letter Word: Riding the Emotional Rollercoaster of Illness Management." *Sociology of Health & Illness* 38(6):899–915.

Nugus, Peter. 2019. "Re-structuring the Negotiated Order of the Hospital." *Sociology of Health & Illness* 41(2):378–94.

Payton, Andrew R. and Peggy A. Thoits. 2011. "Medicalization, Direct-to-Consumer Advertising, and Mental Illness Stigma." *Society and Mental Health* 1(1):55–70.

Perry, Brea L. 2011. "The Labeling Paradox: Stigma, the Sick Role, and Social Networks in Mental Illness." *Journal of Health and Social Behavior* 52(4):460–77.

Ritzer, George and Jeffrey Stepnisky. 2018. *Sociological Theory*, 10th ed. Los Angeles, CA: Sage.

Ritzer, George and William Yagatich. 2012. "Contemporary Sociological Theory," in George Ritzer (ed.), *The Wiley-Blackwell Companion to Sociology*. Oxford: Wiley-Blackwell, pp. 98–118.

Rohall, David E. 2020. *Symbolic Interaction in Society*. Lanham, MD: Rowman and Littlefield.

Rosenhan, D. L. 1973. "On Being Sane in Insane Places." *Science* 179:250–8.

Saunders, Benjamin. 2017. "'It Seems Like You're Going Around in Circles': Recurrent Biographical Disruption through Past, Present and Anticipated Future in the Narratives of Young Adults with Inflammatory Bowel Disease." *Sociology of Health & Illness* 39(5):726–40.

Scambler, Graham. 2012. "Health-related Stigma." *Sociology of Health & Illness* 31(3):441–55.

Scheff, Thomas J. 1974. "The Labeling Theory of Mental Illness." *American Sociological Review* 39(3):444–52.

Scheff, Thomas J. 1999. *Being Mentally Ill: A Sociological Theory*, 3rd ed. Chicago, IL: Aldine.

Schnittker, Jason. 2013. "Public Beliefs About Mental Illness," in Carol Aneshensel, Jo Phelan, and Alex Bierman (eds.), *Handbook of the Sociology of Mental Health*, 2nd ed. Dordrecht: Springer, pp. 75–94.

Stepney, Melissa, Susan Kirkpatrick, Louise Locock, Suman Prinjha, and Sara Ryan. 2018. "A Licence to Drive? Neurological Illness, Loss and Disruption." *Sociology of Health & Illness* 40(7):1186–99.

Strauss, Anselm (ed.). 1964. *George Herbert Mead on Social Psychology*. Chicago, IL: University of Chicago Press.

Strauss, Anselm. 1975. *Chronic Illness and the Quality of Life*. St. Louis, MO: Mosby.

Strauss, Anselm, Leonard Schatzman, Danuta Ehrlich, Rue Bucher, and Melvin Sabshin. 1963. "The Hospital and its Negotiated Order," in Eliot Freidson (ed.), *The Hospital in Modern Society*. New York: Free Press, pp. 147–69.

Thoits, Peggy A. 2016. "'I'm not Mentally Ill': Identity Deflection as a Form of Stigma Resistance." *Journal of Health and Social Behavior* 57(2):135–51.

Thoits, Peggy A. and Bruce G. Link. 2016. "Stigma Resistance and Well-being among Persons in Treatment for Psychosis." *Society and Mental Health* 6(1):1–20.

Thomas, William I. and Dorothy Swaine Thomas. 1928. *The Child in America: Behavior, Problems, and Programs.* New York: Knopf.

Timmermans, Stefan. 2006. *Postmortem: How Medical Examiners Explain Suspicious Deaths.* Chicago, IL: University of Chicago Press.

Timmermans, Stefan. 2013. "Seven Warrants for Qualitative Health Sociology." *Social Science & Medicine* 77:1–8.

Timmermans, Stefan and Iddo Tavory. 2012. "Theory Construction in Qualitative Research: From Grounded Theory to Abductive Analysis." *Sociological Theory* 30(3):167–86.

Weber, Max. [1922] 1978. *Economy and Society*, 2 vols, Guenther Roth and Claus Wittich (trans. and eds.). Berkeley, CA: University of California Press.

Wouters, Edwin and Katinka De Wet. 2016. "Women's Experience of HIV as a Chronic Illness in South Africa: Hard-earned Lives, Biographical Disruption and Moral Career." *Sociology of Health & Illness* 38(4):521–42.

Wright, Eric, William P. Gronfein, and Timothy J. Owens. 2000. "Deinstitutionalization, Social Rejection, and the Self-Esteem of Former Mental Patients." *Journal of Health and Social Behavior* 44(March):68–90.

Chapter 7

Journey to Postmodernism

French structuralism, poststructuralism and postmodernism begin the trail leading to contemporary theory in medical sociology. Although many contemporary theories reflect the influence of the classics, the theories in this chapter constitute a rupture with the past and an effort to forge new and different interpretations of sociological phenomena in changing times. This group of theories is included as a chapter in this book because they represent a distinct period of theory development in sociology in anticipation of the twenty-first century. French structuralism and poststructuralism were both a prelude to what was to come: postmodern theory. Yet despite a promising beginning, postmodern theory quickly floundered because of some fundamental shortcomings, providing a clear message for subsequent theories in medical sociology.

The leading theorist in both poststructuralism and postmodernism is the French philosopher and social theoretician Michel Foucault. He is of interest in medical sociology as he included concepts of mental illness and medical practice in his theorizing and influenced the development of social constructionism and a new sociological specialty, the sociology of the body. This chapter will first discuss French structuralism and the reaction to it that fueled the rise of poststructuralism and the work of Foucault, followed by a discussion of the emergence of sociological interest in the physical human body, and the rise and fall of postmodern theory in medical sociology.

French Structuralism

French structuralism was a short-lived theoretical perspective in the 1960s. While interest in it was not limited to France, the perspective dominated the country's intellectual agenda so thoroughly at that time it became known as French structuralism and part of the national effort in the country to regain its pre-World War II theoretical influence in a variety of academic disciplines (Heilbron 2015). The structures that French structuralists were initially interested in were primarily linguistic, not social, but debate about its merits spilled over into theoretical discourse in the social sciences. In reaction to the joyless individual freedom of existentialist thinking espoused by the French philosopher, novelist, and playwright Jean-Paul Sartre (1905–1980) and his followers, French structuralism looked beyond what it considered the surface appearances of an individual-centered world emphasizing self-direction to focus instead on what it maintained were "deep" structures shaping what people think, what they know, and how they behave. In this context, people were not free agents; rather, their thoughts and actions were invariably guided by structure. The origins of this perspective were in the semiotic (sign systems) theory of the Swiss linguist Ferdinand de Saussure (1857–1913) and carried forward by the French structural anthropologist Claude Lévi-Strauss (1908–2009).

According to de Saussure ([1916] 1966), people are not free to think outside the rules of their own language; that is, one's language *requires* that person to organize and express his or her thoughts in a specific format. This is because the way people think and understand their world is structured by language. The meaning of the words expressed, what de Saussure referred to as the "sound-image or signifier," and the concept or psychological image it evokes ("the signified") is determined by the configuration of the language used and the culture that produced it. He argued that two properties of language are particularly important. First, there is no natural link between the signifier and the signified, only a conditional cultural designation. For example, calling a "cow" a "cow" has no effect upon a cow whatsoever; rather, the meaning of the word "cow" is the meaning people have assigned to it in whatever language they speak and the human activity that results in reaction to it. Second, however, is de Saussure's claim that words have no meaning by themselves. Words acquire meaning only in reference to what they are not; that is, their meaning is based upon how they differ from other words. Important in this regard is the concept of binary opposites in which the meaning of a word is best understood in relation to its opposite (such as good or bad, hot or cold, early or late, and so on). The basic message that de Saussure's semiotic theory delivers is that language forces a person into its patterns of use if they desire to communicate effectively with others. In this way, language constitutes a deep structure in society shaping patterns of thought according to its rules of grammar, as people are not free to think outside of the language they speak.

This so-called "linguistic turn" from language as a source of creativity and spontaneity to the structuralist claim that the individual is not autonomous but constrained by discourse attracted considerable attention, some positive and some negative. According to the late historian Tony Judt (2005:398), the 1960s were "the great age of Theory" in the social sciences and humanities.

This was because of a widespread interest in theories, generally on the part of a large and receptive audience in newly expanded universities in North America and Western Europe experiencing a surge in student enroll-ment, and on the part of academic journals seeking publishable material. Theories of structuralism were popular, not just those of de Saussure and his colleagues, such as Roland Barthes in linguistics, but also Émile Durkheim and Talcott Parsons in sociology, Louis Althusser in structural Marxism, Fernand Braudel and the Annales School in history, and Lévi-Strauss in structural anthropology.

What these theories had in common was an overemphasis on structure as *the* determining force in human social affairs. Structuralism depicted social meanings as fixed, not free, and maintained by traditional and universal structures (deep structures) that formed a stable and self-contained system. Individuals were given little or no credit for creativity or being a catalyst for social change. "What counted," said Judt (2005:399), "was not surface social practices or cultural symptoms but [understanding] the inner essences, the deep structures of human affairs."

Judt (2005:400) implies that an advantage of French structuralism was that it was untestable and therefore above rejection, as he says:

> It was thus not subject to empirical testing or disproof—there was no sense in which structuralism could ever be demonstrated to be wrong—and the iconoclastic ambition of its assertions, allied to this imperme-ability to contradiction, guaranteed it a wide audience. Anything and everything could be explained as a combination of "structures".

However, being empirically untestable is a major disadvantage in sociology as untestable abstract theories sooner or later encounter skepticism as their logic is met with a counter logic. As it turned out, it was just a matter of time until structuralism's demise. The end was not long in coming as French structuralism was essentially dead by the 1970s (Giddens 1987). A major weakness was that it was unable to explain how structures, deep or on the surface, are produced, reproduced, or transformed and, like its American rela-tive, structural-functionalism, it had clear difficulty accounting for change. Also, according to Judt, the notion that everything is "structured" leaves something vital unexplained. What French structuralism left uncovered was the elephant in the room: agency. It was missing. Therefore, Judt (2005:400–1) surmises that: "As an interpretation of human experience, any theory dependent on an arrangement of structures from which human choice had been eliminated was thus hobbled by its own assumptions."

This is not to say that structuralism did not have any "triumphs." According to Johan Heilbron (2015:157), as a sociologist working in France at the time: "Structuralism to me meant the idea that everything has an underlying structure waiting to be discovered. It was fantastic." The notion that there are "deep" structures (deeply embedded norms?) below the surface appearance of everyday life shaping social interaction and relationships *is* indeed intriguing to a sociologist (or should be). It could explain much about patterns of social behavior, including those in medical sociology. However, this notion has yet to be succinctly conceptualized and remains relatively unexplored. Consequently, as Heilbron (2015:157) observed: "The fashion of structuralism had little impact on sociology."

Poststructuralism

Poststructuralism is not a unified theory with statements, propositions, and testable hypotheses, but consists of various theoretical concepts that emerged in the 1960s in opposition to structuralism. What poststructuralist thinking generally had in common was a rejection of the idea that there are central unifying rules operating as deep structures in society organizing language and social phenomena into stable systems, meanings, and relationships. Rather, it took the position that rules change; systems can be unstable. One of the two major figures among the poststructuralists (the other was Foucault) was the French philosopher Jacques Derrida (1930–2004) who argued that the meaning of written words was not socially constraining or fixed, nor always stable and orderly. Depending upon the context in which they are used, meanings found in writing can and do change in his view. Derrida (1978) introduced the term "deconstruction" that could be considered as a practical method for analyzing texts, which in writing meant breaking down parts of complex sentences into small groups of related phrases, analyzing them as a separate grouping to determine their meaning, and then incrementally putting them back together in order to better understand the whole.

In a poststructuralist sense, however, deconstruction in research meant figuratively taking (i.e., "tearing") apart written texts and looking within them for contradictions, inconsistencies, repressed meanings, and evidence of questionable validity. This method does not involve determining what causes something, but seeks to understand a whole in terms of its parts and its parts in terms of what they contribute to the meaning of the whole. This approach can mean deconstructing previous deconstructions. It can begin and end with "writers writ[ing] about writers for other writers" (Castoriadis 1992:16, as quoted in Alvesson 2002:29), which is not particularly useful in sociology and, moreover, "strongly discourages empirical work" (Alvesson 2002:29). In sociology empirical research linked to theory is clearly preferred over analyzing written texts in a search for meanings, hidden or otherwise.

Deconstruction or "decentering" could be considered a methodological tactic in sociology to turn society "inside-out" by making marginalized groups the focus instead of those in the mainstream. Understanding social interaction on the margins would take priority over analyzing the center (i.e., power structures) but such an approach would be incomplete without considering the center's role in creating and structuring marginalization. However, the larger problem with poststructuralism generally for medical and other sociologists is that it is highly abstract, largely philosophical, and untestable because it lacks methodologies for collecting and analyzing data representative of the empirical world. At some point, theories must be testable in order to demonstrate their scientific validity; otherwise, as noted earlier, they can only rely on their unverified surface logic as evidence of their authenticity. As a result, poststructuralism was not of great use to sociology and its contribution to sociological theory appears limited to providing a background for postmodern theory and the work of Foucault (Ritzer and Stepnisky 2018). It has subsequently disappeared, having faded into postmodernism and, for that matter, into history.

Foucault and Medical Sociology

The leading representative of poststructuralism, as noted in the introduction, is Michel Foucault (1926–1984), initially a structuralist, though he later denied it, but he adjusted his views over time to reflect a poststructuralist approach that was unique in its originality (Judt 2005; Merquior 1985; Ritzer and Stepnisky 2018). He did not acknowledge the existence of "some deep, ultimate truth" or "formal rule-governed model of behavior" (Ritzer and Stepnisky 2018:631). Rather, he turned his attention to an analysis of knowledge which, by itself, is usually considered to be objective and neutral, but Foucault (1969, 1979) characterized it instead as closely intertwined with power. He described his methods of historical analysis as "archaeology" in which the past is analyzed in discontinuous segments rather than as a uniform whole and as "genealogy" when past epochs are compared to the present. Foucault provided social histories of the way knowledge produced expertise over time that empowered professions and institutions—such as medicine, religion, and the state—to control social behavior. Knowledge and power were depicted as being so closely interconnected that an extension of one meant a simultaneous expansion of the other, prompting Foucault to use the term "knowledge/power" as one word to express this tight unity (Turner 1996). He did not consider modern power to be hierarchical (exercised from the top down) as typically thought, but instead portrayed it as "localized," meaning that it was everywhere (that is, both vertical and horizontal) and inescapable.

Foucault (1979) notes that traditionally power had indeed been monolithic, hierarchical, and visible, expressed in law, recorded in writing, and negative in that it was intended to punish. But in the nineteenth and twentieth centuries, new methods of power emerged through new techniques, namely the use of power in the hands of experts whose opinions and findings were generally accepted as truth and widely believed to be positive and utilized for the good of society. The knowledge/power link was pervasive throughout society because people voluntarily accepted it. While repressive, it could also be productive and enabling. Foucault, however, focused on repression. He portrayed knowledge/power as subtle in its expression and difficult to resist as it had become normalized. Instead of behavior being molded by deep structures, it was controlled by voluntary acceptance of the knowledge/power of expert groups. This is seen in Foucault's (2007) use of the term "governmentality" which he utilized to express different things, but one prominent meaning refers to governments systematically using the rationality of the governed as a form of power to manage their freedom and choice (Dean 2018).

Box 7.1 Michel Foucault

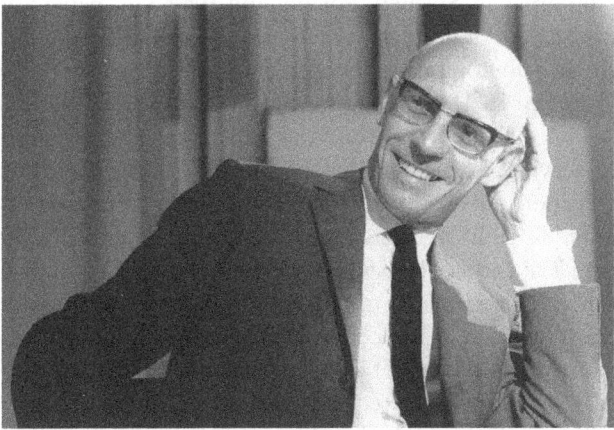

Image 7.1 Michel Foucault

Foucault was born on October 26, 1926 in Poitiers, France in an upper-middle-class family. Both his father and grandfather were surgeons, but he rebelled against his father's wishes to also become a physician by deciding to study philosophy. He additionally changed his first name when older from Paul-Michel (Paul was his father's name) to simply Michel because he considered his father to be a bully. He began school at the age of four because he could not bear being separated from his older sister and, as a teenager during World War II, attended a Catholic Jesuit secondary school while his city was under occupation by the German Army.

After the war ended, he transferred to a boarding school in Paris to prepare for the qualifying examinations at France's prestigious *École normale supérieure*, scoring fourth among all students in the country taking the exam. One of his professors was Louis Althusser, the structural Marxist, who was an early influence. At the *École*, Foucault was allegedly unpopular, socially isolated, and attempted suicide on more than one occasion. He nonetheless graduated in 1949 with a master's level degree in philosophy. His father had arranged for him to have psychiatric help and the experience likely initiated an interest in mental health. This led him to also complete a BA in psychology in 1948 from the University of Paris, followed by a Diploma in Psychotherapy in 1952. Foucault joined the French Communist Party in 1950 and quit in 1953, but remained friends with Althusser who had helped secure a position for him at the *École* as an instructor where he taught psychology both there and part-time at the University of Lille.

From 1955 to 1960, Foucault worked out of French embassies as a cultural diplomat in Sweden, Poland, and West Germany teaching French language and culture at various universities and institutes, and working on his doctorate in philosophy at the University of Paris, which he finished in 1960. His dissertation became a book, *Madness and Civilization* (1965). He then began a full-fledged academic career, first serving as the head of philosophy at the University of Clermont-Ferrand in northwest France and then spent two years at the University of Tunis in Tunisia. His well-received book on French structuralism, *The Order of Things*, published in 1966, gave him prominence as a scholar. He returned to Paris in 1968, teaching at a suburban campus, the University of Vincennes, before negotiating an appointment as chair of the history of systems of thought at the Collège de France in 1970 where he stayed until his death on June 25, 1984 at the age of 58 from HIV/AIDS. In addition to his books, teaching, and popular public lectures, he was active in various human rights, gay rights, anti-racist, and penal reform movements.

Of Foucault's several books, two had the most direct relevance for medical sociology: *Madness and Civilization: A History of Insanity in an Age of Reason* (1965) and *Birth of the Clinic* (1973). Foucault (1973) used the example of the medical profession in both of these books to illustrate how medical know-ledge functioned as a means to regulate madness and illness. In *Madness and Civilization* (1965), he argues that mental illness did not officially exist until the seventeenth century, when it was defined by the medical profession as a public threat that needed to be controlled. Prior to this time, during the Middle Ages and the Renaissance, Foucault observed that people who were mentally ill or retarded were generally regarded as "fools" and "village idiots" and tolerated by their communities for amusement, sadism, or charity, or because they were harmless and not a bother. If violent or angry, they might be killed or chased away. Some were kept at home by their families, some-times in chains if they could not be controlled, and others were driven away and forced to wander over the countryside, surviving as best they could. Some were allegedly placed on boats or ships, the so-called "ships of fools," in which the crews had been bribed to put them ashore in some distant place. Foucault found that these ships of fools stimulated the imagination of certain early Renaissance writers and artists, such as the German satirist Sebastian Brant (1458–1521) and the Dutch painter Hieronymus Bosch (1450–1560). Both created symbolic works featuring mad people adrift in search of their reason in a sea of unreason.

However, the deliberate removal of mentally ill persons from their com-munities signified considerably more than just the idea of the mad going forth in search of normality but marked an initial step to separate the insane from the sane. As the medical profession gained more knowledge, separation began featuring confinement in mental hospitals under the jurisdiction of psychiatrists as experts in the control of madness. Foucault's analysis can be extended to current public policies of deinstitutionalization and community care. The relocation of mental patients from psychiatric hospitals back into communities with the use of medications, while preferable to many patients, continues this process of regulation and control, but in a different form—namely the use of drugs to confine the mind instead of the body's confine-ment. The more knowledge produced by psychiatry, the more its power to control the mentally ill.

Madness and Civilization was Foucault's first major book. Its tone was anti-psychiatric and its approach influential in forming a branch of social constructionism, to be discussed in Chapter 9. The basic goal of social constructionism is to understand the processes by which certain behaviors are defined as medical conditions and the way in which these definitions function as a form of social control (Conrad and Barker 2010). Social constructionist theory maintains that mental illness is based on socially con-structed rules defining norms for normal and abnormal behavior. These rules are not rigid. They can change according to the dominant modes of thinking in particular historical periods and are dependent upon who has the power to designate and enforce prevailing concepts of abnormality (Horwitz 2013). The most publicized example of a mental illness being reclassified is the American Psychiatric Association's repudiation of homosexuality as a mental disorder in the 1970s. Any mental illness that can be voted out of existence opens a host of questions about what constitutes a mental illness in the first place and lends support to a social constructionist perspective along the lines suggested by Foucault.

Foucault's second work of direct relevance to medical sociology is *Birth of the Clinic* (1973) in which he again focused on power relations to show how the medical profession defined normality and abnormality through surveillance (what he called the medical or clinical "gaze"). He noted two distinct trends emerging in the history of medical practice: (1) "medicine of the species" (the classification, diagnosis, and treatment of disease) and (2) "medicine of social spaces" (the prevention of disease through public health measures). Medicine of the species made the human body an object of study subject to medical intervention and control, while medicine of social spaces made the health of the general public subject to medical and civil regulation. In this social history, not just the mind, but also the body comes under the monitoring and jurisdiction of medical experts on behalf of society.

Foucault also wrote a three-volume *The History of Sexuality* (1980) which, despite its subject matter, seems to have had less impact on medical sociology than his books on madness and the clinic. He had found that contrary to what is commonly believed, the expression of sexuality was not repressed in Western societies after the Victorian era. Instead, discourse about it literally exploded and sexuality became subject to increased scrutinization, control, and policing by the medical profession, the state, and the Church. While this had the appearance of discouraging "unproductive sexualities," what was actually produced in Foucault's (1980:45) view was more attention to what he called "perpetual spirals of power and pleasure." Power and pleasure were synchronized as, he argued, there was pleasure in the power of monitoring and pleasure in evading being monitored. He characterized medicine's interest in sexuality as more moral than scientific and primarily oriented toward preventing it. Medicine, in his view, had divided its interest in sex into two components: (1) "a biology of reproduction," directed toward scientific knowledge of sex and (2) "a medicine of sex," geared toward preventing the spread of such knowledge in order to use its power to regulate sexuality.

Western Christianity, expressly the Catholic Church, was depicted by Foucault as a source of sexual repression, particularly the use of confession to elicit (or in his words "extort") sexual transgressions from people and issue the moral admonishments that followed along with the opportunity for redemption. And there was also the interest of the state in regulating sexual behavior and punishing abnormality as a means of controlling population growth and eliminating deviance. The final two volumes of Foucault's treatise on sexuality were focused on ancient Greece and Rome. Both were empires that lacked unified and authoritarian moral codes about sex and were open to homosexuality and other practices. Control over sexuality in these societies stemmed more from self-control and self-practices than the external controls that Foucault saw emerging later under the influence of early Christianity.

Despite past praise for Foucault's ideas in both sociology (Cousins and Hussain 1984) and medical sociology (Petersen 2012; Petersen and Bunton 1997), several criticisms exist. There are rebuttals, for example, claiming that his perspective does not consider possible limits on the exercise of power, nor explain relations between macro-level power structures other than dwell on their mechanisms for reproduction; moreover, as stated earlier, there was a general disregard of agency in poststructuralism, especially by Foucault (Giddens 1987; Münch 1993). Anthony Giddens (1987:98) found that Foucault's history tends to have no active subjects at all, people are simply passive; and he goes on to say that the "individuals who appear in Foucault's analyses seem impotent to determine their own destinies." Giddens (1987:98) concludes: "It is history with the agency removed."

As for medical sociology, an assessment of Foucault by British medical sociologist David Armstrong (1997) is instructive. Armstrong (1997:15) highlighted the objectivity of his evaluation by asking:

> Who is Foucault? I do not know and I do not really care. I confess that I have not read any of the biographies that have been written about him and I have no interest in his personal life. Indeed, if, as in some Shakespearean authorship mystery, I was told that he never really existed and that the books bearing his name were written by a number of different people it would not bother me.

Armstrong's intent was simply to explore the effect Foucault's major books had on himself as a reader without knowing anything about him. His review helps to determine Foucault's importance in medical sociology in the late 1990s that can be used as a comparison to his status today. Armstrong found Foucault's works on madness and the clinic more applicable at that time to the interests of history than sociology. It is true Foucault's social histories are just that: histories. Armstrong nevertheless observed that some of Foucault's ideas influenced medical sociology, primarily his analysis of the relationship between medical knowledge and professional power, as well as the historical trends he identified in medical practice. These concepts were incorporated into social constructionist thinking. The impact of Foucault's book on sexual history, however, was depicted as "relatively slight," perhaps because sexuality is not one of medical sociology's major topics.

If Foucault's influence some twenty-plus years ago in medical sociology appears modest in Armstrong's review, what is it today? The answer seems to be that it has lessened even further with the passage of time. Foucault is seldom cited in American literature on medical sociology and the last major British work was published in 1997 with Armstrong's critical review the first chapter (Petersen and Bunton 1997). The prospect of significant revival is limited. His treatise on madness does not reflect the current mental health emphasis on community care. His accounts of medical practice do not consider the greater participation of patients in decision-making with doctors about their medical procedures, nor the status of physicians as employees in large health care corporations, the role of the marketplace in health care, the controls on care and costs by insurance companies and government agencies, and federal and state policies reducing the professional power of physicians—what George Ritzer and David Walczak (1988) refer to as "deprofessionalization." For the present, Foucault's marriage of knowledge/power remains of interest in medical sociology because it can be extended to explain the continuing translation of technological knowledge into medical power and this seems to be his major theoretical legacy.

Sociology of the Body

Foucault deserves credit in sociology, not just for his knowledge/power typology, but also for helping to establish the sociology of the body as an academic subject. Bryan Turner's book, *The Body and Society* (1984), was the catalyst for what became a new area of study. The field already existed in a limited capacity at the time, but Turner's book provided the critical mass for solidifying its basis as a sociological subspecialty. Foucault's deep imprint on *The Body and Society* is readily apparent when reading it, even though Turner (1992:230) pointed out that Foucault was more influential for his later book, *Regulating Bodies* (1992) that elaborated on medicine's role as a form of social control over the body. Turner (1996:38) was critical of the lack of originality in some of Foucault's ideas in the second edition of *The Body and Society*, where he notes how closely Foucault's discussion of reasoning on the part of medicine and the church in *The History of Sexuality* (1980) paralleled Max Weber's ([1922] 1978) earlier concept of "rationalization." Nevertheless, Foucault's work on the regulation of the body by social institutions provides the theoretical foundation for Turner's analysis.

In *The Body and Society*, Turner focused on the transfer of the social control and monitoring of the human body from religion to medicine and the control of women's bodies by men in patriarchal systems of authority which easily fit into a Foucauldian background. As the social control over the use of bodies by the church decreased, control by medicine increased. Turner concluded that all societies are confronted with four essential tasks: (1) the *reproduction* of the population over time (controlling population pressures); (2) the *regulation* of bodies in space (controlling behavior); (3) the *restraint* of the "interior" body (controlling desire) through disciplinary measures (religion, medicine); and (4) the *representation* of the "exterior" body in social space (dressing and adorning the body to signify status). The link to medical sociology through these four societal tasks was the connection to medicine's monopoly on supervision of the physical and social body. Turner (1984:50–1) therefore relied on Foucault's perspective on the control of the body to place his own social history of the body squarely within the parameters of medical sociology making it a subspecialty of a specialty. "A sociology of the body," says Turner (1984:51), "is thus fundamentally an exercise within medical sociology."

Other work followed in British medical sociology that echoed this theme, including Turner's two subsequent books, *Medical Power and Social Knowledge* (1987) and *Regulating Bodies* (1992), followed by new editions of *The Body and Society* (1996, 2008), along with Simon Williams' treatise, *Medicine and the Body* (2003), and Sarah Nettleton's textbook *The Sociology of Health and Illness* (2013). Nettleton (2013:93) noted that illness can obviously have profound effects upon the body, psychologically and socially, that health is increasingly conceptualized through bodily maintenance activities or lifestyles, and that medicine can alter the body through reconstruction, transplants, genetics, and assisted reproduction. Because of these connections, the study of the body seemed to be on its way to becoming a central topic in medical sociology. But this has yet to happen.

Why? As Turner (2008) observed, two distinctive approaches to the sociology of the body evolved. One examined how the body is socially constructed (i.e., defined and socially treated) and the other focused on the phenomenology (i.e., perception) of the experience of the body in everyday life. Though clearly related to medical sociology, the sociology of the body—as it has developed so far—became expressly concerned with the study of emotions and the sociological understanding of the control, use, and phenomenological experience of the body. The latter consists of inquiry about the dialectical relationship between the physical body and the mind that focuses on human subjectivity and the "lived" or phenomenological experience of both *having* and *being* in a body. Emphasis was therefore placed on understanding "embodiment" which refers to "the ways in which individuals understand and experience physical sensations and locate themselves in social space, how they conceptualize themselves as separated from other physical phenomena, how they carry themselves, how they distinguish outside from inside and invest themselves as subject or object" (Lupton 1998:85). This approach reflects the view that individual experience is invariably embodied, whether or not the individual is conscious of it (Nettleton 2016).

By going in this direction, the sociology of the body developed more externally to medical sociology than within it, as the phenomenological approach to explaining the experience of the body as interpreted by the mind became the dominant viewpoint. This perspective did not stray far from its base in philosophy established by the French philosopher Maurice Merleau-Ponty (1962, 2004) and lacked a focus on health and illness. According to the British sociologist Nick Crossley (2012:87), Merleau-Ponty is "above all, a philosopher of embodiment," but his insights can nevertheless be relevant for medical sociology through the utilization of his philosophical account of mind and body to explain health-related activities, the experience of illness, and the embodied nature of medical practice. Yet Crossley (2012:100–2) also notes that "Merleau-Ponty has nothing to say [directly] about these practices." Consequently, the usefulness of his perspective would appear to be limited to philosophical discourse.

In general sociology, these abstractions about the "lived" experience of the body were picked up in social theory as subjective descriptions of various types of naturalistic, socially constructed, and civilized bodies (Schilling 2003). One focus was on examining the manner in which people shape, decorate, present, manage, and socially evaluate bodies. Class position, for example, is held to have a profound influence on how people develop their bodies and apply symbolic values to particular body forms. As Chris Schilling (1993:140) observes, bodies represent physical capital with their value determined by "the ability of dominant groups to define their bodies and lifestyles as superior, worthy of reward, and as, metaphorically and literally, the embodiment of class."

However, the turn toward phenomenology resulted in less interest in the sociology of the body from medical sociology, particularly in the U.S., since health-related interests were underrepresented and the subject matter became generally abstract, descriptive, and reliant on analyzing subjective and intuitive bodily experiences. Consequently, the sociology of the body has not become prominent in American medical sociology; only in British medical sociology has it gained a niche foothold (Bury 2004). The low level of interest in it in the U.S. is predictable, given the emphasis in American sociology on the empirical verification of theories and the absence of empirical research associated with the sociology of the body. Its use in medical sociology is foremost that of philosophical conjecture about how people experience their body and relate to those of others in regard to health and disease, along with the role of medical practice as a structural entity exercising control over the body on behalf of society. The best option for going beyond the current singular framework of subjectivity would appear to be the use of phenomenology to construct testable hypotheses about the "lived" experience of being ill, injured, or disabled. This approach has not yet materialized.

Postmodern Theory

Postmodern theory evolved out of poststructuralism in the 1960s, as an oppositional counter-culture emerged among various groups in Western countries critical of conventional authority and morality. Political authority was challenged by a wave of protests, especially in France in May 1968 where a major student and worker revolt caused considerable social upheaval and demonstrated to many intellectuals, including Foucault and other poststructuralists, that society was undergoing significant social and cultural change (Ashley 1997). Although the protests accomplished little of practical value, postmodern thought offered the idea that modernity and its postindustrial social system was breaking up as the twenty-first century was arriving and being replaced by new conditions. The attraction was its contention that modern society was undergoing a transition from the recent past (the latter part of the twentieth century) and postmodernism could provide a useful theoretical framework for explaining the changes. Given the growing popularity of this theory as the twenty-first century was readily approaching, and the repeated tendency of human societies to view an oncoming new century with hope, excitement, and the expectation of positive change, postmodern theory offered a fresh lens for perceiving what some thought would be a new social world.

Postmodernism had been generally ignored by sociologists until the mid-1980s when primarily British social scientists decided it was worthy of serious attention and began showing interest in it (Bertens 1995). Postmodernism in sociology presented itself as a critique of modern sociological theory and grand theoretical narratives making sweeping generalizations about society as a whole; it rejected notions of continuity and order and called for new concepts explaining the disruptions of late modern social change (Best and Kellner 1991). Its central argument was that no single coherent rationality existed in society and the framework for social life had become fragmented, diversified, and decentralized. Its sociological relevance rested in its depiction of the destabilization of society and the requirement to adjust theory to explain new social realities—although these new realities were never precisely identified.

Ideas about the postmodern spanned a number of disciplines and there are a variety of concepts associated with it. The term "postmodern" can be taken to mean "just after the modern." A general definition is that postmodernism is "a modification or change in the way(s) in which we experience and relate to modern thought, modern conditions, and modern forms of life, in short to modernity" (Smart 1993:39). The visual arts, architecture, literary criticism, and philosophy all produced works reflecting postmodern themes by the late 1960s before sociologists considered the perspective applicable to their field. Contributions to sociological thinking about postmodernity came from scholars in several disciplines, some of whom considered themselves postmodernists and others who did not. Among the most influential in this group of predominantly French intellectuals were Foucault, Derrida and other philosophers such as Jean-François Lyotard and Gilles Deleuze, psychoanalyst Félix Guattari, and sociologist Jean Baudrillard. The exception was the American neo-Marxist literary critic Fredric Jameson.

The sociological version of postmodern theory started with the premise that postindustrial society's traditional centers of authority were disintegrating and giving way to the emergence of a new social modernity—the postmodern. Modern assumptions about social coherence, stability, and macro-level (structural) explanations of causality were rejected in favor of notions of multiplicity, plurality, indeterminacy, and fragmentation (Best and Kellner 1991; Denzin 1991). Postmodern social theory mandated a turning away from theorizing in terms of grand systems (meta-narratives) that conceptualized the social as a totality, along with the negation of formal, positivist (scientifically based) conceptions of social theory and the belief that the sociological classics speak to the current era (Denzin 1991). The classical legacies of Durkheim, Weber, and Marx were considered exhausted. Sociology needed to focus instead on the analysis of a fragmenting and deconstructing society evolving toward a new social form.

The Rise of Postmodern Theory

While there was a lack of agreement about the exact nature and definition of postmodernity across the various disciplines, postmodern sociology maintained that the social conditions emerging from the rupture with modernity was bringing new sociological principles with it (Baudrillard 1988; Featherstone 1991; Smart 1993). Far-reaching social change was indeed prevalent as the twenty-first century approached. These changes stemmed from the economic and cultural globalization spread by Western capitalism, the deindustrialization of the West, the explosion of information technology, the increasing use of knowledge as a commodity, the collapse of state socialism in the former Soviet Union and Eastern Europe and its capitalist modification in China and Vietnam, the expanding multiculturalization of Western Europe and North America, changing patterns of social stratification, the rise of cultural and sexual identity politics, and the multiplicity of family forms.

According to Bernice Pescosolido and Beth Rubin (2000:58), postmodernism contributed two critically important points to the sociological analysis of social life: it illustrated the limits of (1) a "modern" metaphor for understanding contemporary circumstances, and (2) the research methods developed under that metaphor for studying those circumstances. The most lasting contribution of postmodern social theory may lie in its methodological approach that rejected both the search for absolute truths or grand narratives and a focus on finding the centers or foundations of social phenomena. Instead, postmodern theory claimed that the influence of former postindustrial centers of authority and power needed to be deconstructed in order to concentrate on the margins of society, thereby uncovering the social situations of marginalized groups. This meant, as Michael Ryan (2007:3570) observed, that postmodern theory "represents the death of the grand narrative" in social thought. Sweeping generalizations about society as a whole and their inability to account for diversity were discredited. As Pescosolido and Rubin (2000:52) concluded, postmodern theory seemed "right on target in capturing the spirit of rapid social change that characterizes the present era."

Many of the main features of postmodern culture are expressed in the observations of Zygmunt Bauman (1992:31) and others (Baudrillard 1994; McQuaide 2005; Ritzer 1997). What was forecasted included the following:

- enhanced pluralism (diversity)
- constant change
- no universal authority
- leveling of social hierarchies
- multiple interpretations of society
- dominance of the media and its messages
- increasingly realistic simulations of reality

The presence in society to varying degrees of these features of contemporary culture in the late twentieth and early twenty-first centuries lent a certain amount of credence to postmodernist claims. The theory reached its highest level of popularity in sociology during the early 1990s and momentarily seemed poised to also have an important future in medical sociology. But this did not occur. Instead, as Ryan (2007:3571) notes: "Few theories have had as meteoric a rise and fall in sociology as postmodern social theory."

Postmodern Medical Sociology

Little work in medical sociology ever expressed explicit postmodern themes and the theory appeared only briefly. The first and only monograph was

Nicholas Fox's *Postmodernism, Sociology and Health* (1993), which focused on discourse in health care settings, what he called health-talk. This was a pioneering effort, highly abstract and faithful to postmodern terminology, notably that of Deleuze and Guattari (1988), and used their concepts of "territorializing" and "de-territorializing" the "Body-without-Organs (BwO)" in analyzing definitions of the body and texts of conversations about it. The Body-without-Organs referred not to a physical body, but in this instance a political body whose surface is inscribed (territorialized) with discourses of medical knowledge which can be changed and become something other than what it is (deterritorialized). Deleuze and Guattari's jargon likely had limited appeal for attracting a new readership in medical sociology, but had a role in studies of discourse conceptualizing differences between the social and the biological bodies in the sociology of the body (Fox 2012).

Among the papers appearing in major medical sociology journals were Barry Glassner's (1989) essay on fitness and the postmodern self that described how people pursued physical fitness to achieve a degree of independence from the medical profession and medical technology, avert risks to their health and sense of self, and protect themselves from obesity, drug abuse, and depression. Glassner (1989:187) concluded that contemporary modes of fitness activities, with its practical beliefs, behavioral prescriptions, and use of technology, were indicative of an elemental postmodern form of culture.

The author and his colleagues (Cockerham, Rütten, and Abel 1997) noted how the authority and status of the medical profession had declined consistent with the postmodern message about the deconstruction of traditional centers of postindustrial authority. This was seen in medicine with increases in government regulation, the rise of managed care organizations (HMOs) monitoring decision-making by physicians on their staff to limit costs, the rise of large health care corporations in which physicians became employees, and greater participation of patients in treatment decisions (Cockerham 2017). With growing public realization that medical practice had limitations and that the individual is ultimately responsible for his or her own health, more widespread participation in healthy lifestyles was seen to result. However, health lifestyle choices were found not to be simply a deliberate product of independent "postmodern" individuals, but served to anchor individuals in particular class-based structures of style and activity. Adopting such collective forms of health behavior was depicted as promoting a sense of purpose, stability, and connection to other people through the maintenance of personal health in a period of uncertain social change.

Additionally, Pescosolido and Rubin (2000) linked postmodern conditions to the deinstitutionalization of the mentally ill in the United States and the expansion of community care. Michael McQuaide (2005) connected a postmodern view of culture to the rise of complementary and alternative forms of medicine (CAM). McQuaide finds that changing relationships between physicians and patients, skepticism about medicine's curative power, greater privatization of purpose, and a corresponding decline in the quality of civic culture promoted individual efforts at self-improvement and the use of alternative forms of health care.

Overall, the application of postmodern theory in medical sociology was relatively meager and it failed to gain a wide audience. By the late 1990s, the use of postmodern concepts abruptly declined and a strong foothold in medical sociology never materialized (Cockerham 2007). Postmodern theory had offered little of practical utility to medical sociologists other than its notion of the fragmentation of postindustrial society and the decline in authority, which could be extended to include medicine. Its demise tells us something about the use of theory generally in medical sociology. In order to be a success it is necessary for any theory in medical sociology to meet two obvious and fundamental conditions. The theory must (1) relate to health matters and (2) be applicable to the empirical world. That is, the theory must specify a direct and *verifiable* connection to the realm of health and disease that has some practical relevance for understanding and explaining the effects of these biological phenomena on the human social condition or, conversely, the effects of social factors on these phenomena. And, at the same time, it must be tested with empirical data validating its propositions. Postmodern theory could not meet the criterion.

The Fall of Postmodern Theory

As Pescosolido and Rubin (2000) pointed out, the postmodernist embrace of disruption resulting from late twentieth-century changes and the interpretation of it as a new social form rather than a social transition was misguided. There were three possible responses to the postmodernist scenario: (1) agreement that a rupture with modernity had occurred and we are indeed living in a new era; (2) disagreement that such a rupture had taken place as continuities with the past persist; or (3) the assertion that a dialectic of continuity and discontinuity is causing both change from and continuity with modernity (Best and Kellner 1991). The notion that an absolute break with the past has occurred has been solidly rejected by most sociologists, as no postmodern theorist was able to identify the exact point of rupture between modernity and postmodernity (Best and Kellner 1991; Cockerham 2007; Pescosolido and Rubin 2000). For example, Steven Best and Douglas Kellner (1991:277) found that

> Baudrillard and his followers dramatically proclaim a fundamental break in history and the end of a historical era without providing a clear

account of the transition to postmodernity and without specifying the
continuities between the previous era and the allegedly new one.

This shortcoming influenced skeptical mainstream sociologists to avoid the
term "postmodern" and opt instead for descriptions like "high modernity,"
"late modernity," or "second modernity" to describe the social changes
characteristic of the current stage of modernity (Beck 1992; Giddens 1991).

While the strength of postmodern theory was its depiction of the type of
social change taking place at the turn of the millennium, its greatest shortcoming was its failure to explain social conditions after the replacement of
modernity. What this society was actually going to be like was a question
that the postmodernists did not (or could not) answer; they only called
attention to the nature of the changes taking place. To sustain itself, postmodernism needed to offer exact accounts of what constituted new social
conditions and social forms—and it was unable to do so. Thus its strength
in describing the style of late modern social change dissipated in the face
of continuing requirements to account for the overall form of society the
postmodernists claimed was coming. According to Pescosolido and Rubin
(2000:64): "Postmodernism fails to provide the kinds of compelling interpretations of what follows the postmodern transition in terms of new social
structures, with their attending opportunities and limitations."

There were other criticisms, including the complaint that postmodern
concepts were too abstract, too ambiguous, lacked an adequate concept
of agency, and did not provide clear conceptualizations; also, there was an
inability to account for social causation and the relative significance of causal
factors like the economy or the state in the change process, not having
empirical confirmation (just conjecture), and there was a tendency to be
superficial—focusing only on surface descriptions of social change and
missing the influence of potentially deeper structures (Best and Kellner 1991;
Cockerham 2007; Ritzer 1997; Ritzer and Stepnisky 2018; Ryan 2007).

As Jonathan Turner (1992:160) pointed out years ago, notions of causality
are missing in postmodern theory and "... the question of causality cannot
be ignored, if only because Western thought in general, as well as specific
engineering applications of theoretical ideas, encourage thinking in terms of
cause and effect." He was also uncomfortable with the philosophical nature
of postmodern theorizing, expressing his own "bias that philosophizing is
best left to the philosophers—they are certainly better trained for it and certainly need the work," while noting that practicing sociologists as scientists
have a different agenda than philosophers and historians of ideas which is to
determine how the social world *actually* works (Turner 1992:156).

Ultimately, this means formulating theories that explain the social causes
of health, disease, and related topics, along with the effects or outcomes of

those causes in ways that can be tested to determine their validity in the empirical world.

Another problem was that postmodern theory rejected the theories of Durkheim, Weber, Marx, and others in classical sociology by claiming they had worn out their usefulness. Consequently, the postmodern perspective entered into theoretical discourse in sociology by subtracting the very foundation upon which sociological theorizing was dependent. Given its other defects, it now seems unlikely to think that postmodern theory could have had long-term success in sociology since it required abandonment of its legacies without a more convincing rationale for doing so.

In addition to these problems, postmodern theory also invariably featured the use of an obtuse jargon that only its dedicated adherents found meaningful and others regarded as prattle. While some terms like Baudrillard's (1994) notions of hyperreality (signs/images of the real substituted for the real) and simulation-simulacra (copies of which there are no originals become more real than the real) and Derrida's (1978) idea of deconstruction had some novel utility in sociology, use of postmodern terminology could be off-putting for readers. New terms and vocabularies such as, but not limited to, Deleuze and Guattari's Body-without-Organs and Body-with-Organs or Baudrillard's (1994:2) description of "a hyperreal produced from a radiating synthesis of combinatory models in a hyperspace without atmosphere" were not unusual. Such language was "supposed to awaken us" (Hoy 1994:46), but reading it could be more of a punishment than a reward. While postmodern theorists might feel a certain intellectual superiority in mastering and practicing postmodern discourse, the nonsensical nature of much of the jargon undermined the capacity of a larger, non-partisan audience to take it seriously.

The language not only inhibited wider acceptance of the perspective but subjected the field at times to ridicule. Although some scholars, for example, could see Baudrillard as playful, ironic, and fanciful (Albright 2019), others described him as writing crescendos of nonsense and using scientific terms to obscure trite observations (Sokal and Bricmont 1998). It became easy to dismiss postmodern theory, especially after Alan Sokal (1996) published a cleverly devised paper on postmodern physics ("Transgressing the Boundaries: Towards a Transformative Hermeneutics of Quantum Gravity") as a joke in a postmodernist journal Social Text. The journal editors accepted this paper as a serious attempt to apply a postmodern interpretation to a query in physics, while the author skillfully used postmodern jargon to discuss quantum gravity using examples theoretical physicists would recognize as farce. Some sociologists like Denzin (1991), Ashley (1997), and Charles Lemert (1997) produced serious subsequent works on postmodernism concerning its intellectual merits, but the damage had been done. Postmodern theory suddenly faded from active use in sociology and is now little more than an artifact of a recent past in social thought (Ryan 2007). Ironically, the theory was essentially dead by the time the twenty-first century arrived (Cockerham 2007).

Summary

So what is there to make of theoretical significance for contemporary medical sociology out of the debris remaining from French structuralism, poststructuralism, and postmodernism? From French structuralism comes the notion of deep structures underlying and shaping the surface appearance of everyday social life. In this case, however, the deep structure was language's effects on structuring thinking and, by extension, possibly social behavior. Yet, considerations of this possibility were grounded solely in discourse and not carried forward in sociology in any meaningful way, nor were there considerations of other possible deep structures such as ingrained and powerful social norms. This potential contribution to sociological theory remains unrealized.

Structuralism sank under the weight of the poststructuralist attack, also a French invention, as Derrida argued that written language was not rigid but creative and innovative, and he put forth the technique of deconstruction as a method for deciphering texts. While useful in analyzing writing, deconstruction has not proven itself helpful in analyzing the health-related actions of people in real life. Poststructuralism, in turn, morphed into postmodernism with Foucault straddling both as the most prominent theorist of each. Foucault's social histories of the surveillance and control of the body by religion, medicine, and the state provided a foundation for (1) a subspecialty of the sociology of the body and (2) a branch of social constructionist theory, both of which are linked to medical sociology. His third contribution was insight into the unity of knowledge/power in which the expansion of one meant an escalation of the other and helps us to conceptualize how medical power has evolved and functioned in society.

A particular shortcoming to Foucault's approach is that agency is missing; additionally, it is untestable but has survived as a method by which past histories (archaeologies) have been used to explain conditions in the present (genealogies). As for postmodernism, it had a meteoric rise in the late twentieth century with its abstract conjectures about the fragmentation of society and postindustrial centers of authority, and with the rise of various forms of diversity and constant change. Postmodern theory also had a meteoric collapse as it failed on several fronts and is not even a zombie theory today—but fully dead.

Guide to Critical Thinking

1. What does the term "deconstruction" mean?
2. How does Foucault's concept of knowledge/power apply to medical practice?
3. What was the attraction of postmodern theory? Why did it fail?

Suggested Reading

Scambler, Graham (ed.). 2012. *Contemporary Theorists for Medical Sociology*. London: Routledge.
Provides additional reading on Foucault, Merleau-Ponty, Deleuze, and Guattari.
Turner, Bryan S. 2008. *The Body and Society*, 3rd ed. Oxford: Blackwell.
A pioneering work on the sociology of the body.

References

Albright, Julie M. 2019. "Postmodernism and Poststructuralism," in J. Michael Ryan (ed.), *Core Concepts in Sociology*. Oxford: Wiley Blackwell, pp. 215–18.
Alvesson, Mats. 2002. *Postmodernism and Social Research*. Buckingham: Open University Press.
Armstrong, David. 1997. "Foucault and the Sociology of Health and Illness," in Alan Petersen and Robin Bunton (eds.), *Foucault, Health and Medicine*. London: Routledge, pp. 15–30.
Ashley, David. 1997. *History Without a Subject: The Postmodern Condition*. Boulder, CO: Westview Press.
Baudrillard, Jean. 1988. *Selected Writings*, M. Poster (ed.). Stanford, CA: Stanford University Press.
Baudrillard, Jean. 1994. *Simulacra and Simulation*. Ann Arbor, MI: University of Michigan Press.
Bauman, Zygmunt. 1992. *Intimations of Postmodernity*. London: Routledge.
Beck, Ulrich. 1992. *The Risk Society: Towards a New Modernity*. London: Sage.
Bertens, Hans. 1995. *The Idea of the Postmodern*. London: Routledge.
Best, Steven and Douglas Kellner. 1991. *Postmodern Theory*. New York: Guilford Press.
Bury, Michael. 2004. *Health and Illness*. Cambridge: Polity.
Cockerham, William C. 2007. "A Note on the Fate of Postmodern Theory and its Failure to Meet the Basic Requirement for Success in Medical Sociology." *Social Theory & Health* 5(4):285–96.
Cockerham, William C. 2017. *Medical Sociology*, 14th ed. New York: Routledge.
Cockerham, William C., Alfred Rütten, and Thomas Abel. 1997. "Conceptualizing Health Lifestyles: Moving Beyond Weber." *Sociological Quarterly* 38(2):321–42.
Conrad, Peter and Kristin K. Barker. 2010. "The Social Construction of Illness: Key Insights and Policy Implications." *Journal of Health and Social Behavior* 51(extra issue):S50–S79.

Cousins, Mark and Athar Hussain. 1984. *Michel Foucault*. New York: St. Martin's.

Crossley, Nick. 2012. "Merleau-Ponty, Medicine and the Body," in Graham Scambler (ed.), *Contemporary Theorists for Medical Sociology*. London: Routledge, pp. 87–103.

Dean, Mitchell. 2018. "Governmentality," in Bryan Turner (ed.), *The Wiley Blackwell Encyclopedia of Social Theory*. Oxford: Wiley Blackwell, pp. 1000–2.

Deleuze, Gilles and Félix Guattari. 1988. *A Thousand Plateaus*. London: Athlone.

Denzin, Norman K. 1991. *Images of Postmodern Society: Social Theory and Contemporary Cinema*. London: Sage.

Derrida, Jacques. 1978. *Writing and Difference*. Chicago, IL: University of Chicago Press.

Featherstone, Mike. 1991. *Consumer Culture and Postmodernism*. London: Sage.

Foucault, Michel. 1965. *Madness and Civilization: A History of Insanity in an Age of Reason*. New York: Pantheon.

Foucault, Michel. 1969. *The Archaeology of Knowledge and the Discourse on Language*. New York: Harper Colophon.

Foucault, Michel. 1973. *Birth of the Clinic*. London: Tavistock.

Foucault, Michel. 1979. *Discipline and Punish: The Birth of the Prison*. New York: Vintage.

Foucault, Michel. 1980. *The History of Sexuality, Vol. 1: An Introduction*. New York: Vintage Books.

Foucault, Michel. 2007. *Security, Territory, Population: Lectures at the Collège de France, 1977–1978*. London: Palgrave Macmillan.

Fox, Nicholas J. 1993. *Postmodernism, Sociology and Health*. Buckingham: Open University Press.

Fox, Nick. 2012. "Deleuze and Guattari," in Graham Scambler (ed.), *Contemporary Theorists for Medical Sociology*. London: Routledge, pp. 150–66.

Giddens, Anthony. 1987. *Sociology and Modern Sociology*. Stanford, CA: Stanford University Press.

Giddens, Anthony. 1991. *Modernity and Self-Identity*. Stanford, CA: Stanford University Press.

Glassner, Barry. 1989. "Fitness and the Postmodern Self." *Journal of Health and Social Behavior* 30(2):180–91.

Heilbron, Johan. 2015. *French Sociology*. Ithaca, NY: Cornell University Press.

Horwitz, Allan V. 2013. "The Sociological Study of Mental Illness: A Critique and Synthesis of Four Perspectives," in Carol Aneshensel, Jo Phelan, and Alex Bierman (eds.), *Handbook of the Sociology of Mental Disorder*, 2nd ed. Dordrecht: Springer, pp. 95–112.

Hoy, David. 1994. "Jacques Derrida," in Quentin Skinner (ed.), *The Return of Grand Theory in the Human Sciences*. Cambridge: Cambridge University Press, pp. 43–64.

Judt, Tony. 2005. *Postwar: A History of Europe Since 1945*. New York: Penguin.

Lemert, Charles. 1997. *Postmodernism Is Not What You Think*. Oxford: Blackwell.

Lupton, Deborah. 1998. *The Body in Everyday Life*. London: Routledge.

McQuaide, Michael M. 2005. "The Rise of Alternative Health Care: A Sociological Account." *Social Theory & Health* 3(4):286–301.

Merleau-Ponty, Maurice. 1962. *The Phenomenology of Perception*. London: Routledge.

Merleau-Ponty, Maurice. 2004. *The World of Perception*. London: Routledge.

Merquior, J. D. 1985. *Foucault*. Berkeley, CA: University of California Press.

Münch, Richard. 1993. *Sociological Theory*, Vol. 3. Chicago, IL: Nelson-Hall.

Nettleton, Sarah. 2013. *The Sociology of Health and Illness*, 3rd ed. Cambridge: Polity.

Nettleton, Sarah. 2016. "The Sociology of the Body," in William Cockerham (ed.), *The New Blackwell Companion to Medical Sociology*. Oxford: Wiley Blackwell, pp. 47–68.

Pescosolido, Bernice S. and Beth Rubin. 2000. "The Web of Group Affiliations Revisited: Social Life, Postmodernism, and Sociology." *American Sociological Review* 65(1):52–76.

Petersen, Alan. 2012. "Foucault, Health and Healthcare," in Graham Scambler (ed.), *Contemporary Theorists for Medical Sociology*. London: Routledge, pp. 7–19.

Petersen, Alan and Robin Bunton. 1997. *Foucault, Health and Medicine*. London: Routledge.

Ritzer, George. 1997. *Postmodern Social Theory*. McGraw-Hill: New York.

Ritzer, George and Jeffrey Stepnisky. 2018. *Sociological Theory*, 10th ed. Los Angeles, CA: Sage.

Ritzer, George and David Walczak. 1988. "Rationalization and the Deprofessionalization of Physicians." *Social Forces* 67(1):1–22.

Ryan, J. Michael. 2007. "Postmodern Social Theory," in George Ritzer (ed.), *The Blackwell Encyclopedia of Sociology*, Vol. 7. Oxford: Blackwell, pp. 3569–72.

Saussure, Ferdinand de. [1916] 1966. *Course in General Linguistics*. New York: McGraw-Hill.

Schilling, Chris. 1993. *The Body and Social Theory*. London: Sage.

Schilling, Chris. 2003. *The Body and Social Theory*, 2nd ed. London: Sage.

Smart, Barry. 1993. *Postmodernity*. London: Routledge.

Sokal, Alan. 1996. "Transgressing the Boundaries: Towards a Transformative Hermeneutics of Quantum Gravity." *Social Text* 46/47:217–52.

Sokal, Alan and Jean Bricmont. 1998. *Fashionable Nonsense*. London: Picador.

Turner, Bryan S. 1984. *The Body and Society*. Oxford: Blackwell.

Turner, Bryan S. 1987. *Medical Power and Social Knowledge*. London: Sage.

Turner, Bryan S. 1992. *Regulating Bodies: Essays in Medical Sociology*. London: Routledge.

Turner, Bryan S. 1996. *The Body and Society*, 2nd ed. Oxford: Blackwell.

Turner, Bryan S. 2008. *The Body and Society*, 3rd ed. Oxford: Blackwell.

Turner, Jonathan. 1992. "The Promise of Positivism," in Steven Seidman and David Wagner (eds.), *Postmodernism & Social Theory*. Oxford: Blackwell, pp. 156–78.

Weber, Max. [1922] 1978. *Economy and Society*, 2 vols, Guenther Roth and Claus Wittich (trans. and eds.). Berkeley, CA: University of California Press.

Williams, Simon J. 2003. *Medicine and the Body*. London: Sage.

Chapter 8

The Stress Process

Contemporary theorizing in medical sociology continues with this chapter on the stress process. Stress can be defined as a heightened mind–body reaction to stimuli inducing fear or anxiety in the individual. It is a topic investigated extensively by American medical sociologists because of its potentially harmful health effects. In fact, so many papers on stress were published in the American Sociological Association's *Journal of Health and Social Behavior* that it was once dubbed "the stress journal" (Clair et al. 2007). This is no longer the case, but the study of stress has nonetheless continued to be a major area of research in medical sociology in the United States though attracting little attention elsewhere.[1] The relevance of medical sociology in stress studies lies in the stress process in which certain social situations trigger adverse psychological reactions on the part of someone experiencing them to the extent that a harmful physiological reaction is provoked in the mind and/or body. Essentially, the stress response chain consists of: (1) a social response eliciting (2) a psychological response, which elicits (3) a physiological response.

As Leonard Pearlin (1989:241) put it, "sociologists have an intellectual stake in the study of stress" because it affords an opportunity to investigate how the repeated experiences people have with the structural arrangements in their lives can put unhealthy pressure on them. This is seen in a summary of what we know in medical sociology from past research on stress provided by Peggy Thoits (2010). She determined that (1) the impact of stress on health is substantial, (2) some people and groups experience more of it than others, (3) members of racial [and sexual minority] groups are burdened by additional stress from discrimination, (4) stress can continue over the life course contributing to differences in health between disadvantaged and advantaged social groups, and (5) the impact of stress is reduced for people who possess high levels of personal mastery (being in control), self-esteem, and social support. It is from this body of research findings that stress-oriented concepts and theories have been developed with Pearlin's 1989 paper on the sociological study of stress in the forefront.

Stress is one of the few areas that lack roots in classical theory; its study originated in medical sociology in the late twentieth century. Few theoretical papers on stress have had a lasting impact in medical sociology with Pearlin's (1989) paper the leading exception. This paper contained his concept of the stress process, which has changed little since its inception and has yet to be superseded by another theory or theories (Aneshensel 2015; Aneshensel and Avison 2015; Pearlin and Bierman 2013). As Carol Aneshensel and William Avison (2015:67) point out: "First published when stress research was in its infancy, this model became the most influential theory guiding sociological research on stress and mental health, especially research concerned with the disproportionate concentration of mental health problems in some social strata." It was the single most cited theoretical article in all of American medical sociology in the early twenty-first century (Cockerham 2007) and provides the basis for the discussion of stress theory in this chapter.

The Stress Process Model

Even though Pearlin (1924–2014) presented his ideas as an overview of concepts rather than a formal theory with propositions and testable statements, it nevertheless became the most influential theory on stress and health in medical sociology (Aneshensel 2015; Aneshensel and Avison 2015; McLeod 2012). This is because its organization and content sets forth the social structural parameters and sequencing of the stress experience in the form of a model. Pearlin's approach, as William Avison and Stephanie Thomas (2016:244) observed, "assumed that the origins of stress are in the social world" and guided medical sociologists toward placing a greater emphasis on the social context of stress rather than on individual histories or biology. Pearlin had determined that most research on stress involves examining a demanding situation whose experience of it is perceived as threatening or burdensome. In his view, stress originates in situations, but what is also important is how people react to them in the *context* of their lives. Consequently, there is much more to stress research than simply looking at how people respond to certain stressors, such as life events, but also the social circumstances of stressed people. Pearlin (1989:242) illustrates this point with a distinctly sociological assessment when he says that:

> Many stressful experiences, it should be recognized, don't spring out of a vacuum but typically can be traced back to surrounding social structures and people's locations within them. The most encompassing of these structures are the various systems of stratification that cut across societies, such as those based on social and economic class, race, ethnicity, gender, and age. To the extent that these systems embody the

unequal distribution of resources, opportunities, and self-regard, a low status within them may itself be a source of stressful life conditions.

Pearlin (1989; Pearlin and Bierman 2013) maintained that the stress process consists of three components: (1) *stressors*, which he defines as any condition having the potential to arouse the adaptive capacity of the individual; (2) *moderators*, which consist of coping abilities, sense of mastery, and sources of social support; and (3) *outcomes*, the health effects of the distress experienced by the person. He identified two major types of social stressors: life events and chronic strain. The theory holds that not all people react to these stressors the same way because of differences in stress moderators which, in turn, influence different outcomes. According to Aneshensel (2015:72), medical sociologists "embraced the stress process model because it gives prominence to the social structural origins of all aspects of stressful life experience, from exposure to stressors through access to resources, to the manifestations of psychological distress."

What Pearlin accomplished with his stress process model was to provide a distinctly sociological approach to stress research that separated it from other disciplines, principally psychiatry and psychology, which primarily focused on the individual's stress reactions. Instead, Pearlin's model emphasized the relevance of social structures—namely stratification hierarchies—in shaping the experience of stress. Previously researchers in various health-related fields had concentrated on investigating the stressors people deal with, not the possible structural origins of those stressors that fell within the purview of sociological inquiry. The basic message that Pearlin (1989:242) delivered was that "the structural contexts of people's lives are not extraneous to the stress process but are fundamental to that process," which signified that structure rather than agency was the focus of the stress process model.

Others, such as Thoits (2013) and Jane McLeod (2012), applied symbolic interaction theory to provide a role for agency in the stress process model by pointing out that whether or not a stressful situation produces physiological or psychological damage depends upon an individual's perception of that situation and the personal meaning it holds for that person. Symbolic interaction, as discussed in Chapter 6, maintains that people act toward objects and circumstances on the basis of the meanings those things have for them and that such meanings arise through interaction with other people (Blumer 1969; McLeod 2012). It also maintains that situations defined as real are real in their consequences (Thomas and Thomas 1928). Therefore, as McLeod (2015:151) points out:

> Stressors that threaten valued roles, goals, and ideals; and self-conceptions (our identities or how we define ourselves); and self-evaluations

(our sense of ourselves as valuable or worthless and efficacious or not) matter more than others. This implies that in order to understand how positions in social hierarchies influence mental health, we must understand their associations with these kind of threats.

Not all stressors matter. And when they do, a person's responses may correspond to the reality of the threat that a stress stimulus represents or an individual may overreact or underreact to the situation. The exercise of agency does not mean that people necessarily make good choices; sometimes they make bad ones (Thoits 2006:313). Ultimately, however, an individual's subjective interpretation of a social situation is the trigger that produces physiological responses regardless of whether a stress stimulus is derived from either structure or agency. Stress can result from either structural situations beyond individual control (e.g., economic downturns) or a lack of personal resources (e.g., heavy debt) or have its origin in agency by way of unpleasant interpersonal relationships (e.g., divorce, animosity, trouble with others at work), thereby suggesting that both structure and agency are involved in stress reactions and may overlap (e.g., debt causing divorce). Not only is agency central in the origin of stressors, but also in the exercise of personal mastery as a mediator in containing them (Hitlin, Erickson, and Brown 2015). Nonetheless, the stress process model is weighted more heavily toward structure than agency as its emphasis is on how stratified systems of social relationships relate to stress.

Box 8.1 Leonard Pearlin

Leonard I. Pearlin was born December 26, 1924 in Quincy, Massachusetts. His parents were immigrants from Ukraine and Latvia. He served in the Army during World War II in the South Pacific and was awarded the Purple Heart before returning to the United States under the sole surviving son policy after his two older brothers were killed in combat. He attended the University of Oklahoma and graduated with a BA in sociology in 1949. Allegedly he had intended to major in social anthropology but signed up for sociology instead because the registration line was shorter and his wife Gerrie was outside waiting on him. He went on to receive his Ph.D. from Columbia University in 1956, spent a year at Ohio State University, and then accepted a position as a Research Scientist at the Laboratory of Socio-Environmental Studies at the National Institute of Mental Health (NIMH) where he was employed until he retired in 1982. While at NIMH, he worked on a number of studies and began developing his stress process model.

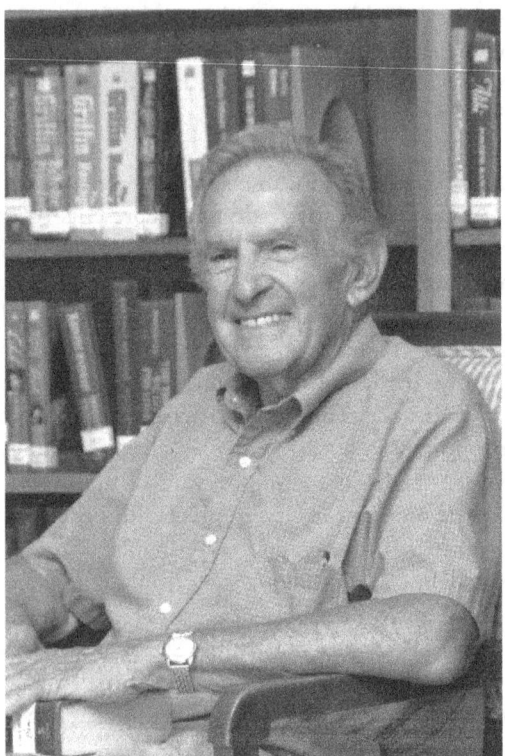

Image 8.1 Leonard Pearlin

Pearlin, known to his friends as Len, then accepted a professorial position at the University of California at San Francisco in the Human Development and Aging Program where he stayed for a dozen years (1982–1994), publishing his stress process model in 1989. He next moved to the Washington, D.C. area and became graduate professor and senior research scientist in the sociology department at the University of Maryland from 1994 until his final retirement in 2007.

He was a prolific scholar, authoring or co-authoring four books, 39 book chapters, and 55 journal articles, as well as editing the *Journal of Health and Social Behavior* (1982–1984) and chairing both the Medical Sociology and Sociology of Mental Health Sections of the American Sociological Association at different times. He was the 1991 recipient of ASA's Leo G. Reeder Award for Distinguished Scholarship in Medical Sociology. To those who knew him, he was welcoming and friendly, noted for being an outstanding mentor of graduate students. He died at Virginia Beach, Virginia on July 23, 2014, at the age of 89.

When Pearlin began his research, sociological investigations of stress were focused more or less exclusively on the analysis of life events. However, Pearlin introduced the notion of chronic strain as another important social stressor, pointing out that chronic strains were often interconnected (e.g., divorce and economic hardship, being fired from one's job and a change in sleeping habits) and linked to a person's location in a status (class, race, etc.) hierarchy (Aneshensel and Avison 2015; McLeod 2015). People at the bottom of society who have less of the good things in life and more of the bad, are likewise the most disadvantaged in regard to stress because they are exposed to greater amounts of it and are more vulnerable since they have the most limited moderators, namely less social and psychological coping capabilities and socioeconomic resources (Lantz et al. 2005).

In addition to life events and chronic strain, there have been suggestions that other types of stressors are also important, such as daily hassles and trauma. However, there is a lack of evidence showing daily hassles, while irritating and frustrating, are likely to induce major stress-based physical and mental symptoms. As for trauma, a pattern that emerges in studies of natural disasters is that the experience, though severe, is usually short in duration and the effects tend to be short term and self-limiting. Yet there are exceptions such as highly traumatizing events like the terrorist attack on the World Trade Center in New York City in 2001 (Brackbill et al. 2013) and when whole communities are destroyed by an earthquake or tsunami (Frankenberg, Nobles, and Sumantri 2012). Among survivors of the World Trade Center attack, the impact of the trauma on many of those most intensely exposed was still apparent five to six years later (Brackbill et al. 2013). Consequently, the level of exposure to a trauma makes a difference with respect to the duration of symptoms. Much more common than trauma in the everyday lives of most people, however, are life events and chronic strain.

Life Events

Life events research has a well-established history in medical sociology. By the 1980s, more than 16 different life events inventories had been published (Avison and Thomas 2016). They largely consisted of checklists used in survey research querying whether or not certain events had been experienced within specified periods of time and were commonly used in life events research. Pearlin (1989) and others (Avison and Thomas 2016) note that the theoretical basis for life events research can be traced to the early work of American physiologist Walter Cannon (1871–1945) and Hungarian-Canadian endocrinologist Hans Selye (1907–1982). Cannon (1932) refined the concept of *homeostasis* in physiology, which in Greek means "staying the same," through his research on the role of the adrenal gland in the human body's adaptation to changes in the weather and the effects of microorganisms, chemical irritants, pollutants, and psychological stress on physiological functioning. Cannon had noted that when the body is threatened by bacteria, antibodies are produced to fight the germs or when the body is stressed, it prepares itself through hormonal secretions for a vigorous "fight or flight" response. Most threats in modern society, however, do not result in a physical confrontation, which leaves the body in an internal state of physiological readiness that goes unresolved until it dissipates on its own.

Building on Cannon's work, Selye (1956) formulated what he called the *general adaptation syndrome* in 1936, which maintained that the energy to adapt to stress is limited and the body's ability to maintain homeostasis decreases over time if stress is prolonged. Selye found that after an initial alarm reaction, there is a second stage of resistance to bodily harm through increased activity on the part of the pituitary and adrenal glands (although we now know the entire endocrine system is involved in reacting to stress). Once hormonal defenses are consumed, Selye indicated that a person would then enter a third stage of exhaustion that resembles a form of premature aging (i.e., "weathering") due to wear and tear on the body. Selye went on to hypothesize that any type of life change, either positive or negative, requiring the individual to adapt to it can produce a specific stress response.

One of the most popular measures of stress supporting his theory was Thomas Holmes and Robert Rahe's Social Readjustment Rating Scale (1967), which listed various life events generally considered stressful and assigned each a numerical value (life change units). These values ranged from 100 for the death of a spouse to 13 for taking a vacation. A divorce had a value of 73, a marriage 50, pregnancy 40, moving to another residence 20, Christmas 12, and so forth. The higher the total score, the greater the probability of having a stress-induced illness, especially if a person experiences several life change units within a short period of time or accumulates 200 or more units within a year. Thus stress researchers, as Pearlin (1989) noted, had both a theory (Selye) and a method of measurement (Holmes and Rahe).

However, as it turned out, both the theory and the method had flaws. A theoretical shortcoming was Selye's (1956) assertion that any type of change, either pleasant or unpleasant, produces stress. But, as Pearlin (1989) observed, sociologists found this difficult to accept because change is a *normal* feature of social life and the ensuing research overwhelmingly came down on the side of unpleasant life events as being of prime importance in causing life event stress-related illnesses and mental difficulties (Mirowsky and Ross 2004; Thoits 2010). Some changes, in fact, are pleasant. Weddings, for example, can be stressful for those managing them, but the stress is short-lived and the outcome usually engenders positive feelings for all concerned. Losing one's job can be stressful, but finding another can be positive and offset the stress caused initially by unemployment (Tausig 2013). Yet in this latter example, the Social Readjustment Rating Scale would have assigned more change value units indicative of more stress to losing a job and finding another, than for just losing the job even though any stress may have dissipated without lasting effects with the new job. Left unemployed, the person's change value score would have remained lower, but their stress would likely be greater.

Furthermore, some life events in the Social Readjustment Rating Scale, such as divorce or losing a job, may result from stress rather than cause it. That is, the stressed individual causes the event rather than the event causing the stress. This possibility can obviously confound what is being measured. Also the meaning of the various events (and level of stress associated with it) may differ in relative importance to different people and groups (McLeod 2012, 2015). What determines the impact of life events on health is the perception of the nature of the change by the individual, which can vary. Additionally, the scale is based on the assumption that the accumulation of several events in a person's life eventually builds up to a physiological impact. However, what types of events, in what combinations, over what periods of time, and under what circumstances life events actually promote stress-induced health problems is not clear; instead, the prediction of poor health rests only on counting life change units.

Another problem is that the scale does not consider intervening variables, such as social support from other people, which might modify the effects of stress for many individuals. While interaction with others can be stressful because of personal conflicts, conflicting expectations, or excessive demands to achieve or maintain a certain level of performance, supportive interpersonal influences have the potential to reduce stressful feelings. Moreover, as noted, life events that are successfully resolved may not be stressful. That is, it may be the case that mastery of an event provides a buffer to stress because successful resolution constitutes a personally meaningful positive experience and may substantially counterbalance any stress associated with it (Reynolds and Turner 2008).

Does this mean that life events research should be abandoned? The answer is no. Life events remain in Pearlin's stress process model. This is because life events do generate stress despite methodological challenges when a sociological perspective is applied. Death of a spouse or loved one, for example, is a potent life events stressor (Young and Foy 2013). Therefore, as Pearlin (1989:245) observed: "Some events under some conditions are powerful stressors that affect people's lives directly and indirectly; research in these stressors should not be abandoned, only rethought." From a sociological standpoint, research on life events and the theories/concepts that explain them, are complex and not easily explained by simple cause-and-effect explanations. Rather, such research needs to also incorporate socioeconomic variables into their analysis, such as class, gender, race, and age, that are experienced differently in events in one's life because of these master statuses.

Chronic Strain

Chronic strains are the second major stressor. Chronic strains are best understood as relatively enduring conflicts, problems, and threats that people face on a daily basis. Pearlin (1989) emphasized social roles (e.g., family roles, work roles) in particular as a source of chronic strains. This is because incumbency in such roles persist over time, are repeated, and involve other people in mutual complementary roles forming a larger role set around which personal relationships are formed and structured. For these reasons, conflict in such roles can be highly stressful. As Pearlin (1989:245) explained:

> … problems rooted in institutionalized social roles are often enduring, for the activities and interpersonal relationships they entail are enduring. Moreover, when problems—or strains, as I refer to them—occur within roles, they are likely to affect their incumbents, because typically we attach considerable importance to our major roles. Difficulties in job, marriage, or parenthood have important effects because the roles themselves are important.

Chronic strain includes role overload, such as the strain associated with work and being a parent while trying to advance one's career. It also involves conflicts within role sets, such as those between husbands and wives or workers and supervisors, inter-role conflict where a person has too many roles, role captivity in which a person is an unwilling incumbent of a role such as being trapped in an unpleasant job or marriage, or role restructuring in which a person changes relationships within roles. Some research maintains that chronic strain may be a more negative influence on health than negative life events (Turner and Avison 2003).

Chronic strains also emanate from racial discrimination (Geronimus et al. 2006, 2015; Grollman 2012; Miller, Rote, and Keith 2013; Williams 2012; Williams and Mohammed 2009), heavy debt and financial strain (Bierman 2014; Drentea and Reynolds 2012; Hughes, Kiecolt, and Keith 2014; Kahn and Pearlin 2006), unpleasant working conditions (Burgard and Ailshire 2009; Schieman, Whitestone, and van Gundy 2006; Siegrist 2010, 2016; Tausig 2013), unhappy marriages (Umberson et al. 2006), and the long-term effects of incarceration (Schnittker and John 2007).

However, chronic strain can also be intertwined with negative life events when the stress associated with those events is long-lasting. Life events can produce chronic strains and chronic strains can generate life events (Pearlin 1989). Both can be either objective or subjective. Although chronic strain tends to have stronger effects on health than a life event since it constitutes a stressful burden that continues over time, such strain can nevertheless be caused by life events and this is especially the case if the life events have negative consequences for the people experiencing them (Thomeer et al. 2018; Turner and Avison 2003). Consequently, both chronic strain and life events can be interrelated as well as stressful and operate together as major social stressors in Pearlin's model.

The cumulative wear and tear on the body's organic systems as it repeatedly adapts to chronic stressors is what is known as an "allostatic load." As the body's allostatic load becomes heavier, its defenses against persistent stress are worn down over time. Teresa Seeman and her colleagues (2008) determined that long-term stresses associated with low socioeconomic status were consistently and negatively associated with increased allostatic loads that, in turn, promoted the risk of cardiovascular, metabolic, and inflammatory problems in the body. Other research has found that lower SES persons carry a significantly greater allostatic load in late life than higher SES individuals and their adverse life experiences in the lower class have a cumulative negative effect on their health (Gruenewald et al. 2012). There is other evidence showing that chronic strain associated with disadvantaged social circumstances initiates differences in cell aging much earlier among low SES children, thereby triggering premature aging long before the onset of old age (Needham et al. 2012).

Signs of premature aging due to high allostatic loads have been described as "weathering" by public health researcher Arline Geronimus (1992). Geronimus and her colleagues (2006, 2015) found support for the weathering hypothesis among a sample of disadvantaged African Americans subjected to racial discrimination and also in a multiracial sample of distressed neighborhoods in Detroit experiencing poverty. In the latter study, the length of telomeres in the body were shorter for the poor than the nonpoor, indicating greater stress–related biological aging. Telomeres are protein caps at the end of each strand of DNA that function to protect chromosomes. As cells are replenished by copying themselves, telomeres naturally become shorter over time causing cells to age. However, telomeres can also be shortened prematurely by stress resulting in early aging or weathering, thereby serving as an indicator of exposure to chronic stress.

Racial disparities in weathering from greater low-grade chronic inflammation has also been found among black and Hispanic school children, especially those with foreign-born parents, as compared to white children in a national sample (Schmeer and Tarrence 2018). Canadian sociologist Aniruddhas Das (2013) additionally found chronic inflammation from "weathering" was prevalent among a nationwide sample of older American black men as a result of stress that was cumulative (built up over time) and multidimensional (occurring in multiple life situations). These long-term stresses emanating from multiple life situations leading to chronic inflammation were depicted as a way that race gets "under the skin" through discriminatory experiences.

Primary and Secondary Stressors

The stresses generated by life events and chronic strains can be either primary or secondary stressors. This is because serious stressors rarely occur as just one stressor in Pearlin's model, but usually involve others in combinations or clusters such as problems at work causing problems at home or vice versa. Stress can impact on multiple aspects of a person's life and that person's problems can come to be shared by other persons in mutual relationships or role sets. In order to determine how the overall organization of people's lives is disrupted by stressors, Pearlin says it is necessary to distinguish between stressors that are primary and secondary. Primary stressors are those that occur first in someone's stress experience and secondary stressors occur as a consequence of the primary stressors. That is, an initial stressor can lead to follow-on stressors as an example of stress proliferation. Primary stressors are primary simply because they are first; secondary stressors may actually be more potent than those that are primary when their effects on the body are stronger. In such instances, it is necessary to determine how stressors are connected and operate together, even though some stressors came first (primary) and others later (secondary), and how some (either primary or secondary) are more threatening to the individual than others.

Mediators

Pearlin (1989:250) maintains that mediators govern or mediate the effects of stressors on stress outcomes. It is the ability to buffer or resolve the effects of stress that ultimately determines the extent of its impact on the body. Pearlin selected the mediators for his model—coping, sense of mastery, and social support—that have attracted the most attention from stress researchers. Coping is the action that people take to avoid or lessen the impact of stressful circumstances. It is a major mediator often learned in families and schools that prepares the individual to deal with problems in life. Some people have better coping skills and styles than others as well as differing personal resources that can used to offset stress. As Thoits (2006) found in her research, people are not necessarily passive when confronted with stressful situations but employ what skills and resources they have to resolve what is causing them stress with varying degrees of success and failure. In analyzing any particular stress situation, an observer must not only consider individual differences in threat assessments, but likewise recognize the coping skills and resources that keep stressors within manageable bounds.

Also important is an individual's sense of mastery in handling stressful situations. Mastery is an individual's perception of his or her ability to control the situations that confront that person (Pearlin and Schooler 1978). It is acquired through social interaction and significantly influenced by the socialization occurring in families (Conger et al. 2009). Several studies find that persons of higher social status and ample resources, along with a personal history of success, have greater confidence in handling problems and find stressors less alarming because of an evaluated sense of mastery (Avison and Thomas 2016; Pearlin and Bierman 2013). Moreover, people who master a crisis have been found to benefit from the experience by feeling good about themselves afterward (Reynolds and Turner 2008).

Social support consists of subjective feelings of belonging, being accepted, loved, cared for, valued, and needed by others and is another key variable in mitigating symptoms of stress (Avison, Ali, and Walters 2007; Thoits 2010, 2011, 2013). Social support is typically provided within families, and also by close friends and associates in one's friendship networks. Such support can be emotional, companionable, informational, and instrumental or contributory as in the case of providing financial assistance. Social support tends to function as a buffer between an individual and his or her stressors by reducing that stress or making it more tolerable. It has attracted the most research as a stress mediator in medical sociology, and is often measured by determining a person's level of perceived support in adjusting to stressful circumstances. Both the presence and effectiveness of social support has been found to vary by a person's position in a social hierarchy and marital status (Thoits 2011).

Outcomes

Pearlin (1989) refers to outcomes as manifestations of organismic stress. That is, stress affects the body organically and in different ways, resulting in different, sometimes multiple, outcomes. Outcomes depend upon how well a person eliminates or adapts to his or her stressors. There is considerable evidence that many people successfully adjust to stressful situations and do not suffer physical or mental change, while others succumb to its effects and their health is harmed (Thoits 2013; Wheaton et al. 2013). The most vulnerable persons are those whose physiological responses are easily elicited and likely to be more pronounced and prolonged. Consequently, the most studied outcome is emotional distress, which can range from very mild to very serious, even traumatic. Some outcomes involve substance abuse and dependence as individuals self-medicate with drugs or alcohol to reduce stress. Some people become argumentative and even violent when stressed. Prolonged stress can lead to a psychophysiological reaction causing changes in bodily tissues that stimulate the onset of physical disorders such as heart disease, hypertension, peptic ulcer, muscular pain, and migraine headaches, and is able to activate a genetic predisposition toward a mental disorder, or a triggering of biochemical abnormalities causing emotional problems. Outcomes therefore vary.

Strengths and Weaknesses

The merit of Pearlin's stress process model is that it connects the experience of stress directly to patterns of social stratification or other status hierarchies through its depiction of the origins of stress, its mediators, and outcomes. It also introduces the concept of chronic strains as separate and more pervasive than stress emanating from a life event and observes that some stressors (secondary stressors) depend upon the prior occurrence of other stressors and may be even more powerful in a follow-up capacity than primary stressors (Aneshensel 2015). Thus stressors are not disconnected from one another in his model but operate together in a process of stress proliferation over time as one stress can easily lead to another. The notion of time is important in this conceptualization of stress as a process because strains are depicted as interconnected and occurring over the life course (Kahn and Pearlin 2006; Pearlin et al. 2005).

What makes this model novel is that it moves sociological stress research away from a focus on a particular life event to an analysis of how the stress process is experienced and plays out over time in relation to status hierarchies, namely SES, age, gender, and race/ethnicity. People in all social strata experience multiple stressors inherent in stressful life events and situations of chronic strain in the course of their lives (Koltai and Schieman 2015; Schieman et al. 2006). However, the higher one's position in a social hierarchy, the better one deals with stress and its effects on the body. This advantage decreases proportionally the lower one goes down the social ladder, with the lower class characterized as being subject to the most stress and having the fewest resources to cope with it (Avison and Thomas 2016; Downey and van Willigen 2005; Grzywacz et al. 2004; Lantz et al. 2005; McLeod 2012; Thoits 2010). This finding is consistent with other research showing that lower SES persons have higher allostatic loads and greater weathering or premature aging (Geronimus et al. 2015; Seeman et al. 2008).

Other examples of chronic strain emanating from structural variables include age with job insecurity (the perception of being threatened by job loss) over the life course, especially worrying for older workers with histories of such insecurity during the late stages of their working life (Burgard and Seelye 2016). Financial strains can also occur over the life course and affect health late in life, with such strains stronger among women and the less educated (Bierman 2014; Kahn and Pearlin 2006). As for gender, men have been shown to be more vulnerable to stressors related to their jobs and breadwinner role, along with being more likely to show externalizing outcomes by way of drinking, drug use, and aggressive behavior, while women are more vulnerable to stressors in their family roles and internalizing their feelings through worry, depression, psychological distress, and feeling sick (Elliott 2013; Longest and Thoits 2012). Transgendered persons and same sex couples also face discriminatory stressors (Grollman 2012), whereas studies of race highlight racial discrimination as a chronic stressor, especially for low-income minorities (Bratter and Gorman 2011; Brown, O'Rand, and Atkin 2012; Miller, Rote, and Keith 2013; Williams 2012; Williams and Mohammed 2009). Consequently, the strength of Pearlin's stress process model rests in analyzing stressors within the social context of people's lives, showing how the origins, mediators, and outcomes of stress are unequally distributed in society.

There have not been significant critiques of the stress process model, but a few shortcomings can be observed. For example, a role for agency in the model is not clearly specified and needs to be more fully developed as reactions to stressors vary according to the perceptions of those stressed and the effectiveness of the mediators—coping, sense of mastery, and social support—employed. There is also a lack of consensus in the literature about the perceived effectiveness of the different mediators in buffering stress and it is not known how the use of mediators may vary among individuals with different social statuses and resources (Hatteberg 2014). Nevertheless, the stress process model currently dominates theorizing about the stress experience in medical sociology.

Measuring Stress: Biomarkers and Genes

It is obvious to say that theories are made more reliable and reflective of reality if they are based on the sound analysis of empirical data. However, accurately measuring the origins and types of stressors, their interrelationships, the effectiveness of mediators, and outcomes is a complex and challenging undertaking. It is made even more difficult because so much of the stress experience is subjective. The early research on stress in medical sociology largely relied upon self-reports about feeling stressed, psychological distress scales, and life event inventories in which respondents would list the ones they experienced. However, sociological stress research is changing by an increasing use of biomarker methods. Biomarkers are medical measures of blood pressure, urine, cholesterol, c-reactive protein, and waist-hip ratios of individuals independent of their self-reports and perhaps even awareness that stressors are affecting their health. An individual may be unaware of high blood pressure, inflammation, or some other adverse physiological response to stress or allostatic load that biomarkers uncover. Biomarkers can be utilized in combination with self-reports or independently of them, but their use forecasts more accurate stress studies leading to increased support of the stress process model or perhaps the formulation of new theories.

An example of the latter is found in the research of medical sociologist Johannes Siegrist (2010, 2016) who formulated the effort–reward imbalance model after researching the origins of stress and the onset of cardiovascular disease among German male blue-collar workers and middle managers. His research team took blood and urine samples and blood pressure readings, as well as measures of life satisfaction, work-load, job security, coping styles, emotional distress, and sleep disturbances. Siegrist found that high personal effort (competitiveness and work-related overcommitment) and low gain (poor promotion prospects, no merit raises, and a blocked career) resulted in a lack of balance between having to work hard and not having that effort rewarded. Workers and managers whose jobs required strong effort that resulted in little reward were most likely to develop cardiovascular disease because of the stress inherent in this situation.

"The effort-reward imbalance model," says Siegrist (2011:254), "claims that failed reciprocity in terms of high cost and low gain elicits strong negative emotions with special propensity to sustained autonomic and neuroendocrine activation and their adverse long-term consequences for health." The model is based on the concept of social reciprocity that can be described as an interpersonal contractual exchange in which one party agrees to perform certain tasks in return for specified rewards (money, job security, advancement). But when the efforts required are more than the agreed-upon rewards, emotional dissatisfaction can become normative for the persons providing the labor. Such workers and managers may have no other choice but to continue because of the labor market (job dependency) or continue in order to improve their future opportunities (strategic choice), or they keep working without equitable rewards because of a psychological need for approval or esteem (overcommitment). Although high-status employees can have demanding jobs, exposure to a high effort–low reward situation and its effects on health was greatest among low-status workers with low levels of education.

The use of biomarkers in this study of stress, along with the work of other sociologists (Das 2013; Schmeer and Tarrance 2018), suggests that sociological stress studies are entering a period of research featuring the availability of more advanced methodologies that can be used to reinforce the stress process model or, alternatively, lead to the development of new theories as seen in the effort–reward imbalance model. A developing area of research on stress and biomarkers is on the physiological effects of racism, as seen in instances of discrimination stimulating the hypothalamic–pituitary–adrenal (HPA) axis controlling reactions to stress involving digestion, immune system secretions, moods, emotions, sexuality, and energy storage and release, along with increasing physiological wear and tear ("weathering"), and elevated cardiometabolic risks (Goosby, Cheadle, and Mitchell 2018).

Another promising new sector of research on stress in medical sociology is gene-environment interaction concerning the sensitivity of genes to environmental influences and environmental effects on genetic expression (Bliss 2018; Boardman, Blalock, and Pampel 2010; Boardman, Daw, and Freese 2013; Daw et al. 2013; Perry 2016). The fact that stressful situations in a person's life can stimulate genetic predispositions toward mental and physical health problems has long been known, but studies of gene-environment interaction in medical sociology have appeared in greater frequency since the completion of the Human Genome Project in 2003. The seminal paper with respect to stress was that of Avshalom Caspi and colleagues (2003) who determined that when the short allele (a variant or alternate form of a gene) of the 5-HTTLPR gene is affected by stressful environments (e.g., childhood deprivation), a person with one or two copies of it is more prone to depression than those without it. Among people who had experienced four or more stressful life events, some 43 percent with two short alleles and 33 percent with one short allele suffered a major depression. Persons with two long alleles, however, were more or less immune to genetic influences associated with stressful life events. This study provided solid initial evidence of a genetic variation affected by the social environment and led to more research in this area.

Bernice Pescosolido and her colleagues (2008), for example, examined the interaction between the GABRA2 gene and social environmental factors, focusing on stress from childhood (maternal) deprivation and the availability of a safety net of family-based social support, in relation to alcohol dependence. They found the GABRA2 gene was not operative in women nor had significant effects generally on African Americans. The gene seemed to cause alcohol dependence only in certain men who were deprived of a mother in childhood, thereby suggesting that "a history of deprivation during childhood may trigger the genetic tendency, reinforcing the power of stress theory and previous transdisciplinary findings" (Pescosolido et al. 2008:S192). Family social support, however, even from families with a history of alcohol dependence, appeared to decrease the genetic predisposition. These findings thus line up on the side of the stress process model, illustrating the effects of environmental stressors (material deprivation) and mediators (family social support) on genetic tendencies toward alcoholism.

Studies such as this suggest that biomarker and gene-based research is the next likely focus of sociological theorizing about stress in medical sociology. Pescosolido et al. (2008:S191) put it this way: "Genes matter. Social structure and experiences matter."

Summary

The study of the relationship between social factors and stress-related diseases is a major area of research in medical sociology. It is clear from existing studies that the experience of stress is a subjective response on the part of an individual as a result of exposure to certain social experiences and environments. The most widely used model to explain stress in medical sociology is Pearlin's stress process model that consists of (1) stressors (any condition having the potential to arouse the adaptive capacity of the individual), (2) moderators (coping abilities, sense of mastery, and sources of social support), and (3) outcomes. The two major types of social stressors identified by Pearlin are: life events and chronic strain. The theory holds that not all people react to these stressors the same way because of differences in stress moderators which, in turn, influence different outcomes. The use of biomarkers and genetic measures in stress research represents an advance over previous measures of the stress process.

Guide to Critical Thinking

1. Define stress and explain how it affects the body.
2. Describe the stress process model.
3. In what ways are social situations stressful? Do ordinary life events cause stress, even those that are positive like weddings and vacations?
4. What are the strengths and weaknesses of the life events' approach to explaining stress?
5. How do ordinary life events differ from chronic strains?
6. What is the difference between primary and secondary stressors?
7. What is "weathering?"
8. Explain the effort–reward imbalance model.

Note

1   Major exceptions are George Brown (2002) in Britain who studied the effects of stress on depression and Johannes Siegrist (2010, 2016) in Germany who formulated effort–reward imbalance theory.

Suggested Reading

Aneshensel, Carol S., Jo C. Phelan, and Alex Bierman (eds.) (2013) *Handbook of the Sociology of Mental Health*, 2nd ed. Dordrecht: Springer.
Contains updated chapters on the stress process with a focus on mental illness.
Bliss, Catherine. 2018. *Social by Nature: The Promise and Peril of Sociogenomics*. Stanford, CA: Stanford University Press.
A book on social genomics based on interviews with sociologists and others working in this relatively new field.
Moore, David S. 2015. *The Developing Genome: An Introduction to Behavioral Epigenetics*. New York: Oxford University Press.
An award-winning book on behavioral epigenetics written from the perspective of psychology.

References

Aneshensel, Carol S. 2015. "Sociological Inquiry into Mental Health: The Legacy of Leonard I. Pearlin." *Journal of Health and Social Behavior* 56(2):166–78.
Aneshensel, Carol S. and William R. Avison. 2015. "The Stress Process: An Appreciation of Leonard I. Pearlin." *Society and Mental Health* 5(2):67–85.
Avison, William R. and Stephanie S. Thomas. 2016. "Stress," in William Cockerham (ed.), *The New Blackwell Companion to Medical Sociology*. Oxford: Wiley-Blackwell, pp. 242–67.
Avison, William R., Jennifer Ali, and David Walters. 2007. "Family Structure, Stress, and Psychological Distress: A Demonstration of the Impact of Differential Response." *Journal of Health and Social Behavior* 48(3):301–17.
Bierman, Alex. 2014. "Reconsidering the Relationship between Age and Financial Strain among Older Adults." *Society and Mental Health* 4(3):197–214.
Bliss, Catherine. 2018. *Social by Nature: The Promise and Peril of Sociogenomics*. Stanford, CA: Stanford University Press.
Blumer, Herbert. 1969. *Symbolic Interaction*. Englewood Cliffs, NJ: Prentice-Hall.
Boardman, Jason D., Casey L. Blalock, and Fred C. Pampel. 2010. "Trends in the Genetic Influences on Smoking." *Journal of Health and Social Behavior* 51(1):108–23.
Boardman, Jason D., Jonathan Daw, and Jeremy Freese. 2013. "Defining the Environment in Gene-Environment Research: Lessons from Epidemiology." *American Journal of Public Health* 103:S61–S72.
Brackbill, Robert M., Steven D. Stellman, Sharon E. Perlman, Deborah J. Walker, and Mark R. Farfel. 2013. "Mental Health of Those Directly Exposed to the World Trade Center Disaster: Unmet Mental Health Care Need, Mental Health Service Use, and Quality of Life." *Social Science & Medicine* 81:110–14.
Bratter, Jennifer L. and Bridget K. Gorman. 2011. "Is Discrimination an Equal Opportunity Risk? Socioeconomic Status and Health Status among Blacks and Whites." *Journal of Health and Social Behavior* 52(3): 365–82.
Brown, George W. 2002. "Social Roles, Context and Evolution in the Origins of Depression." *Journal of Health and Social Behavior* 43(3):255–76.

Brown, Tyson H., Angela M. O'Rand, and Daniel E. Atkin. 2012. "Race-ethnicity and Health Trajectories: Test of Three Hypotheses across Multiple Groups and Health Outcomes." *Journal of Health and Social Behavior* 53(3):359–77.

Burgard, Sarah A. and Jennifer Ailshire. 2009. "Putting Work to Bed: Stressful Experiences on the Job and Sleep Quality." *Journal of Health and Social Behavior* 50(4):476–92.

Burgard, Sarah A. and Sarah Seelye. 2016. "Histories of Perceived Job Insecurity and Psychological Distress among Older U.S. Adults." *Society and Mental Health* 7(1):21–35.

Cannon, Walter B. 1932. *The Wisdom of the Body.* New York: W.W. Norton.

Caspi, Avshalom, Karen Sugden, Terrie E. Moffitt, Alan Taylor, Ian W. Craig, HonaLee Harrington, Joseph McClay, Jonathan Mill, Judy Martin, Anthony Braithwaite, and Richie Poulton. 2003. "Influence of Life Stress on Depression: Moderation by a Polymorphism in the 5-HTT Gene." *Science* 301(5631):386–9.

Clair, Jeffrey M., Cullen Clark, Brian P. Hinote, Caroline O. Robinson, and Jason A. Wasserman. 2007. "Developing, Integrating, and Perpetuating New Ways of Applying Sociology in Health, Medicine, Policy, and Everyday Life." *Social Science & Medicine* 64:248–58.

Cockerham, William C. 2007. "A Note on the Fate of Postmodern Theory and its Failure to Meet the Basic Requirements for Success in Medical Sociology." *Social Theory & Health* 5(4):285–96.

Conger, Katherine Jewsbury, Shannon Tierney Williams, Wendy M. Little, Katherine E. Masyn, and Barbara Shebloski. 2009. "Development of Mastery during Adolescence: The Role of Family Problem-solving." *Journal of Health and Social Behavior* 50(1):99–114.

Das, Aniruddhas. 2013. "How Does Race Get 'Under the Skin'? Inflammation, Weathering, and Metabolic Problems in Late Life." *Social Science & Medicine* 77:75–83.

Daw, Jonathan, Michael Shanahan, Kathleen Mullan Harris, Andrew Smolen, Brett Haberstick, and Jason D. Boardman. 2013. "Genetic Sensitivity to Peer Behaviors: 5HTTLPR, Smoking, and Alcohol Consumption." *Journal of Health and Social Behavior* 46(3):289–305.

Downey, Liam, and Marieke van Willigen. 2005. "Environmental Stressors: The Mental Health Impacts of Living Near Industrial Activity." *Journal of Health and Social Behavior* 46(3): 289–305.

Drentea, Patricia and John P. Reynolds. 2012. "Neither a Borrower nor a Lender Be: The Relative Importance of Debt and SES for Mental Health among Older Adults." *Journal of Aging and Health* 24(4):673–95.

Elliott, Marta. 2013. "Gender Differences in the Determinants of Distress, Alcohol Misuse, and Related Psychiatric Disorders." *Society and Mental Health* 3(2):96–113.

Frankenberg, Elizabeth, Jenna Nobles, and Cecep Sumantri. 2012. "Community Destruction and Traumatic Stress in Post-Tsunami Indonesia." *Journal of Health and Social Behavior* 53(4): 498–514.

Geronimus, Arline. 1992. "The Weathering Hypothesis and the Health of African-American Women and Infants: Evidence and Speculations." *Ethnicity & Disease* 2(3):207–21.

Geronimus, Arline T., Margaret Hicken, Dayna Keene, and John Bound. 2006. "Weathering and Age Patterns of Allostatic Load Scores among Blacks and Whites in the United States." *American Journal of Public Health* 96:826–33.

Geronimus, Arline T., Jay A. Pearson, Erin Linnenbringer, Amy T. Schulz, Angela G. Reyes, Elissa S. Epel, Jue Lin, and Elizabeth H. Blackburn. 2015. "Race-Ethnicity, Poverty, Urban Stressors, and Telomere Length in a Detroit Community-based Sample." *Journal of Health and Social Behavior* 56(2):199–224.

Goosby, Bridget, Jacob E. Chaedle, and Colter Mitchell. 2018. "Stress-Related Biosocial Mechanisms of Discrimination and African American Health Inequities." *Annual Review of Sociology* 44:319–40.

Grollman, Eric Anthony. 2012. "Multiple Forms of Perceived Discrimination and Health among Adolescents and Young Adults." *Journal of Health and Social Behavior* 53(2):199–214.

Gruenewald, Tara L., Arun S. Karlamangla, Perry Hu, Sharon Stein-Merkin, Carolyn Crandall, Brandon Koretz, and Teresa Seeman. 2012. "History of Socioeconomic Disadvantage and Allostatic Load in Later Life." *Social Science & Medicine* 74:75–83.

Grzywacz, Joseph G., David M. Almeida, Shevaun D. Neupert, and Susan L. Ettner. 2004. "Socioeconomic Status and Health: A Micro-level Analysis of Exposure and Vulnerability to Daily Stressors." *Journal of Health and Social Behavior* 45(1):1–16.

Hatteberg, Sarah J. 2014. "Stress, Coping, and Social Support Processes," in William Cockerham, Robert Dingwall, and Stella Quah (eds.), *The Wiley Blackwell Encyclopedia of Health, Illness, Behavior, and Society*, Vol. 5. Oxford: Wiley Blackwell, pp. 2277–83.

Hitlin, Steven, Lance D. Erickson, and J. Scott Brown. 2015. "Agency and Mental Health: A Transition to Adulthood Paradox." *Society and Mental Health* 5(3):163–81.

Holmes, T. H. and R. H. Rahe. 1967. "The Social Readjustment Rating Scale." *Journal of Psychosomatic Research* 11:213–25.

Hughes, Michael, K. Jill Kiecolt, and Verna M. Keith. 2014. "How Racial Identity Moderates the Impact of Financial Stress on Mental Health among African Americans." *Society and Mental Health* 4(1):38–54.

Kahn, Joan, and Leonard I. Pearlin. 2006. "Financial Strain over the Life Course and Health among Older Adults." *Journal of Health and Social Behavior* 47(1):17–31.

Koltai, Jonathan and Scott Schieman. 2015. "Job Pressure and SES-contingent Buffering: Resource Reinforcement, Substitution, or the Stress of Higher Status?" *Journal of Health and Social Behavior* 56(2):180–98.

Lantz, Paula M., James S. House, Richard P. Mero, and David R. Williams. 2005. "Stress, Life Events, and Socioeconomic Disparities in Health: Results from the Americans' Changing Lives Study." *Journal of Health and Social Behavior* 46(3): 274–88.

Longest, Kyle C. and Peggy A. Thoits. 2012. "Gender, the Stress Process and Health: A Configurational Approach." *Society and Mental Health* 2(3):187–206.

McLeod, Jane D. 2012. "The Meaning of Stress: Expanding the Stress Process Model." *Society and Mental Health* 2(3):172–86.

McLeod, Jane D. 2015. "Why and How Inequality Matters." *Journal of Health and Social Behavior* 56(2):149–65.

Miller, Byron, Sunshine M. Rote, and Verna M. Keith. 2013. "Coping with Racial Discrimination: Assessing the Vulnerability of African Americans and the Mediated Moderation of Psychosocial Resources." *Society and Mental Health* 3(2):133–50.

Mirowsky, John, and Catherine E. Ross. 2004. *Social Causes of Psychological Distress*, 2nd ed. New York: Aldine de Gruyter.

Needham, Belinda L., Jose R. Fernandez, Jue Lin, Elissa S. Epel, and Elizabeth H. Blackburn. 2012. "Socioeconomic Status and Cell Aging in Children." *Social Science & Medicine* 74: 1948–51.

Pearlin, Leonard I. 1989. "The Sociological Study of Stress." *Journal of Health and Social Behavior* 30(3):241–56.

Pearlin, Leonard I. and Alex Bierman. 2013. "Current Issues and Future Directions in Research into the Stress Process," in Carol Aneshensel, Jo C. Phelan, and Alex Bierman (eds.), *Handbook of the Sociology of Mental Health*, 2nd ed. Dordrecht: Springer, pp. 325–40.

Pearlin, Leonard I., Scott Schieman, Elena M. Fazio, and Stephen C. Meersman. 2005. "Stress, Health, and the Life Course: Some Conceptual Perspectives." *Journal of Health and Social Behavior* 46(2):205–19.

Pearlin, Leonard I. and Carmi Schooler. 1978. "The Structure of Coping." *Journal of Health and Social Behavior* 19(March):2–21.

Perry, Brea L. 2016. "Gendering Genetics: Biological Contingencies in the Protective Effects of Social Integration for Men and Women." *American Journal of Sociology* 121(6):1655–97.

Pescosolido, Bernice A., Brea L. Perry, J. Scott Long, Jack K. Martin, John I. Nurnberger, Jr., and Victor Hesselbrock. 2008. "Under the Influence of Genetics: How Transdisciplinarity Leads Us to Rethink Social Pathways to Illness." *American Journal of Sociology* 114(Supplement):S171–202.

Reynolds, John R. and R. Jay Turner. 2008. "Major Life Events: Their Personal Meaning, Resolution, and Mental Health Significance." *Journal of Health and Social Behavior* 49(2): 223–37.

Schieman, Scott, Yuko Kurashina Whitestone, and Karen van Gundy. 2006. "The Nature of Work and the Stress of Higher Status." *Journal of Health and Social Behavior* 47(2):242–57.

Schmeer, Kammi K. and Jacob Tarrence. 2018. "Racial-ethnic Disparities in Inflammation: Evidence of Weathering in Childhood?" *Journal of Health and Social Behavior* 59(3):411–20.

Schnittker, Jason. 2010. "Gene-Environment Correlations in the Stress–Depression Relationship." *Journal of Health and Social Behavior* 51(2):229–43.

Schnittker, Jason and Andrea John. 2007. "Enduring Stigma: The Long-term Effects of Incarceration on Health." *Journal of Health and Social Behavior* 48(2):115–30.

Seeman, T., S. Merkin, E. Crimmins, B. Koretz, S. Charnette, and A. Karlamanga. 2008. "Education, Income, and Ethnic Differences in Cumulative Risk Profiles in a National Sample of US Adults: NHANES III (1988–1994)." *Social Science & Medicine* 66:72–97.

Selye, Hans. 1956. *The Stress of Life*. New York: McGraw-Hill.

Siegrist, Johannes. 2010. "Effort–Reward Imbalance at Work and Cardiovascular Disease." *International Journal of Occupational Medicine and Environmental Health* 23:279–85.

Siegrist, Johannes. 2011. "Social Determinants of Health—Contributions from European Health and Medical Sociology." *Politica y Sociedad* 48(2):249–58.

Siegrist, Johannes. 2016. "Stress in the Workplace," in William Cockerham (ed.), *The New Blackwell Companion to Medical Sociology*. Oxford: Wiley-Blackwell, pp. 268–87.

Tausig, Mark. 2013. "The Sociology of Work and Well-being," in Carol Aneshensel, Jo C. Phelan, and Alex Bierman (eds.), *Handbook of the Sociology of Mental Health*, 2nd ed. Dordrecht: Springer, pp. 433–56.

Thoits, Peggy A. 2006. "Personal Agency in the Stress Process." *Journal of Health and Social Behavior* 47(4):309–23.

Thoits, Peggy A. 2010. "Stress and Health: Major Findings and Policy Implications." *Journal of Health and Social Behavior* 51(extra issue):S41–S53.

Thoits, Peggy A. 2011. "Mechanisms Linking Social Ties and Support to Physical and Mental Health." *Journal of Health and Social Behavior* 52(2):145–61.

Thoits, Peggy A. 2013. "Self-identity, Stress, and Mental Health," in Carol Aneshensel, Jo Phelan, and Alex Bierman (eds.), *Handbook of the Sociology of Mental Health*, 2nd ed. Dordrecht: Springer, pp. 357–78.

Thomas, William I. and Dorothy Swaine Thomas. 1928. *The Child in America: Behavior, Problems, and Programs*. New York: Knopf.

Thomeer, Mieke Beth, Allen J. LeBlanc, David M. Frost, and Kayla Bowen. 2018. "Anticipatory Minority Stressors among Same-sex Couples: A Relationship Timeline Approach." *Social Psychology Quarterly* 81(2):126–48.

Turner, R. Jay and William R. Avison. 2003. "Status Variations in Stress Exposure: Implications for the Interpretation of Research on Race, Socioeconomic Status, and Gender." *Journal of Health and Social Behavior* 44(4):488–505.

Umberson, Debra, Kristi Williams, Daniel A. Powers, Hui Liu, and Belinda Needham. 2006. "You Make Me Sick: Marital Quality and Health Over the Life Course." *Journal of Health and Social Behavior* 47(1):1–16.

Wheaton, Blair, Marisa Young, Shirin Montazer, and Katie Stuart-Lahman. 2013. "Social Stress in the Twenty-first Century," in Carol Aneshensel, Jo Phelan, and Alex Bierman (eds.), *Handbook of the Sociology of Mental Health*, 2nd ed. Dordrecht: Springer, pp. 299–324.

Williams, David R. 2012. "Miles to Go before We Sleep: Racial Inequities in Health." *Journal of Health and Social Behavior* 53(3): 279–95.

Williams, David R. and Selina A. Mohammed. 2009. "Discrimination and Racial Disparities in Health: Evidence and Needed Research." *Journal of Behavioral Medicine* 32:20–47.

Young, Wendy B. and Steven L. Foy. 2013. "The Influence of Meaning-making after Spousal Loss on Trajectories of Psychological Distress." *Society and Mental Health* 3(3):187–202.

Chapter 9

The Social Construction
of Gender and Race

Although there are multiple versions of social constructionism, the discussion in this chapter will examine its application to medical sociology with a focus on gender and race. These two variables are standard measures in virtually every quantitative study in medical sociology, are often important in qualitative research, and have shown themselves to be leading predictors of health outcomes. They are typically used as components of theories in medical sociology, rather than as theories themselves, but relevant theoretical statements exist about each and both gender and race are considered by most sociologists to be social constructions of biological differences.

Social Constructionism

At its core, social constructionism, as a micro-level theory like symbolic interaction, is based on the perception that reality is socially constructed by people interacting with one another, defining their world as they see it, and producing knowledge about it. In medical sociology, this perspective takes "the view that scientific knowledge and biological discourses about the body, health, and illness are produced through subjective, historically determined human interests, and are subject to change and reinterpretation" (Gabe, Bury, and Elston 2004:130). This perspective stands in sharp contrast to those in the physical and biological sciences that maintain that phenomena found in nature are independent of human actions, decisions, and history. Instead of falling in line with this viewpoint, social constructionism places its emphasis on claiming that the meanings of phenomena are not inherent in the phenomena themselves but instead develop through interaction in a social context (Conrad and Barker 2010:S67). As Icelandic medical sociologist Sigrun Olafsdottir (2013:41) explains: "Social constructs are viewed as the by-products of countless human choices, rather than laws that result from divine will or nature."

This means that phenomena are not discovered but socially produced (Turner 2004). That is, things are what they are defined as, even illness.

The social construction of illness, for example, is based on the assertion that the expression of physiological symptoms is shaped by cultural and moral values, experienced through interaction with other people, and influenced by particular beliefs in society about what constitutes health and illness (Lorber 1997; Nowakowski and Sumerau 2019). As Alexandra Nowakowski and J. E. Sumerau (2019:724) explain:

> Put simply, the social construction of health and illness in a given case relies heavily upon the ways medical authorities and patients, individually and collectively, define and label an illness by assigning meaning to a set of symptoms in relation to existing medical hypotheses and understandings about a given set of biological phenomena.

The result is a transformation of symptoms into a diagnosis which produces socially appropriate illness behavior and a modified social status as a result of a person's defined ill condition.

Several different lines of thought provide a foundation for social constructionism. One strand can be traced to Émile Durkheim's perspective in *The Rules of Sociological Method* ([1895] 1964) where he maintains that deviant behavior is a violation of social rules and has no reality apart from these rules. Without rules to be broken, there is no deviance. Other links can be made to the symbolic interactionist assertion that objects have no intrinsic meanings in themselves but are what people define them as and that what is defined as real is real in its consequences (Blumer 1969). There is also labeling theory's claim that deviance is not found in the quality of an act committed by an individual but results from the definition of that act applied to it by other people (Becker 1973), along with the notion of residual rule breaking maintaining that mere rule breaking is not enough to label a person mentally ill but depends upon the extent to which the behavior in question is defined as unnatural by those who have knowledge of it (Scheff 1999). Drawing on this type of thinking, two major branches of social constructionism emerged in medical sociology. One is grounded in agency and symbolic interaction largely through the work of Peter Berger, Thomas Luckmann, and Eliot Freidson. The other developed in a different direction showcasing the relevance of structure as presented by Michel Foucault.

Agency: Berger, Luckmann, and Freidson

With respect to agency, Berger and Luckmann provide an account in *The Social Construction of Reality* (1967) of how the reality of everyday life is created through social interaction. The two authors (Berger and Luckmann 1967:129) maintain that society has both an objective and subjective reality and that any adequate theoretical understanding of it must take both of these aspects into consideration. They note the means by which frequently repeated forms of social behaviors, actions, and roles become routine and habitual patterns of social interaction, forming a distinct body of knowledge. This knowledge is continuously reaffirmed in the events of everyday life and becomes institutionalized by society over time as an objective reality passed on to future generations. Institutionalization is considered inherent in every social situation that continues in time and "by the very fact of their existence, institutions control human conduct by setting up predefined patterns of conduct, which channel it in one direction as against the many other directions that would theoretically be possible" (Berger and Luckmann 1967:55).

However, the objective reality of everyday life is also subjectively meaningful to the individual as a coherent social world (Berger and Luckmann 1967:19). The experience of society as a subjective reality is attained through primary and secondary socialization, with the former more important than the latter. Primary socialization involves being given an identity and a specific place in society. As Berger and Luckmann (1967:132) explain: "The child learns that he [or she] *is* what he [or she] is called." Primary socialization is carried out by significant others (usually parents and other family members) who interpret the objective reality of society, construct it to make it meaningful from their point of view, and transmit it to the child as a subjective reality to be internalized in the mind as a guide for social behavior. This is accomplished through language which provides a means by which concepts about how the world is structured and experienced can be explained, become a taken-for-granted subjective reality, and be potentially reconstructed or referred to at some future time. As for secondary socialization, it is the internalization of institutional "subworlds," such as training for a particular occupation or profession, including the assimilation of medical knowledge and procedures by medical students that inducts them into the professional world of medicine. For Berger and Luckmann, the social construction of reality is about the role of knowledge in society in creating patterns of social interaction.

Freidson picks up on a similar theme in *The Profession of Medicine* (1970) where he treats illness and disease as social constructions. Freidson (1970:206) observes "that, just like law and religion, the profession of medicine uses normative criteria to pick out what it is interested in, and that its work constitutes a social reality that is distinct from (and on occasion virtually independent of) physical reality." While he recognizes that illness as a biophysical state exists independently of human knowledge, illness as a social state is created and shaped by human knowledge and evaluation. A diagnosis of an illness, for example, can have behavioral consequences independent of its biological ramifications. That is, simply naming something an illness affects behavior as biological abnormalities have social and cultural meanings associated with them (Nowakowski and Sumerau 2019; Olafsdottir 2013). Thus the biological realities of disease are not denied; rather, they have implications beyond their biological basis that are social. This is because medicine has jurisdiction over deciding what is and is not illness and "by virtue of being the authority on what illness 'really' is, *medicine creates the social possibilities for acting sick*" (Freidson 1970:206, original emphasis).

Moreover, Freidson and others (Barker 2005; Conrad and Barker 2010; Nettleton 2013; Olafsdottir 2013) all observed that medical concepts and definitions change over time, which for some, reinforces the social constructionist argument that diseases and their definitions are socially constructed. For instance, hysteria and neurasthenia no longer exist as mental illnesses, while homosexuality as previously noted was considered a mental disorder by psychiatrists in the early 1970s but this is no longer the case today as the gay rights movement and prevailing civil rights norms led to the medical profession's conclusion that a non-heterosexual orientation is not a form of insanity. This opens up the question of whether or not an illness is actually an illness in the first place if political activism can remove it as a diagnostic category.

When it comes to mental illness, people have traditionally been labeled as such when they violated taken-for-granted understandings of normality in ways that cannot be explained except as mental disorder. Consequently, whether an individual is determined to be mentally ill according to social constructionism is not dependent on his or her symptoms, but on how those symptoms match the rules or norms for normal and abnormal behaviors. However, these rules are not rigid; sometimes they can change according to the dominant modes of thinking in particular historical periods.

Additionally some illnesses are "contested" in that while called an "illness" (e.g., fibromyalgia syndrome, irritable bowel syndrome, chronic fatigue syndrome), as Peter Conrad and Kristin Barker (2010:570) nonetheless note, "they are medically suspect because they are not associated with any known physical abnormality." They are illnesses because the medical profession regards them as such. Other diseases are "stigmatized" as is the case with epilepsy and HIV/AIDS (Scambler 2009). Overall, when these various viewpoints are combined under the umbrella of social constructionism, this body of work is intended to illustrate "how illness is shaped by social interactions, shared cultural traditions, shifting frameworks of knowledge, and relations of power" (Conrad and Barker 2010:S69).

Structure: Foucault

The second branch of social constructionism in medical sociology stems from the influence of Foucault (1965, 1973) who focused on the utilization of power to show how the medical profession was able to determine normality and abnormality through surveillance (the medical or clinical "gaze") and use its definitions to establish professional control over the human body. As noted in Chapter 7, he stressed the relationship between knowledge and power and argued that they were so closely linked that an extension of knowledge meant a simultaneous expansion of power. Foucault (1965) provided a social history of how knowledge produced expertise that was used by medicine to extend its power to regulate human behavior and repress deviance and abnormality. He argued that mental illness, for example, did not officially exist until the seventeenth century, when it was defined by the medical profession as a threat to the general public that needed to be controlled. As knowledge of mental illness increased, the power of psychiatry to control the mentally ill likewise increased. This argument fit into the parameters of social constructionism which looks at how categories of knowledge, such as mental illness, evolve and change from one era to another and examines who has the power to enforce definitions of normality and abnormality (Horwitz 2013).

Social constructionism criticized not only psychiatry's efforts to expand its classification of various behaviors as abnormal by defining more and more behaviors as illness, but the classification system itself. Allan Horwitz (2002) relates how a group of research-oriented psychiatrists captured the most powerful positions in their profession in the 1970s and became proponents of diagnostic psychiatry. This group, favoring a biomedical model as a result of their training and experience, developed a disease-based classification system for mental illness that became the dominant perspective in psychiatry as the basis for diagnosis in the first edition of DSM-I published in 1980. Social constructionists responded that mental illness is itself a social construction in that its diagnostic categories were created by psychiatrists who use medical terminology to disguise the fact that these afflictions are not diseases. This application of psychiatric knowledge was considered to be a political exercise in the maintenance of professional power instead of a technically neutral decision. In this context, the social constructionist perspective sought to explain how a medically based classification system of mental illnesses was developed and persists without strong clinical evidence of disease supporting many of its basic assumptions (Horwitz 2002, 2013; Horwitz and Wakefield 2012).

Strengths and Weaknesses

The strength of social constructionism appears to be in explaining how social factors and cultural adaptations help shape our understanding of health, illness, and medical treatment and in this way remains a useful theory in medical sociology. Given the significant differences between Berger and Luckmann in comparison to Foucault, it is obvious that social constructionism lacks a single, unified doctrine. According to Bryan Turner (2004:43), "These different types of constructionism present very different accounts of human agency and thus have different implications for an understanding of the relationship between patients, doctors, and disease entities." The more social constructionist work is influenced by Berger and Luckmann, the more agency-oriented it is; the closer to Foucault, the less agency has a role.

However, even though the use of social constructionism has expanded in medical sociology, its acceptance has not been universal. Mike Bury (1986), for one, noted many years ago that social constructionism does not fully incorporate into its perspective the biological reality of pain and suffering that people experience when ill—regardless of how their affliction is socially defined and constructed. To claim that the body can only or best be understood by the various discourses concerning it, overlooks the fact that it has *both* a physical and social reality and social constructionism does not explain the physical side. Horowitz (2002:9), in turn, accurately notes that if all behaviors are socially constructed, they have no meaning "outside of the culture-bound rules that define them" which limits its application and, moreover, that "phenomena such as the distorted thought processes of schizophrenia, massive and continual alcohol consumption, or depleted levels of serotonin can have consequences regardless of the social definitions placed on them."

Additionally, Bury (1986) finds that social constructionism has not recognized the advances made in medical science for the common good and this still seems to be the case. This is because its general approach in medical sociology is that of criticism, largely of the medical profession. Also its contention that knowledge is relative and no one form of it is more valid than another, if taken literally, implies that social constructionism itself cannot be considered more valid than any other theory (Gabe et al. 2004). Finally, Olafsdottir (2013) adds that while it can be shown that certain phenomena are socially constructed, it sometimes is not made clear why and how it matters. As a theory, social constructionism remains in a state of development.

Gender

Many sociologists consider the term "gender" to be a social construction in that the biological differences in anatomy, hormones, and chromosomes between males and females come under the heading of "sex" and the cultural and social differences between the two sexes refer to "gender" (Epstein 2007). As British sociologist Elizabeth Frazer (2018:914) points out: "In social theory, gender refers most often to the social role of masculinity or femininity that is played by human beings of male or female sex." Gender represents the social roles and rules that determine how sex is socially expressed and enacted (Frazier 2018:915). According to the feminist theorist Judith Butler (1990), a role implies a performance and therefore gender roles are performative in that they are produced, staged, acted out, and reproduced along socially constructed lines of behavior. But unlike actors, people who perform gender roles usually do so on a lifelong basis.

Applicable studies pertain to variabilities in the roles, forms of labor, tasks, benefits, burdens, sexual identities, identity politics, and, of course, health and mortality of the two genders. The overall pattern of health and life expectancy for men and women shows a "paradox" in that women are sick more often, report poorer health, have more depression and anxiety, and use more health services on average than men—but live longer (Cockerham 2017a, 2017b). Women, with the exception of exercise, also live healthier lifestyles. Men, in comparison, have less sickness or morbidity, report better health, and visit physicians less often and generally do not live as long as their female counterpart. Men also have more personality disorders, substance abuse, drink more alcohol and smoke more, eat less healthy diets, are employed in much greater numbers in hazardous occupations, and when they are subject to illness or chronic disease, the affliction is likely to be more life-threatening. The role of gender in health matters is therefore substantial.

For example, John McKinlay (1996) pointed out years ago that the "fact" that women were not likely to have heart disease until menopause was accepted knowledge within the medical community. Gender differences in the onset of heart disease, however, were an artifact of incorrect medical observations. The symptoms produced by heart disease among premenopausal women can be more atypical, subtle, and vague than in men, causing them to be attributed instead to flu, fatigue, stomach, or emotional problems. As a consequence, the statistical data (rates of heart disease by gender and age) that physicians used to guide their diagnostic process were based on wrongful assumptions. McKinlay suggested that thousands of women were systematically misdiagnosed due to socially constructed physiological profiles that were, at least in part, grounded in a gendered ideology in medicine where the male body was traditionally viewed as the diagnostic norm. However, as Steven Epstein (2007:4) notes, the normative standard for medical research was not just males, but white, middle-aged males whose results from clinical trials "could simply be generalized to the entire population."

This meant, of course, that women, racial and ethnic minorities, and older adults were generally not included in medical research. A new paradigm eventually emerged beginning in the mid-1980s where the inclusion of previously excluded groups became essential in any medical research project that was to be taken seriously. This represented a transformation in medical thinking away from the assumption that the findings for middle-aged white men apply to everyone in the same way—a so-called "orthodoxy of sameness" (Epstein 2007:4). In determining that differences matter in medical research, as clinical findings showed that "one size does not fit all," a new normative standard of inclusion in clinical investigations was achieved. Yet Epstein discovered that this inclusion had the unintended consequence of sorting people into social categories almost exclusively on the basis of biological differences, thereby reinforcing the significance of physical over social diversity.

From a physician's point of view, the social may not matter as long as the biological is known and can provide a physiological cure or method of control. Yet it may be the social that causes the biological affliction to originate in the first place, affects not only the onset but also the progress of the biologically based disease, and provides the day-to-day living environment which the illness begins in, and the ill person returns to, following whatever treatment is rendered. What is key to optimal health is the interaction between the social and the biological. Therefore, as several sources suggest, simply including women and racial minorities in medical research without also linking the ways in which the biological and the social intersect with one another in causing disease provides an incomplete understanding of what is really meant by "health" and how it can be effectively maintained by both genders and all races and social classes (Bird and Rieker 2008; Epstein 2007; Shim 2014). In her study of social differences in heart disease, Janet Shim (2014:210), for example, concludes that "nominal reforms cannot hope to answer fundamental questions of why inequalities in cardiovascular risk and disease occur and how they are produced."

Knowledge produced about race and gender has as much to do with social issues, problems, and circumstances as it has with biology. Clinical trials contributing to medical knowledge illustrate that the construction of such knowledge is embedded within a specific social context where certain groups have power to define what is an illness and how it should be treated, whereas other groups are largely or exclusively just the subject of the medical gaze (Foucault 1973). This circumstance underscores the fact that different systems of knowledge can differ in the interpretation of disease, which has implications for how we understand and respond to health problems in society. This is consistent with the social constructionist argument that scientific knowledge and biological discourses about the body, health, and illness are produced through subjective, historically determined human interests, and are subject to change and reinterpretation.

Most studies of gender in medical sociology have feminist roots and focus more on women than men, especially in regard to social constructionist accounts of the health of the female body and its regulation in a male-dominated society. Social and cultural assumptions are held to influence our perceptions of the body, including the use of the male body as the standard for medical training and research, the assignment of less socially desirable physical and emotional traits to women, and the ways in which women's illnesses are socially constructed (Annandale and Clark 1996; Lorber 1997). Other feminist theory is grounded in conflict theory or symbolic interaction, and deals with the sexist treatment of women patients by male doctors and the less than equal status of female physicians in professional settings and hierarchies (Hinze 2004; Riska 2016). There is, however, no unified perspective among feminist theorists other than a "woman-centered" perspective that examines the various facets of women's health and seeks an end to sexist orientations in health and illness and society at large (Annandale 2014, 2016; Annandale and Clark 1996; Bradby 2012).

Intersectionality Theory

When it comes to theories of gender and health, intersectionality theory has been one of the more promising theoretical perspectives expanding into medical sociology. Intersectionality theory originated among American black feminist scholars seeking to call attention to the multiple forms of social inequality that affect disadvantaged individuals, especially black women (Collins, 1993, 2000, 2004, 2015, 2019; Crenshaw 1989). While legal scholar Kimberlé Williams Crenshaw (1989) is credited with naming intersectionality theory, the leading theorist in sociology is Patricia Hill Collins. Intersectionality theory has an activist orientation in that some of its "core ideas" are connected to views found in community organizing, identity politics, coalition politics, and social justice (Collins 2015, 2019). The theory was developed as a way of understanding and analyzing the complexity of human experience in which social inequality is shaped by several factors in diverse and mutually influencing ways (Collins and Bilge 2016:2). The approach focuses on examining forms of discrimination and inequality stemming from gender, race, ethnicity, class, age, nation, and sexual orientation, and makes the key point that such variables are not simply individual characteristics but operate *simultaneously* at multiple levels in people's lives. These variables, observes Collins (2015:2), "operate not as unitary, mutually exclusive entities, but as reciprocally constructing phenomena that in turn shape complex social inequalities."

Intersectionality theory also holds that individual and group characteristics cannot be fully understood by prioritizing one variable (e.g., class) over another (e.g., gender) since all such variables combine to disadvantage some people in relation to others at the same time. That is, people do not experience social life—and instances of inequality or, for that matter, equality—only from the standpoint of one social characteristic but undergo all of them concurrently. Intersectionality theory therefore provides a perspective intended to investigate the interaction of numerous characteristics of a population, not only at the individual level but also at structural levels in order to capture the multiple factors that influence individual lives.

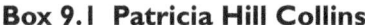

Box 9.1 Patricia Hill Collins

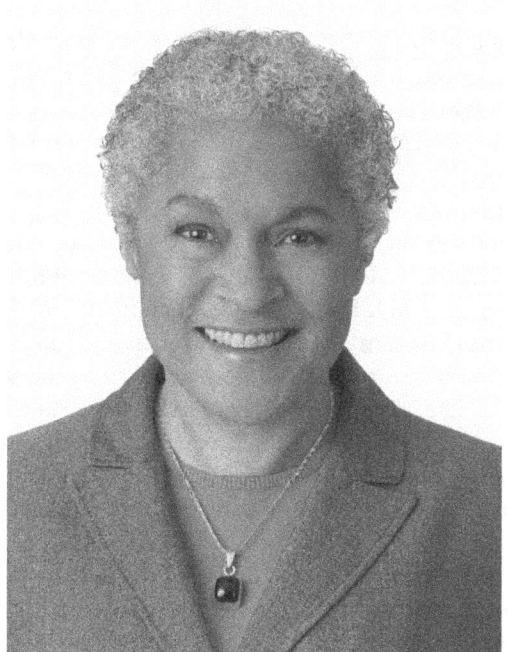

Image 9.1 Patricia Hill Collins

Patricia Hill Collins was the 100th President of the American Sociological Association (2009) and is Distinguished University Professor Emerita at the University of Maryland, as well as Charles Phelps Taft Emeritus Professor of Sociology in the Department of African American Studies at the University of Cincinnati. She was born in 1948 and grew up in an African American working-class neighborhood of Philadelphia, PA. Her father, Albert Hill, was a World War II Army veteran and factory worker, while her mother, Eunice Randolph Hill, worked as a secretary. She was an only child, attended public schools, and coped with being a racial minority. In an often-cited quote, Collins (2000:vii) says:

Beginning in adolescence, I was increasingly the "first," "one of the few," or the "only" African American and/or woman and/or working class person in my schools, communities, and work settings. I saw nothing wrong with being who I was, but apparently many others did. My world grew larger, but I felt I was growing smaller. I tried to disappear into myself in order to deflect the painful, daily assaults designed to teach me that being an African American, working-class woman made me lesser than those who were not. And as I felt smaller, I became quieter and eventually was virtually silenced.

After high school, she not only regained her voice, but expanded it to an international audience by focusing on race, black feminism, and social theory as a sociologist. First, she obtained a BA in sociology from Brandeis University and an MA in education in social science teaching from Harvard University. This was followed by a teaching stint in the Boston schools and serving as the director of the African-American Center at Tufts University. She married Roger Collins, an education professor, had a daughter Valerie in 1979, and earned a Ph.D. in sociology from Brandeis in 1984. Earlier, in 1982, she had joined the African American Studies Department at the University of Cincinnati and remained there until 2005, at which time she moved to the sociology department at the University of Maryland in College Park.

She gained prominence with the first of her many books, the award-winning monograph *Black Feminist Thought*, initially published in 1990. The book presented her early version of intersectionality, arguing that race, class, gender, and sexuality were all forms of oppression occurring simultaneously within a pervasive system of power. She maintained that black women, because of their experiences of race and gender, are uniquely positioned in society to understand and explain systematic discrimination and oppression. And this she has undertaken to do and encourage others in the process. Another book, *Black Sexual Politics: African Americans, Gender, and the New Racism* (2004), won the 2007 American Sociological Association Distinguished Publication Award.

Associated with intersectionality theory is the double disadvantage (or double jeopardy) hypothesis that maintains persons with more than one disadvantaged social status have worse health than those with a single disadvantage or a privileged status (Ferraro and Farmer 1996). This is because they are subjected to multiple forms of discrimination more frequently due to their multiple statuses, which accentuate health-related stresses. This outcome is seen in research showing that individuals with more than one stigmatized social status (i.e., race, ethnicity, gender, sexual orientation, obesity, religion) have more psychological distress, lower self-rated health, and more functional limitations with respect to walking, climbing stairs, bathing, and other physical difficulties (Grollman 2014).

While intersectionality theory does not provide a set of propositions that together form a precise theoretical statement, it does offer a loose set of principles to guide researchers (Landry 2007). Intersectionality theory's central assumptions are that (1) human lives cannot be reduced to single characteristics; (2) experiences cannot be accurately understood by prioritizing any one single factor or constellation of factors; (3) the social categories of race/ethnicity, gender, class, and sexuality are socially constructed, fluid and flexible; (4) these categories are inseparable and shaped by interacting and mutually constituting social processes and structures, which, in turn, are molded by power and influenced by both time and place; and (5) the promotion of social justice and equity are paramount (Hankivsky 2011, 2012; Hankivsky and Cormier 2009). Although intersectionality theory, unlike most sociological theories, has an activist agenda (to achieve social justice and an end to inequality), arguably it can be applied objectively to social problems and offers the advantage of a multidimensional orientation with respect to uncovering unequal relationships, including those that affect health.

While most accounts of intersectionality's intellectual origins are traced back to various forms of feminism (Collins and Bilge 2016; Hankivsky and Grace 2015), Polish sociologist Joshua Dubrow (2010) finds that its orientation can reach even further back to Max Weber's ([1922] 1978) multidimensional view of social stratification. Although seldom acknowledged by intersectionality theorists, Weber's argument that class, status, and power are analytically distinct characteristics, yet combine in the individual in varying contexts to reflect that person's overall social position, provides a link to classical sociological theory. However, intersectionality's primary focus has not been directed toward analyzing class imbalances, but the total experience of women of color in oppressive patriarchal hierarchies as expressed in the various civil rights and black feminist movements beginning in the 1960s and 1970s (Collins and Bilge 2016). It is intended to be a critical social theory (Collins 2019).

While the influence of intersectionality has increased in recent years, discussions continue about how to best operationalize the theory because of its methodological complexity (Bauer 2014; Bauer and Scheim 2019; Choo and Ferree 2010; Gkiouleka et al. 2018; Green, Evans, and Subramanian 2017; Hancock 2007; Hinze, Lin, and Andersson 2012; McCall 2005; Richardson and Brown 2016; Scheim and Bauer 2019a, 2019b; Veenstra 2009). It has proven quantitatively difficult to separate the effects of all intersecting social variables acting simultaneously on those being studied and this complexity has hampered its development. Most of the research has been qualitative or historical and interpreted subjectively, and some have suggested this is the best methodology for studying intersectionality (Bowleg 2008). Others recommended approaches using mixed qualitative and quantitative methods (Choo and Ferree 2010; Hankivsky and Grace 2015) and some quantitative assessments have been successful (within statistical limits) using interaction terms (Bauer 2014; Dubrow 2010; Veenstra 2009, 2013).

Interaction terms are a statistical technique utilized in multiple or logistic regression analysis to determine the simultaneous effect of two or more independent variables on at least one dependent variable. However, interaction terms require large data sets, are limited in the number of interactions that can be performed, and require additional steps when performing regression analysis (Bauer and Scheim 2019). More complex multi-level models, such as hierarchical linear modeling (HLM), can perform a larger number of interactions but have yet to be a common methodology in intersectionality studies since data are required specific to each level (i.e., individual, household, neighborhood, community, and so on) of analysis.

In Canada, medical sociologist Gerry Veenstra (2013), utilizing interaction terms, determined that wealthy black men and South Asian women, women with less than a high school education, and wealthy bisexuals were more likely to report hypertension. In contrast, poor black men, poor South Asian women and men, and women with a university degree reported less hypertension. In another study, Veenstra (2011) found that low-income gay men and South Asian women were most likely to self-report fair or poor health. In the U.S., Susan Hinze and her associates (Hinze et al. 2012) used interaction terms and found that older black women with less than a high school education were especially disadvantaged with respect to health in that they were more likely than all other adults in a national sample to be obese, smoke, have a chronic illness, experience depression, not be married, have smaller networks of friends, and not exercise.

The author and his colleagues (Cockerham et al. 2017) used intersectionality theory and interaction terms to determine the combined effects of socioeconomic status and gender on self-rated health and system barriers to health care in Ukraine. The sample was racially homogeneous, so the interaction of gender and class was the key measure. It was found that low SES women rated their health worse than all other women and men generally, including low SES men; these women also faced the greatest barriers to health care until older ages when an upsurge in the ailments of men caused them to likewise face the same obstacles—the most important of which were out-of-pocket costs for care in a health system that was officially free. Consequently, despite limitations, intersectionality theory can be utilized in quantitative research, but to date there are few specific measures (i.e., statistical methods, scales) that can be applied directly to its concepts (Bauer and Scheim 2019; Richardson and Brown 2016; Scheim and Bauer 2019a, 2019b).

The strength of intersectionality theory lies in its assertion that gender, class, race, and sexual orientation operate simultaneously at multiple levels in constructing identity and influencing perceptions and behavior. The theory holds that these variables cannot be fully understood by prioritizing one, for example, gender, over another, such as class, since all variables are mutually constructing systems of power that combine to affect people in relation to others at the same time. However, while people bring *all* of their identities to every social situation, not all of them may be relevant in every instance (Veenstra 2011). Therefore, an unanswered question in intersectionality research pertains to whether all identities and social positions are of equal or sufficient value to warrant study (Bauer 2014). The answer is that they may not be and it is therefore more analytically precise to concentrate on those that are relevant. It is also common that variables with more predictive strength emerge during data analysis and treating all variables as equal is neither accurate nor desired if identifying the most important social determinant is the goal. When quantitative studies invariably find that certain sociodemographic variables, primarily class, have more powerful associations with health and disease than other variables, such as gender and race, intersectionality does not yet provide a fully sufficient theoretical or methodological approach.

Also, as mentioned earlier, intersectionality theory has an activist agenda oriented toward achieving social justice and equality. This means its research focus is on inequalities "as socially constructed consequences of structures beyond the individual, and as the consequences of power differences between dominant and subordinate groups" (Varcoe, Pauly, and Laliberte 2011:332). The theory's orientation therefore centers on analyzing the "underlying power structures that produce inequalities" (Green, Evans, and Subramanian 2017:214). Most studies focus on some form of discrimination (Scheim and Bauer 2019a). Consequently, the emphasis in intersectionality studies is not generally on investigating the more immediate causes of health inequities (i.e., a lack of resources, poor health behaviors, or limited access to health care), but the structural causes of inequities (i.e., sexism, racism, discrimination, poverty, social institutions, social policies, and power imbalances). In more or less exclusively concentrating on oppression/discrimination, intersectionality theory limits itself to one central topic. If it were to be utilized more broadly, such as generally including analyses of a range of differences in social identities and positions, such as adding some that are not inherently oppressive or discriminatory and making more direct comparisons to the experiences of all categories of people—including socially and economically advantaged persons, heterosexual males, and racial majorities—the theory could likely provide even greater explanatory power (Landry 2007).

Race and Ethnicity

Race, like gender and social class, serves as a variable in practically every study in medical sociology. A definition of race is that of "a human group defined by itself or others as distinct by virtue of perceived common physical characteristics that are held to be inherent" (Cornell and Hartmann 2007:25). The concept of race in relation to health, however, is not simply a matter of biology, but the convergence of external physical traits, most conspicuously skin color, with geographic origins and multiple social, cultural, economic, and political circumstances, including discrimination, on health outcomes (Bradby and Nazroo 2016; Monk 2015). Many sociologists therefore consider race to be a social construction, since its relevance in everyday life is primarily social, not biological.

What makes race a social construction is that the characteristics used to define a "race" are *choices* that people make about themselves and others, not some form of biological predeterminism or natural law (Cornell and Hartmann 2007). Its meaning resides almost entirely in socially constructed perceptions and definitions, rather than in human physiology. This is not to say that race does not have its basis in biology because it does. It is why people come in different sizes and colors. Race as a biological term refers to a person's observed physical characteristics, with skin color the single most important determinant of an individual's racial identity (Monk 2015). But the social is relevant as well, as even among darker-skinned people, a lighter skin tone has higher social status (Keith and Herring 1991; Monk 2015). Hair, eye color, and facial features are also major racial characteristics and these are socially ranked as well.

Although all humans have the same anatomy and physiology and their biological similarities far outweigh any differences, social beliefs about racial differences cause people to be treated unfairly. Such beliefs have typically resulted in social constructions of racial hierarchies in which certain races are subjectively rated as superior and others as inferior with respect to morals, intelligence, culture, values, and the like. This type of social construction constitutes racism in which certain races are valued more than others, despite a general biological sameness and the realistic recognition that skin color does not determine character or other human social traits.

Michael Omi and Howard Winant in their book *Racial Formation in the United States* (2015) point out that even though race is socially attached to particular bodies, there is no biological basis for doing so and that race is a complex, socially mediated construct that marginalizes people and is used to justify social, economic, and health inequalities. Omi and Winant conceptualize race as a central factor in all social relationships, saying that race establishes the identity of humans, shapes conflict and cohesion, and is a key aspect of social life. They suggest that American society is so completely racialized that not to have a racial identity puts a person in jeopardy of not having any identity at all. Omi and Winant also note that the meaning of race is unstable and subject to change through political struggles which is also consistent with a social constructionist perspective.

An ethnic group is identified largely on a cultural rather than physical basis. Ethnic groups may belong to the same race or a different race, but their culture, religion, national origin, and customs set them apart. Members of an ethnic group have a common ancestry, a shared historical past, and a specific cultural focus with respect to religious affiliation, language or dialect, nationality, or some other factor that reflects their social connection. The dominant racial/ethnic group in a society is typically the majority group with respect to two key variables: size and power. The majority group is usually the most numerous, although there are exceptions, and typically has the most political power. Therefore, a minority group can be defined as one that (1) is physically, culturally, or behaviorally different from the majority, (2) has less power, and (3) is usually fewer in number than the majority. LGBT persons, the physically handicapped, and others not in the majority in regard to a particular social identity can also meet this definition, as a minority group is not limited to classifications based solely on race or ethnicity. It can include any group whose members are singled out from others in society because they are different from the majority.

Ethnicity is not as powerful a predictor of health outcomes in medical sociology as race and is seldom used as a measure in contemporary research unless the topic under investigation warrants it. Race, however, is a standard variable and findings of health disadvantages on the basis of race are often associated with racism and racial discrimination (Bradby 2012; Bratter and Gorman 2011; Grollman 2014; Phelan and Link 2015; Williams 2012; Williams and Mohammed 2009, 2013; Williams and Sternthal 2010). Perceived discrimination, for example, has been linked to depression, negative health behaviors, hypertension, and poor self-rated physical and mental health among African Americans (Monk 2015; Sims et al. 2012; Sims et al. 2016).

The most common form of racism is racial prejudice. Prejudice is a feeling or attitude, usually unfavorable or hostile, directed toward a particular person or group and typically learned from others. People can be prejudiced yet not act on their beliefs. If people do act accordingly, they are engaging in discrimination which refers to the differential treatment of people on the basis of prejudice. Usually such treatment is negative. There is such a thing as being prejudiced against a group or being prejudiced in favor of a group. Note that prejudice is a belief, while discrimination is an act. Both keep people and groups socially distant from one another. Both promote situations in which some people find themselves in disadvantaged positions because of the way their group or race has been negatively evaluated by another which can extend to health.

Conflict theory offers an explanation of racism, such as that provided by Robert Blauner (1972) and others (Omi and Winant 2015), who view racial disparities in Marxist terms as a means by which the capitalist ruling class deliberately exploits minorities. Blauner's theory is essentially an "internal colonialism" model in that it explains how whites, as the majority group, exploit racial minorities within the same society. They do this by using the labor of minorities to enrich themselves. In return for their work, minorities are paid low wages. Moreover, by keeping minorities in low-paying jobs, the owners and managers of capitalist enterprises are able to restrict the wages of all workers and maintain a cheap supply of labor. If majority group workers demand higher wages, they can be replaced by minority group persons who are willing to accept lower pay. Racism is therefore seen as a mechanism capitalists use to ensure high profits. Conflict theory thus holds that racism exists primarily because it benefits the ruling socioeconomic class. However, most of the emphasis of conflict theory with respect to health has been on class, not race, and use of the theory to explain racial differences in health never attracted much attention in the U.S. (S. Hill 2016).

The conditions for racism are most clearly evident when different racial groups come into contact with one another as a result of migration under conditions of inequality. Historically, such migrations have occurred through (1) military conquest: one group defeats and dominates an indigenous group (such as European colonization of North and South America, Asia, and Africa); (2) gradual expansion of a nation's frontier: one group pushes out and decimates another group (as Europeans and native-born persons of European descent pushed back the Native Americans in North America and the Aborigines in Australia); (3) involuntary migration: an enslaved or indentured group is sent to a country as a source of forced labor (as when blacks from Africa were sent as slaves to the United States, Brazil, and the West Indies); and (4) voluntary migration: when groups willingly move to another country for political protection or economic opportunity (as in recent Mexican and Central American immigration to the United States and Middle Eastern and North African migration to Europe). These various forms of migration have produced most of the interracial societies in the world where racism is prevalent. Migration is not the whole answer to explaining racism; but in combination with social, economic, and political disadvantages, migration appears to be a major factor in promoting racial prejudice and discrimination.

Gordon Allport (1958) long ago hypothesized that contact between races will not necessarily make relations better but will often make them worse, depending on the circumstances in which the contact takes place. Allport formulated the contact hypothesis, which maintains that prejudice will decrease if two groups with equal status have contact but will increase or intensify if contact occurs under conditions of inequality. Before Allport, many had believed that prejudice flourishes when the races are isolated and would disappear if people only got to know one another. This notion turned out to be simplistic; it is the conditions under which people have contact, rather than contact itself, that determines the likelihood that prejudice will develop. In cases where racial/ethnic groups come into contact in a competitive situation, Allport points out that prejudice will get worse. Conversely, prejudice will lessen if the groups cooperate to pursue common goals.

Shirley Hill (2016) notes that racism has affected the health of blacks most powerfully through the perpetuation of class inequities and poverty. She finds that more than a fourth of all blacks still live in poverty and nearly half of all black children do the same. For most (about 85 percent) of U.S. history, slavery and segregation limited opportunities for blacks while enhancing opportunities for several generations of whites (Feagin and Bennefield 2014). It has only been since the civil rights movement of the 1960s that large numbers of blacks became upwardly mobile in the American class structure and achieved middle-class or higher status. Yet many blacks are on the lower end of the middle class and the overall health profile of African Americans in the U.S. rests on an historical foundation that reflects a legacy of social, economic, and political disadvantage (Erving 2011; Feagin and Bennefield 2014; S. Hill 2016; Hinote and Wasserman 2017; Lemelle 2011; Williams and Sternthal 2010).

Consequently, as seen in the most recent (2016) mortality rates in the U.S. for the leading causes of death by race for all causes, non-Hispanic blacks have the highest death rates of 882.8 per 100,000, followed by non-Hispanic whites (749.0), American Indians/Alaska natives (591.2), Hispanics (525.8), and Asians/Pacific Islanders (392.6). Non-Hispanic blacks also have the highest mortality rates for all major causes of death, except for chronic lower respiratory disease, drug overdoses, and suicide which are higher among non-Hispanic whites, and liver disease and cirrhosis which are higher among American Indians/Alaska natives. Also accidental deaths are higher among American Indians/Native Alaskans and non-Hispanic whites. Particularly striking are the exceptionally high death rates for non-Hispanic blacks for heart disease, cerebrovascular diseases (stroke), cancer, diabetes, AIDS, and homicide that far exceed those of all other racial groups. Asians/ Pacific Islanders, in contrast, have the lowest mortality rates, or close to it, for all causes of death.

Infant mortality tells the same story with blacks having the highest rates by far (11.25 infant deaths per 1,000 live births), followed by American

Indians/Native Alaskans (8.58), Hispanics (4.96), whites (4.90), and Asians/Pacific Islanders (408). To speak of blacks having a health crisis, would be to speak correctly. Longevity is shorter for black females on average than all other females and black male longevity is shorter than anyone. When it comes to theorizing about health and mortality according to race, any theory needs to be able to account for such circumstances.

Theoretical Perspectives on Racism and Health

As pointed out in the introduction to this chapter, race, like gender, is typically a component of theories in medical sociology, not theories themselves. There are, however, a few theoretical statements linked directly to race. And among those that are, they either apply to health differences between all races generally or between non-Hispanic blacks and whites. Theoretical concepts concerning health specific to Hispanics, Asians, Native Americans, or those of mixed races have yet to be formulated.

To begin, there is critical race theory which, although the word "theory" is in its name, is not a theory at all, but a race-equity methodology and social movement originating in legal studies. It is intended to shift discussions about race away from a majority group's perspective to that of racially marginalized groups and their "lived" experience (Delgado and Stefancic 2017; Ford and Airhihenbuwa 2010). Race is held to be a social construction and a particular feature of this method is an individual's critical analysis of his or her own personal story in regard to experiencing race and racism.

There is also systematic race theory which is a concept focused on racism as an inherent feature of U.S. social systems (Feagin 2006; Feagin and Bennefield 2014). The source of racism in American society is initially ascribed to the economic advantages of slavery for whites which is credited for producing lasting racial stereotypes, ideologies, and practices disadvantaging blacks which have been passed on throughout the country's history. As a concept, systemic racism is portrayed by Joe Feagin (2006) as responsible for maintaining (1) a dominant racial hierarchy, (2) white framing (pro-white notions of racial distinctiveness), (3) individual and collective discrimination, (4) race-based material inequities, and (5) racist institutions. Systematic race theory holds that health care is racialized and discriminatory because it is controlled by white decision makers and others subscribing to white racial framing (stereotypes) of negativity about other races (Feagin and Bennefield 2014).

Intersectionality theory, discussed in the previous section on gender, focuses not only on the effects of sexism, but racism and other forms of discrimination affecting health. As pointed out, the theory was developed by black feminists as a method of analyzing the various forms of social inequality resulting from the intersection of gender, race, ethnicity, class, age, and sexual orientation (Collins and Bilge 2016:2). Although intersectionality theory is still in a formative stage with respect to formulating precise theoretical propositions and a quantitative methodology, earlier in this chapter studies were discussed in which the intersection of race and gender helped explain the health disadvantages of low SES black women in the U.S. (Hinze et al. 2012) and South Asian women in Canada (Veenstra 2011, 2013). Other U.S. studies show similar findings for black women with respect to hypertension (Richardson and Brown 2016) and diabetes (Sims et al. 2011), and higher blood lead levels among children in black segregated neighborhoods in Detroit (Moody, Darden, and Pigozzi 2018). Consequently, intersectionality theory offers a method for the theoretical modeling of race and other variables subject to discrimination.

Another approach is that of Shirley Hill (2016) who used theoretical concepts with general applicability in medical sociology, namely health lifestyle theory and fundamental cause theory, to explain how racial disparities cause sickness among African Americans. That is, these theories analyze the association of any or all races with healthy or unhealthy lifestyle practices and class-based determinants of disease. Hill (2016:14, 59) found that health lifestyle theory offers a broader framework than the health belief model for exploring obstacles to making healthy choices, and fundamental cause theory shows how social conditions lead to sickness and death. Health lifestyle theory, discussed in the next chapter, uses race/ethnicity as a structural variable, along with age, gender, class circumstances, the influence of collectivities (e.g., religion, social networks), and living conditions, to determine differences in health lifestyle practices in everyday life and how they impact positively or negatively on the maintenance of one's health (Cockerham 2005, 2013). While recognizing that racial differences in health behavior are not always completely explained by SES, the most powerful determinant of health lifestyles in the model has nonetheless been shown to be class circumstances.

Fundamental cause theory, to be discussed in Chapter 12, maintains that SES is a fundamental cause of health inequalities that persists over time despite changes in disease, potential risks of exposure, and types of interventions (Link and Phelan 1995; Phelan and Link 2013, 2015). The role of SES in health matters is its connection with the social and material resources needed to avoid disease, injury, and early mortality. Jo Phelan and Bruce Link (2015) who formulated the theory, subsequently determined that racism is also a fundamental cause of inequities in health because of the way it produces differences in prestige, power, beneficial social connections, and the freedom to control one's life. According to both health lifestyle and fundamental cause theories, what makes race important for health is its close association with class circumstances. That is, being poor and a racial minority often go hand-in-hand and the adverse health conditions that result are often linked more to class disadvantages in health lifestyles, neighborhoods, health care, and the like than the color of a person's skin.

Summary

This chapter examines social constructionist theory, which is the view that definitions of reality are socially constructed. Drawing on this type of thinking, two major branches of social constructionism emerged in medical sociology. One is grounded in agency and symbolic interaction largely through the work of Peter Berger, Thomas Luckmann, and Eliot Freidson. The other developed in a different direction showcasing the relevance of structure as presented by Michel Foucault. Two foci of social constructionist theory—gender and race—are examined in this chapter. Both are held to be social constructions in that their meaning in everyday life is usually based on socially defined criteria or definitions, instead of biological phenomena. Knowledge produced about race and gender has as much or more to do with social issues, problems, and circumstances as it has with biology. This is consistent with the social constructionist argument that scientific knowledge and biological discourses about the body, health, and illness are produced through subjective, historically determined human interests, and are subject to change and reinterpretation. This chapter highlights intersectionality theory, which focuses on examining forms of discrimination and inequality stemming from gender, race, ethnicity, class, age, nation, and sexual orientation, and makes the key point that such variables are not simply individual characteristics but operate simultaneously at multiple levels in people's lives.

Guide to Critical Thinking

1. What is social construction theory?
2. Social constructionism has two main branches. How are they similar and how are they different?
3. Is gender a social construction? Explain.
4. What are the strengths and weaknesses of intersectionality theory?
5. Is race a social construction? Explain.
6. How does racism affect health?

Suggested Reading

Collins, Patricia Hill and Sirma Bilge. 2016. *Intersectionality*. Cambridge: Polity.
A summary of intersectionality theory.
Hill, Shirley A. 2016. *Inequality and African-American Health*. Bristol: Policy Press.
An excellent analysis of the social causes and processes affecting African American
   health from the past until the present.

References

Allport, Gordon. 1958. *The Nature of Prejudice*. Garden City, NY: Anchor.

Annandale, Ellen. 2014. *The Sociology of Health and Medicine*, 2nd ed. Cambridge: Polity.

Annandale, Ellen. 2016. "Health Status and Gender," in William Cockerham (ed.), *The New Blackwell Companion to Medical Sociology*. Oxford: Wiley Blackwell, pp. 97–112.

Annandale, Ellen and Judith Clark. 1996. "What is Gender? Feminist Theory and the Sociology of Human Reproduction." *Sociology of Health & Illness* 18(1):17–44.

Barker, Kristin K. 2005. *The Fibromyalgia Story: Medical Authority and Women's Worlds of Pain*. Philadelphia, PA: Temple University Press.

Bauer, Greta R. 2014. "Incorporating Intersectionality Theory into Population Health Research Methodology: Challenges and the Potential to Advance Health Equity." *Social Science & Medicine* 110:10–17.

Bauer, Greta and Ayden I. Scheim. 2019. "Methods for Intercategorical Intersectionality in Quantitative Research: Discrimination as a Mediator of Health Inequalities." *Social Science & Medicine* 226:225–35.

Becker, Howard. 1973. *Outsiders: Studies in the Sociology of Deviance*. New York: Free Press.

Berger, Peter L. and Thomas Luckmann. 1967. *The Social Construction of Reality: A Treatise in the Sociology of Knowledge*. New York: Anchor.

Bird, Chloe E. and Patricia P. Rieker. 2008. *Gender and Health: The Effects of Constrained Choices and Social Policies*. Cambridge: Cambridge University Press.

Blauner, Robert. 1972. *Racial Oppression in America*. New York: Harper & Row.

Blumer, Herbert. 1969. *Symbolic Interactionism: Perspective and Method*. Englewood Cliffs, NJ: Prentice-Hall.

Bowleg, Lisa. 2008. "When Black + Lesbian + Woman ≠ Black Lesbian Woman: The Methodological Challenges of Qualitative and Quantitative Intersectionality Research." *Sex Roles* 59:312–25.

Bradby, Hannah. 2012. *Medicine, Health and Society*. London: Sage.

Bradby, Hannah and James Y. Nazroo. 2016. "Health, Ethnicity, and Race," in William Cockerham (ed.), *The New Blackwell Companion to Medical Sociology*. Oxford: Wiley Blackwell, pp. 113–29.

Bratter, Jennifer L. and Bridget K. Gorman. 2011. "Is Discrimination an Equal Opportunity Risk? Racial Experiences, Socioeconomic Status, and Health Status among Black and White Adults." *Journal of Health and Social Behavior* 52(3):365–82.

Bury, M. R. 1986. "Social Constructionism and the Development of Medical Sociology." *Sociology of Health & Illness* 8(2):137–69.

Butler, Judith. 1990. *Gender Trouble: Feminism and the Subversion of Identity*. London: Routledge.

Choo, Hae Yeon and Myra Marx Ferree. 2010. "Practicing Intersectionality in Sociological Research." *Sociological Theory* 28(1):129–49.

Cockerham, William C. 2005. "Health Lifestyle Theory and the Convergence of Agency and Structure." *Journal of Health and Social Behavior* 46(1):51–67.

Cockerham, William C. 2013. "Bourdieu and an Update of Health Lifestyle Theory," in William Cockerham (ed.), *Medical Sociology on the Move: New Directions in Theory*. Dordrecht: Springer, pp. 127–54.

Cockerham, William C. 2017a. *Medical Sociology*, 14th ed. New York: Routledge.

Cockerham, William C. 2017b. *Sociology of Mental Disorder*, 10th ed. New York: Routledge.

Cockerham, William C., Bryant W. Hamby, Olena Hankivsky, Elizabeth H. Baker, and Setareh Rouhani. 2017. "Self-rated Health and Barriers to Healthcare in Ukraine: The Pivotal Role of Gender." *Communist and Post-Communist Studies* 50:53–63.

Collins, Patricia Hill. 1993. "Toward a New Vision: Race, Class, and Gender as Categories of Analysis and Connection." *Race, Sex, and Class* 1(1):25–45.

Collins, Patricia Hill. 2000. *Black Feminist Thought: Knowledge, Consciousness, and the Politics of Empowerment*, 2nd ed. New York: Routledge.

Collins, Patricia Hill. 2004. *Black Sexual Politics: African Americans, Gender, and the New Racism*. New York: Routledge.

Collins, Patricia Hill. 2015. "Intersectionality's Definitional Dilemmas." *Annual Review of Sociology* 41:1–20.

Collins, Patricia Hill. 2019. *Intersectionality as Critical Social Theory*. Durham, NC: Duke University Press.

Collins, Patricia Hill and Sirma Bilge. 2016. *Intersectionality*. Cambridge: Polity.

Conrad, Peter and Kristin K. Barker. 2010. "The Social Construction of Illness: Key Insights and Policy Implications." *Journal of Health and Social Behavior* 51(extra issue):S67–S79.

Cornell, Stephen and Douglas Hartmann. 2007. *Ethnicity and Race: Making Identities in a Changing World*, 2nd ed. Thousand Oaks, CA: Pine Forge Press.

Crenshaw, Kimberlé Williams. 1989. "Demarginalizing the Intersection of Race and Sex: A Black Feminist Critique of Anti-discrimination Doctrine, Feminist Theory, and Antiracist Politics." *University of Chicago Legal Forum* 1:132–67.

Delgado, Richard and Jean Stefancic. 2017. *Critical Race Theory*, 3rd ed. New York: New York University Press.

Dubrow, Joshua, 2010. *Why Should Social Scientists Account for Intersectionality in Quantitative Analysis of Survey Data?* Warsaw: Polish Academy of Sciences.

Durkheim, Émile. [1895] 1964. *The Rules of Sociological Method*. Glencoe, IL: Free Press.

Epstein, Steven. 2007. *Inclusion: The Politics of Difference in Medical Research*. Chicago, IL: University of Chicago Press.

Erving, Christy L. 2011. "Gender and Physical Health: A Study of African Americans and Caribbean Black Adults." *Journal of Health and Social Behavior* 52(3):383–99.

Feagin, Joe. 2006. *Systematic Racism: A History of Oppression*. New York: Routledge.

Feagin, Joe and Zinobia Bennefield. 2014. "Systemic Racism and U.S. Health Care." *Social Science & Medicine* 103:7–14.

Ferraro, Kenneth and Melissa Farmer. 1996. "Double Jeopardy to Health Hypothesis for African Americans: Analysis and Critique." *Journal of Health and Social Behavior* 37(1):27–43.

Ford, Chandra L. and Collins O. Airhihenbuwa. 2010. "Critical Race Theory, Race Equity, and Public Health: Toward Antiracism Praxis." *American Journal of Public Health* 100(51):S30–S34.

Foucault, Michel. 1965. *Madness and Civilization: A History of Insanity in an Age of Reason*. New York: Pantheon.

Foucault, Michel. 1973. *Birth of the Clinic*. London: Tavistock.

Frazer, Elizabeth. 2018. "Gender," in Bryan Turner (ed.), *The Wiley Blackwell Encyclopedia of Social Theory*, Vol. II. Oxford: Wiley Blackwell, pp. 914–16.

Freidson, Eliot. 1970. *Profession of Medicine*. New York: Dodd, Mead.

Gabe, Jonathan, Mike Bury, and Mary Ann Elston (eds.). 2004. *Key Concepts in Medical Sociology*. London: Sage.

Gkiouleka, Anna, Tim Huijts, Jason Beckfield, and Clare Bambra. 2018. "Understanding the Micro and Macro Politics of Health: Inequalities, Intersectionality & Institutions—A Research Agenda." *Social Science & Medicine* 200:92–8.

Green, Mark A., Clare R. Evans, and S.V. Subramanian. 2017. "Can Intersectionality Theory Enrich Population Health Research?" *Social Science & Medicine* 178:214–16.

Grollman, Eric Anthony. 2014. "Multiple Disadvantaged Statuses and Health: The Role of Multiple Forms of Discrimination." *Journal of Health and Social Behavior* 55(1):3–19.

Hancock, Ange-Marie. 2007. "When Multiplication Doesn't Equal Quick Addition: Examining Intersectionality as a Research Paradigm." *Perspectives on Politics* 5:63–79.

Hankivsky, Olena (ed.). 2011. *Health Inequities in Canada: Intersectional Frameworks and Practices*. Vancouver: University of British Columbia Press.

Hankivsky, Olena. 2012. "Women's Health, Men's Health and Gender and Health: Implications of Intersectionality." *Social Science & Medicine* 74:1712–20.

Hankivsky, Olena, and Renee Cormier. 2009. *Intersectionality: Moving Women's Health Forward*. Vancouver: Women's Health Research Network.

Hankivsky, Olena and Daniel Grace. 2015. "Understanding and Emphasizing Differences and Intersectionality," in S. Heese-Biber and R. Johnson (eds.), *Oxford Handbook of Mixed and Multimethod Research*. New York: Oxford University Press, pp. 110–27.

Hill, Shirley A. 2016. *Inequality and African-American Health*. Bristol: Policy Press.

Hinote, Brian P. and Jason Adam Wasserman. 2017. *Social and Behavioral Science for Health Professionals*. Lanham, MD: Rowman and Littlefield.

Hinze, Susan W. 2004. "'Am I Being Over-Sensitive?' Women's Experience of Sexual Harassment During Medical Training." *Health* 8(1):107–27.

Hinze, Susan W., Jielu Lin, and Tanetta E. Andersson. 2012. "Can We Capture the Intersections? Older Black Women, Education, and Health." *Women's Health Issues* 22–1:e91–e98.

Horwitz, Allan V. 2002. *Creating Mental Illness*. Chicago, IL: University of Chicago Press.

Horwitz, Allan V. 2013. "The Sociological Study of Mental Illness: A Critique and Synthesis of Four Perspectives," in Carol Aneshensel, Jo Phelan, and Alex Bierman (eds.), *Handbook of the Sociology of Mental Disorder*, 2nd ed. Dordrecht: Springer, pp. 95–112.

Horwitz, Allan V. and Jerome C. Wakefield. 2012. *All We Have to Fear: Psychiatry's Transformation of Natural Anxieties into Mental Disorder*. New York: Oxford University Press.

Keith, Verna M. and Cedric Herring. 1991. "Skin Tone and Stratification in the Black Community." *American Journal of Sociology* 97(3):760–78.

Landry, Bart. 2007. *Race, Gender and Class: Theory and Methods of Analysis.* Upper Saddle River, NJ: Pearson Prentice-Hall.

Lemelle, Anthony J. 2011. "Conceptual, Operational, and Theoretical Overview of African American Health Related Disparities for Social and Behavioral Interventions," in Anthony Lemelle, Wornie Reed, and Sandra Taylor (eds.), *Handbook of African American Health.* New York: Springer, pp. 3–34.

Link, Bruce G. and Jo C. Phelan. 1995. "Social Conditions as Fundamental Causes of Disease." *Journal of Health and Social Behavior* 35(extra issue):80–94.

Lorber, Judith. 1997. *Gender and the Social Construction of Illness.* Thousand Oaks, CA: Sage.

McCall, Leslie. 2005. "The Complexity of Intersectionality." *Signs: Journal of Women in Culture and Society* 30:1771–800.

McKinlay, John. 1996. "Some Contributions from the Social System to Gender Inequalities in Heart Disease." *Journal of Health and Social Behavior* 37(1):1–26.

Monk, Ellis P., Jr. 2015. "The Cost of Color: Skin Color, Discrimination, and Health among African-Americans." *American Journal of Sociology* 121(2):396–444.

Moody, Heather, Joe T. Darden, and Bruce Wm. Pigozzi. 2018. "The Racial Gap in Childhood Blood Lead Levels Related to Socioeconomic Position of Residence in Metropolitan Detroit." *Sociology of Race and Ethnicity* 2(2):200–18.

Nettleton, Sarah. 2013. *The Sociology of Health and Illness,* 2nd ed. Cambridge: Polity.

Nowakowski, Alexandra C. H. and J. E. Sumerau. 2019. "Reframing Health and Illness: A Collaborative Autoethnography on the Experience of Health and Illness Transformations in the Life Course." *Sociology of Health & Illness* 41(4):723–39.

Olafsdottir, Sigrun. 2013. "Social Construction and Health," in William Cockerham (ed.), *Medical Sociology on the Move: New Directions in Theory.* Dordrecht: Springer, pp. 41–59.

Omi, Michael and Howard Winant. 2015. *Racial Formation in the United States,* 3rd ed. New York: Routledge.

Phelan, Jo C. and Bruce G. Link. 2013. "Fundamental Cause Theory," in William Cockerham (ed.), *Medical Sociology on the Move: New Directions in Theory.* Dordrecht: Springer, pp. 105–26.

Phelan, Jo C. and Bruce G. Link. 2015. "Is Racism a Fundamental Cause of Inequalities in Health?" *Annual Review of Sociology* 41:311–30.

Richardson, Liana J. and Tyson H. Brown. 2016. "(En)gendering Racial Disparities in Health Trajectories: A Life Course and Intersectional Analysis." *SSM-Population Health* 2:425–35.

Riska, Elianne. 2016. "Health Professions and Occupations," in William Cockerham (ed.), *The New Blackwell Companion to Medical Sociology.* Oxford: Wiley Blackwell, pp. 337–54.

Scambler, Graham. 2009. "Health-related Stigma." *Sociology of Health & Illness* 41:431–55.

Scheff, Thomas J. 1999. *Being Mentally Ill: A Sociological Theory,* 3rd ed. Chicago, IL: Aldine.

Scheim, Ayden I. and Greta Bauer. 2019a. "The Intersectional Discrimination Index: Development and Validation of Measures of Self-Reported Enacted and Anticipated Discrimination for Intercategorical Analysis." *Social Science & Medicine* 226:225–35.

Scheim, Ayden I. and Greta Bauer. 2019b. "Advancing Quantitative Intersectionality Research Methods: Intracategorical and Intercategorical Approaches to Shared and Differential Constructs." *Social Science & Medicine* 226:235–45.

Shim, Janet K. 2014. *Heart Sick: The Politics of Risk, Inequality, and Heart Disease.* New York: New York University Press.

Sims, Mario, Ana V. Diez-Roux, Shawn Boykin, Daniel Sarpong, Samson Y. Gebeab, Sharon B. Wyatt, DeMarc Hickson, Marinelle Payton, Lynette Ekunwe, and Herman A. Taylor. 2011. "The Socioeconomic Gradient of Diabetes Prevalence, Awareness, Treatment, and Control Among African Americans in the Jackson Heart Study." *Annals of Epidemiology* 21:892–98.

Sims, Mario, Ana V. Diez-Roux, Amanda Dudley, Samson Gebreab, Sharon B. Wyatt, Marino A. Bruce, Sherman A, James, Jennifer C. Robinson, David R. Williams, and Herman A. Taylor. 2012. "Perceived Discrimination and Hypertension among African Americans in the Jackson Heart Study." *American Journal of Public Health* 102(52):S258–65.

Sims, Mario, Ana V. Diez-Roux, Samson Y. Gebreab, Allison Brenner, Patricia Dubbert, Sharon Wyatt, Marino Bruce, DeMarc Hickson, Tom Payne, and Herman Taylor. 2016. "Perceived Discrimination is Associated with Health Behaviours among African-Americans in the Jackson Heart Study." *Journal of Epidemiology and Community Health* 70(2):187–94.

Turner, Bryan. 2004. *The New Medical Sociology.* New York: W. W. Norton.

Varcoe, Collen, Bernadette Pauly, and Shari Laliberte. 2011. "Intersectionality, Justice, and Influencing Policy," in Olena Hankivsky (ed.), *Health Inequities in Canada: Intersectional Frameworks and Practices.* Vancouver: University of British Columbia Press, pp. 112–27.

Veenstra, Gerry. 2009. "Racialized Identity and Health in Canada: Results from a Nationally Representative Survey." *Social Science & Medicine* 69:538–42.

Veenstra, Gerry. 2011. "Race, Gender, Class, and Sexual Orientation: Intersecting Axes of Inequality and Self-rated Health in Canada." *International Journal for Equity in Health* 10:3, https://doi.org/10.1186/1475-9276-10-3.

Veenstra, Gerry. 2013. "Race, Gender, Class, Sexuality (RGCS) and Hypertension." *Social Science & Medicine* 89:16–24.

Weber, Max. [1922] 1978. *Economy and Society*, Vol. 1. Berkeley, CA: University of California Press.

Williams, David R. 2012. "Miles to Go Before We Sleep: Racial Inequities in Health." *Journal of Health and Social Behavior* 53(3): 279–95.

Williams, David R. and Selina A. Mohammed. 2009. "Discrimination and Racial Disparities in Health: Evidence and Needed Research." *Journal of Behavioral Medicine* 32:20–47.

Williams, David R. and Selina A. Mohammed. 2013. "Racism and Health I: Pathways and Scientific Evidence." *American Behavioral Scientist* 57: 1552–73.

Williams, David R. and Michelle Sternthal. 2010. "Understanding Racial-Ethnic Disparities in Health: Sociological Contributions." *Journal of Health and Social Behavior* 51(extra issue): S15–S27.

Chapter 10

Health Lifestyle Theory

The primary means by which individuals manufacture health or, conversely, undermine or destroy it, is through their lifestyle. Whether or not they exercise, what foods and beverages they consume, whether they smoke, drink alcohol, engage in drug abuse, visit physicians for checkups and preventive care, or conduct other health-related activities comprise a person's health lifestyle. Such lifestyles can be either positive or negative or a mixture of these two binary opposites, but over time they either promote or harm health. Health behavior is the activity undertaken by individuals for the purpose of maintaining or enhancing their health, preventing health problems, or achieving a positive body image. It is what individuals do to keep themselves as healthy as possible. The aggregate form of such behaviors constitutes a health lifestyle. Everyone has one.

Health lifestyle theory, formulated by the author (Cockerham 2005, 2013a, 2013b; Hinote 2015), provides a theoretical model of this form of behavior. Previously, no such theory existed. It became apparent, however, that such a theory was needed as the epidemiological transition that had taken place in the twentieth century shifted the major causes of human mortality from communicable to chronic diseases that in many instances were linked to health lifestyle practices. This circumstance carries with it the revelation that the ultimate responsibility for one's health falls on one's own self through healthy living.

In past periods of history, when life expectancy was shorter, a person's health was more or less taken for granted; that is, an individual was either naturally healthy or unhealthy and that was simply the way life had turned out for that person. This situation is now different with a majority of people expecting to live to advanced ages and in the process becoming more susceptible to chronic diseases associated with lifestyles. Chronic diseases—such as heart disease, cancer, and diabetes—cannot be cured by medical treatment and certain negative lifestyle practices can cause these afflictions and end life. Today health can be viewed as an achievement—something that people are supposed to work at to enhance the longevity and quality of their life or risk chronic illness and premature death if they do not. This means that having a healthy lifestyle is not just linked to religious guidelines and health-conscious individuals and groups, but has become a societal norm although not practiced normatively throughout society. Instead there are distinct patterns of health lifestyle participation largely arranged along a social class gradient that brings sociological theorizing into play.

Agency Versus Structure

Of particular importance in constructing theory is the relative influence of agency and structure. When applied to health lifestyles, the question becomes: Are the decisions people make with respect to food, exercise, smoking, and the like largely a matter of unfettered choice or are they principally influenced by social structural variables such as class position and gender? One might think that lifestyle practices are determined by individual choice. That is, a person either chooses to pursue a healthy lifestyle or not, and this is basically the tale to be told. On the surface, such a decision would appear to reside solely in the realm of free will. But is this really the case? Are health and other lifestyles engaged in by individuals without reference to the social structures in their lives? If so, then why do lifestyles tend to cluster in specific patterns reflecting significant differences by class, gender, and other structural variables? Clearly, something in addition to free choice is involved. Therefore, health lifestyle theory takes the position that lifestyles are shaped into distinct configurations from the top down by structural influences that people adopt as their own. In this scenario, structure channels health and other lifestyle practices down particular pathways instead of others. People still retain the option to choose, but such choices are generally made along class lines and in accordance with other structural influences that might be relevant for those choosing.

To assign individuals complete freedom in their lifestyle choices overlooks the pervasive boundaries placed on those choices by the social structures in their lives. As Graham Scambler (2018:95) points out, "there is never a non-structured social world." Individual choices in *all* circumstances are limited by what is available and considered socially appropriate (Bauman 1999). Structure is therefore present as guidelines in every social context. While agency theorists, as discussed in Chapter 1, maintain that agency will never be completely determined by structure, it can be repeated that "there is no hypothetical moment in which agency actually gets 'free' of structure" (Emirbayer and Mische 1998:1004).

Agency is important, but it seems social structural conditions can nevertheless act on individuals and model their lifestyle patterns in particular ways. Agency allows them to accept, reject or modify these patterns, but structure limits the quantity and quality of the options available. Therefore, agency is not the whole story. In some situations, structure is dominant (Stead et al. 2011; Williams 2003). Structure invariably has a role in lifestyle decisions and it is usually the *interaction* between agency and structure as a dialectical process that is decisive in determining a lifestyle's features (Cockerham 2005, 2013a, 2013b).

Consequently, in formulating a sociological theory of health lifestyles, the relative contributions of agency and structure need to be considered. A person's capacity for self-direction underlies the operation of all forms of agency. Symbolic interaction theory describes this very process when it discusses people constructing their social behavior on the basis of their definitions and interpretations of the social situations they find themselves in (Blumer 1969). However, in examining the theoretical logic of the classical theorists in sociology, Jeffrey Alexander (1983, vol. 1:105) found that the basic question for sociology's founders was not how social arrangements are constructed from negotiations among individuals, but rather how social theories that accept the collective character of these arrangements retain a concept of individual freedom. Free will in his view is not irreconcilable with some form of structural determinism. As Alexander (1983:105) puts it:

> The notion of collective order actually need never deny free will in an individual case; it can and usually does refer to the probability that individuals will act in a patterned fashion, not to the certainty that any specific individual will so act. As such, it can accept a notion of determinism as compatible with the widest latitude for any given individual. To believe otherwise is to adopt a reified [misleading] conception of individual freedom.

Therefore, there can be alternative acts on the part of individuals contrary to a general pattern of lifestyles for their particular social group, but that pattern remains in place nonetheless because it is representative of what people in that group commonly do. Knowing a person's lifestyle explains a great deal about that person's social background and identity. In this chapter, the theorizing of Max Weber, Anthony Giddens, and Pierre Bourdieu that health lifestyle theory builds on will be reviewed, followed by a presentation of the theory and the current research associated with it.

Box 10.1 William C. Cockerham

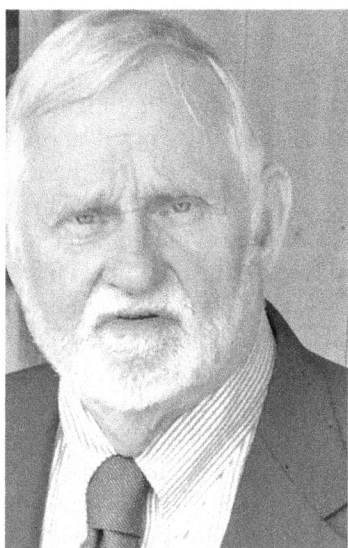

Image 10.1 William C. Cockerham

Health lifestyle theory was born of necessity. One was needed but did not exist even though such lifestyles are an inherent feature of everyday life. While on the sociology and medical school faculties at the University of Illinois at Urbana-Champaign, I started doing research in the late 1980s with a sociology colleague, Günther Lüschen (1930–2015). Initially we conducted a survey in Illinois and another in Northrhine-Westphalia in West Germany (Cockerham, Kunz, and Lüschen 1988), then obtained funding from various sources to extend it in 1990–1991 in West Germany and to four other countries (Belgium, France, Netherlands, and Spain) in the European Union as the Western European Study of Health (WESH) Project (Lüschen et al. 1995). We coordinated the study out of the Technical University of Aachen in Germany where Lüschen had moved to head the Institute of Sports Science. The best theoretical framework available in the beginning was Max Weber's ([1922] 1978) original conceptualization of lifestyles, later incorporating it with Anthony Giddens' (1991) work on identity and lifestyles in late modernity (Cockerham, Abel, and Lüschen 1993).

I first took the view, consistent with Weber, that health lifestyles were a matter of personal choice (agency). People made their own decisions, for example, about whether they wanted to smoke. I didn't smoke and it was my choice, but there was a clue out there that I didn't immediately recognize: No one in my extended family smoked, in the present or near past. No one. Were structural influences like kinship really that important? It turned out they are.

At the University of California at Berkeley, which I attended after getting my undergraduate degree at the University of Oklahoma and active duty in the Army, I studied symbolic interaction theory as a graduate student with Herbert Blumer and Norman Denzin. These two scholars, along with Anselm Strauss, a leading symbolic interactionist and medical sociologist, who worked across the bay in San Francisco at the UC Medical Center and helped with my Ph.D. dissertation—were a strong influence in shaping my view of sociology. Consistent with symbolic interaction, I favored agency over structure.

But there was a problem with an agency approach. Our survey responses of health practices in the Illinois and WESH studies formed distinct constellations of behavior along class lines. That is, class-specific patterns, say those of the middle class or working class in one country, generally matched those of the same class in other countries. If health lifestyles were largely a matter of free choice, such patterns would not be so obvious. It was clear that membership in a particular social class shaped the health lifestyles of the people in that class in powerful ways and different from people in other classes.

This meant structure was decisive. After I moved to the University of Alabama at Birmingham to help start a Ph.D. program in medical sociology, Thomas Abel (University of Bern, Switzerland), Alfred Rütten (University of Erlangen-Nuremberg, Germany), and I published several papers in the 1990s on various dimensions of health lifestyles (Cockerham, Rütten, and Abel 1997). There still was no general theory of health lifestyles anywhere, despite various ideas and approaches.

A theory specific to health lifestyles was clearly needed, so I added Pierre Bourdieu's (1984) notion of habitus to a model and tested it with data obtained in Russia and Eastern Europe from another project (Cockerham 1999) along with data from the Russian Longitudinal Monitoring Survey (Cockerham 2000; Cockerham, Snead, and DeWaal 2002), the Centers for Disease Control and Prevention (CDC) in the United States (Snead and Cockerham 2002), and the Lifestyles, Living Conditions, and Health (LLH) in the Commonwealth of Independent States of the former Soviet Union Project, funded by the Copernicus Program of the European Union (Cockerham, Hinote, and Abbott 2006; Hinote, Cockerham, and Abbott 2009).

The reason Russia was important was because of a long-term (1965–2012) decline in male life expectancy in which unhealthy lifestyles had a key role. Russia was a natural laboratory for the adverse effects of health lifestyles on longevity. The *Journal of Health and Social Behavior* published the theoretical model in 2005.

Lifestyles: Basic Concepts

Although lifestyles are a generally recognized marker of a person's social identity and class position, few theoretical concepts about it previously existed. One reason may have been the influence of Thorstein Veblen's ([1899] 1994) classic, the *Theory of the Leisure Class*, that affixed the term "lifestyle" to modes of leisure adopted by the upper class. The expression "lifestyle" became synonymous with upper-class styles of living and what many considered trivial forms of consumerism by the affluent. Only the wealthy had the time and the money to have a "style" in their lives and so the term was generally applied just to them. As we now know, it was a major oversight to suppose that lifestyles are confined to those in the most advantaged material circumstances. Even the most underprivileged have a lifestyle (Giddens 1991).

Weber

Max Weber ([1922] 1978) provides the deepest insight into the lifestyle concept among the classical theorists and, in doing so, made three lasting contributions. First, he associated lifestyles with status groups, noting that people in such groups shared a similar lifestyle distinct from other groups. To be a member of a group and share its status, a person was expected to also adopt its style of life. Even though an individual has a "lifestyle," lifestyles themselves in his view are a collective phenomenon, reflecting patterns of living characteristic of particular groups or social classes. Although Weber often favored an individualist and agency-oriented view of social action, he did not consider such actions as the uncoordinated practices of disconnected individuals (Kalberg 1994). Instead, he saw social action in terms of regularities and uniformities repeated by numerous actors over time that formed general patterns of behavior. His focus was on the way in which people act in *concert*, not individually.

The bridge from agency to structure for Weber was his notion of "ideal types," consisting of structural entities like his concept of bureaucracy or macro-level processes such as the spread of formal rationality in Western society that allowed him to make general statements about collective forms of social behavior (Kalberg 1994). Ideal types consist of logical constructions of patterned forms of social action that can be used for comparative purposes as examples of social phenomenon in the real world. For instance, in *The Protestant Ethic and the Spirit of Capitalism* (1958), Weber viewed structure in this instance in an essentially "top-down" manner by describing how a social institution (Calvinist religion) and an economic system (capitalism) were powerful forces in shaping the outlook and behavior of individuals (Sibeon 2004). In order for a style of life to emerge that could adapt to the peculiarities of capitalism and come to dominate others, Weber (1958:55) finds "that it had to originate somewhere, and not in isolated individuals alone, but as a way of life common to whole groups of [people]."

Second, Weber pointed out that lifestyles are based not on what people produce, but on what they consume. Consumption is not independent of production, however. As George Ritzer and William Yagatich (2012) note, the distinction between production and consumption is false in that all acts invariably involve both processes. In order to consume something, it has to be first produced and the process of production often requires the consumption of something. In the case of health lifestyles, consumption seems to hold sway over production. Even though it can be argued that positive health lifestyles produce good health, ultimately that health is used or consumed. Therefore, lifestyle differences between groups are primarily based on their relationship to the means of consumption in a society. Moreover, while economic modes of production set the parameters within which styles of consumption occur, it does not determine specific forms of it. This is because the consumption of goods and services conveys a *social* meaning that displays the status and social identity of the consumer. Consumption can therefore be regarded as a set of social and cultural practices that *establish* differences between groups and classes (Bourdieu 1984).

And third, Weber's most important contribution to conceptualizing lifestyles in sociological terms is to note the dialectical interplay between choices and chances (Cockerham, Rütten, and Abel 1997). What Weber calls "life chances" is defined by Ralf Dahrendorf (1979:73) as the probability of finding satisfaction for one's needs, desires, and interests that are anchored in structural conditions. Life chances are therefore a proxy for structure and life choices represent agency. Choices and chances work off each other in tandem to determine a lifestyle. People have necessities, wants, and social identities they match up with their chances in life and select a lifestyle consistent with their social position. Despite the powerful influence of structure as a "normative force" in individual acts, however, Weber accords choice the greater role.

What Weber provides us that is central to formulating a theory of health lifestyles is that: (1) such lifestyles are collective, health-related practices characteristic of particular groups and classes; (2) while lifestyles produce health, the aim of this activity is ultimately one of consumption as people use their health for some end, such as a longer life, work, increased vitality, enhanced enjoyment of their physical body, or a good physical appearance; and (3) the interplay of agency and structure establish and shape the practices that comprise their expression and form.

Giddens

Another major contribution to health lifestyle theory comes from Anthony Giddens who described in *Modernity and Self-Identity* (1991) how late modernity influences contemporary lifestyles by reducing constraints and promoting a diversity of choices. Global transformations of the sense of time, space, and distance, combined with certain disembedding factors (such as increasingly sophisticated and abstract money systems, the widespread availability of rapid social and commercial communications, and the penetration of technical knowledge throughout society), are credited with causing constant change. In such circumstances, people are likely to be pushed by changing social situations into choosing a particular lifestyle that connects their options to a more or less ordered pattern of choices providing consistency for their self-identity. Giddens therefore defines a lifestyle as an integrated set of practices which an individual embraces, not only because such practices satisfy utilitarian needs, but because they give material form to a particular narrative of self-identity.

Giddens also maintains that even persons in the lowest social classes have some choice because no culture, in his view, eliminates choice altogether in day-to-day affairs. The poor have distinctive cultural styles and activities that require choices, such as trying to cope with disadvantaged conditions. While Giddens does not overlook the influence of external sources on the lifestyles of individuals generally, he favors agency over structure in lifestyle selection because of the role of choice in the construction of self-identity. Giddens (1984) contributes to our understanding of structure with his notion of the *duality* of structure, namely that structures are both constraining and enabling at the same time. That is, structures set limits on what people can choose, but they also provide resources (e.g., status, class position, finances) that can help them realize their choices. This constraining and enabling function guides people into lifestyles that are appropriate and realistic for them.

What we primarily gain from Giddens in developing a theory of health lifestyles is recognition of (1) late modernity's role in fostering a diversity of lifestyle choices, (2) the necessity of having to choose, (3) the tendency of choices to cluster in particular patterns, (4) the role of lifestyles in expressing the self-identity of the individual, and (5) the dual function of structure as a constrainer or enabler of choices.

Bourdieu

Unlike Weber and Giddens, Pierre Bourdieu shows a clear preference for structure over agency as seen in his strong emphasis upon the effects of class hierarchies on behavior. The seminal study detailing class as the most decisive variable in the determination of health lifestyles is Bourdieu's book *Distinction* (1984). Based on a survey of French upper-middle-class professionals and working-class respondents that included sports preferences and eating habits, Bourdieu found the working class to be more attentive to maintaining the strength of the male body than its shape, and to favor food that is cheap, nutritious, and abundant. In contrast, the professional class preferred food that is tasty, healthy, light, and low in calories. As for leisure sports such as sailing, skiing, golf, tennis, and horseback riding, he found a stratified system and noted that the working class not only faces economic barriers, but also social barriers in the form of hidden entry requirements of family tradition, obligatory dress and behavior, and childhood socialization. Additionally, these sports were usually practiced in exclusive locations and required investments of money, time, and training that the working class lacked. The working class, in contrast, opted for sports that are popular with the general public and accessible to all classes. These are sports like soccer, wrestling, and boxing that feature strength, endurance, and violence.

Consequently, Bourdieu formulated the notion of "distance from necessity" that emerges as a key explanation of class differences in lifestyles. He points out that the more distant a person is from having to acquire economic necessity, the greater the freedom and time that person has to develop and refine personal tastes in line with a more privileged class status. Lower social strata, in turn, tend to adopt the tastes consistent with their class position, in which obtaining items of necessity (such as inexpensive foods and affordable housing) is paramount. For example, Bourdieu (1984:177) observes that as one rises in class position, the proportion of income spent on food diminishes, and that within the food budget, the proportion spent on heavy, fattening foods, which are also cheap—pasta, potatoes, bacon, and pork— declines, whereas an increasing proportion is spent on leaner, lighter, non-fattening foods and especially fresh fruits and vegetables.

Bourdieu finds that social classes not dominated by the ordinary interests and urgencies of making a daily living claim superiority in social and cultural tastes over those who have only fundamental levels of material well-being. Cultivating a taste in expensive wines, for example, typically signifies higher status. "As the objective distance from necessity grows," states Bourdieu (1984:55), "life-style increasingly becomes the product of what Weber calls a 'stylization of life', a systematic commitment which orients and organizes the most diverse practices—the choice of a vintage or a cheese or the decoration of a holiday home in the country." The greater the social distance from struggling to obtain necessity, the greater the refinement of lifestyle practices. The relevance of the "distance from necessity concept" is seen in health lifestyles where classes higher on the social scale have the time and resources to adopt and cultivate the healthiest practices.

The most important component of Bourdieu's theorizing with respect to lifestyles is his use of the concept of habitus. There is a belief among some in sociology that Bourdieu invented habitus, but this is incorrect (Wacquant 2016). Habitus has a long history. The origin of the term is found in the work of the Greek philosopher Aristotle around 350 B.C. that can be translated as a "disposition" and refers to a psychic urge to do the right thing (Hinote 2014; Wacquant 2016). The medieval scholar Thomas Aquinas in 1269 provided a Latin translation of this concept which established its name as "habitus" and centuries later in 1899, Veblen depicted its meaning as "habits of the mind." The modern notion of habitus originates with the German philosopher Edmund Husserl ([1952] 1989:266–93) who used habitus as a term in 1913 to describe *habitual action* that is intuitively followed and anticipated. Prior to World War II, habitus appears in the work of Weber, Émile Durkheim, Marcel Mauss (Durkheim's nephew), and Norbert Elias in sociology, but was not given special attention, used infrequently, and as a concept was not central to any theoretical perspective (Cockerham 2018).

Bourdieu changed all of this. More than anyone else, he expanded and popularized the notion of habitus in contemporary sociological theory. Among other uses, Bourdieu (1977:72–95; 1984:169–225) employed the notion of habitus to serve as his core explanation for the agency–structure relationship in lifestyle dispositions. Bourdieu (1990:53) defines habitus as

> systems of durable, transposable dispositions, structured structures predisposed to operate as structuring structures, that is, as principles which generate and organize practices and representations that can be objectively adapted to their outcomes without presupposing a conscious aiming at ends or an express mastery of the operations necessary in order to attain them.

Put another way, the habitus serves as a cognitive map or set of perceptions that routinely guides and evaluates a person's choices and options.

According to German sociologists Hans Joas and Wolfgang Knöbl (2009:382–3), people learn a particular schemata of thinking, perceiving, and acting that generally enables them to respond easily to different situations and solve practical tasks. This schemata is the habitus and one of the reasons why social life is so regular and predictable. The habitus provides enduring dispositions toward acting deemed appropriate by a person in particular social situations and settings. Included are dispositions that can be carried out even without giving them a great deal of thought in advance. They are simply habitual ways of acting when performing routine tasks.

The influence of exterior social structures are incorporated into the habitus, as well as the individual's own inclinations, preferences, and interpretations. The dispositions that result not only reflect established normative patterns of social behavior, but they also encompass action that is habitual and even intuitive. Through selective perception the habitus shapes aspirations and expectations into what Bourdieu calls "categories of the probable" that impose perceptual boundaries on dispositions and the potential for action. "As an acquired system of generative schemes," observes Bourdieu (1990:55), "the *habitus* makes possible the free production of all the thoughts, perceptions, actions, inherent in the particular conditions of its production—and only those." Thus the habitus has perceptual boundaries. One can only know what one knows and act accordingly.

When Bourdieu speaks of the internalization of class conditions and their transformation into personal dispositions toward action, he is describing conditions similar to Weber's concept of life chances that determine materially, socially, and culturally what is probable, possible, or impossible for a member of a particular social class or group (Swartz 1997:104). Individuals who internalize similar life chances share the same habitus because, as Bourdieu (1977:85) explains, they are more likely to have similar shared experiences:

> Though it is impossible for *all* members of the same class (or even two of them) to have the same experiences, in the same order, it is certain that each member of the same class is more likely than any member of another class to have been confronted with the situations most frequent for members of that class.

As a result, there is a high degree of affinity in lifestyle choices among members of the same class. Bourdieu maintains that while they may depart from class standards, personal styles are never more than a deviation from a style of a class that relates back to the common style by its difference.

Even though Bourdieu allows agency some autonomy (e.g., agents are determined only to the extent they determine themselves), his emphasis on structure with respect to routine operations of the habitus clearly delineates a lesser role for agency. Some have therefore argued that Bourdieu strips agency of much of its critical reflexive character and is, in fact, determinist even though he denies it (Bohman 1999). Alexander (1995:136) went so far as to label habitus "a Trojan horse of determinism." Yet Bourdieu, in turn, rejected depictions of habitus as exclusively deterministic. He states, for example, that social agents are not "particles" mechanically pushed and pulled about by external forces, nor are they mere structural "*Trägers*" (a German word he used for bearers of heavy loads); rather, it seemed to him

> that the concept of habitus—long outmoded despite a number of occasional uses—was the best one to signify that desire to escape from the philosophy of consciousness without annulling the agent in its true role of practical operator of constructions of the real.
>
> (Bourdieu 1996:180)

Bryan Turner and Stephen Wainwright (2003:273) agree and find that Bourdieu gives "full recognition" to "agency through his notions of strategy and practices," while illustrating the powerful role of institutions and resources "in shaping, constraining, and producing human agency." British medical sociologist Simon Williams (1995) likewise defends Bourdieu by pointing out that the habitus is not a barrier to choice and instead his perspective accounts for the relative durability of differences in lifestyles between social classes.

I would argue that the *process* of experience rescues Bourdieu's concept of habitus from charges of determinism. Through experience, agency acquires new information and rationales for prompting creativity and change by way of the habitus. As Bourdieu (Bourdieu and Wacquant 1992:133) explains, even though experiences confirm habitus, since there is a high probability that most people encounter circumstances that are consistent with those that originally fashioned it, the habitus nevertheless "is an *open system of dispositions* that is constantly subjected to experiences, and therefore constantly affected by them in a way that reinforces or modifies its structures." Thus the habitus can be creative and initiate changes in dispositions, although this potential is not stressed in Bourdieu's work.

While dispositions toward practices originate in the habitus, the practices themselves are carried out in social contexts that Bourdieu conceptualizes as "fields." Fields are networks or configurations of objective relations (domination, subordination, etc.) between social positions (Bourdieu and Wacquant 1992). A field therefore constitutes a structured social space or what Bourdieu describes as an "arena" in which people and institutions use their capital—economic, cultural, and social assets—to maneuver for advantage in a hierarchical structure of relationships. Amounts and types of capital determine positions in the hierarchy relative to others in the same field. Some positions are clearly more powerful and so the power relations of a field typically shape the interaction that takes place within it. Swedish medical sociologist Peter Korp (2008) maintains that healthy lifestyles can be viewed as the habitual practices of groups that dominate social fields where healthy living is considered important. The opposite could be the case in fields with different power dynamics. It is in fields that agency would most likely come into play in Bourdieu's scheme (Veenstra and Burnett 2014).

Bourdieu calls for the rejection of theories that either explicitly or implicitly claim that the weight of structure on individuals takes away their behavioral options. This assertion shows him opposing determinism, although he also maintains that the rejection of mechanistic theories of behavior does not imply that we should bestow exclusive power on some creative free will. The dispositions generated by the habitus tend to be compatible, in his view, with the behavioral parameters set by the wider society; therefore, usual and practical modes of behaving—not unpredictable novelty—typically prevail. Consequently, Bourdieu emphasizes structure more than agency even though he accords agency the capacity to direct behavior; otherwise, his perspective largely accounts for routine behaviors that people enact without having to analyze or even think much about unless deeper attention is required.

Bourdieu's major contributions to our understanding of health lifestyles therefore fall into three major areas: (1) his concept of the "distance from necessity" as the origin of class differences in lifestyle practices, (2) identifying the role of habitus in creating and reproducing lifestyles, and (3) emphasizing how structure, or in Weberian terms, life chances, determine lifestyle choices. He is at his best in analyzing how lifestyles reflect differences between social classes.

The merit of Bourdieu's (1984) approach is that he maintains there is a structural dimension to lifestyle practices rather than individuals making random or uncoordinated choices on their own. What he accomplished was to bring discussions of structure back into the forefront of contemporary theoretical discourse. These structures, especially class position, actively influence and potentially determine behavioral outcomes through a person's subjective interpretation of their circumstances (Swartz 1997). Bourdieu advances a structural theory of social practices that connects individual action to culture, structure, and power relationships with his notions of capital and field that influence the individual externally and habitus that internalizes the influence of external structures within the individual's own behavioral repertoire. From my perspective, Bourdieu's concept of habitus is central to a theory of health lifestyles as it provides the individual with the social context and parameters or boundaries for his or her choices that channel that person along a particular line of behavior as opposed to others that might be chosen.

A Theory of Health Lifestyles

Before presenting a theory of health lifestyles, the first step is to define it. My definition is as follows: health lifestyles are collective patterns of health-related behavior based on choices from options available to people according to their life chances. This view incorporates the dialectical relationship between life choices and life chances proposed by Weber ([1922:531–9] 1978:926–39) and the duality of structure suggested by Giddens (1987:60–1). While health and other lifestyle choices are voluntary, life chances—which represent structure, especially class position—either empower or constrain choices as choices and chances combine to determine lifestyle outcomes. That is, a person has the capability of choosing his or her lifestyle, but the choices are limited by what is possible and strongly influenced by the style common to one's class position, age, gender, and the like. The theory is therefore based on the premise that health lifestyles are not the uncoordinated behaviors of disconnected individuals, but rather are personal routines that merge with those of other people into an aggregate form that is characteristic of specific groups and classes. The theoretical model is shown in Figure 10.1. The arrows between boxes indicate hypothesized causal relationships.

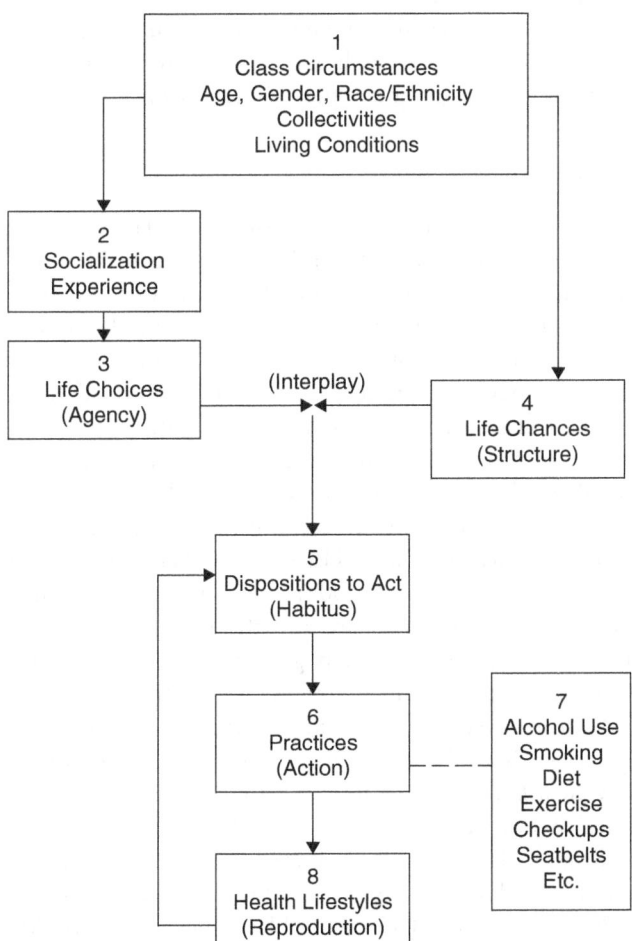

Figure 10.1 Cockerham's Health Lifestyle Model

Beginning with Box 1 in Figure 10.1, four categories of structural variables are listed that have the capacity to shape health lifestyles: (1) class circumstances, (2) age, gender, and race/ethnicity, (3) collectivities, and (4) living conditions. What is meant by "capacity to shape" is that each of these categories can affect the lifestyle choices made by individuals. They do so in ways suggested by Zygmunt Bauman (1999:72) in that they provide an *agenda of choices* (a set of available choices, but the composition of the set itself is not always for the chooser to decide) and the *code of choosing* (social rules or norms that tell the chooser what is appropriate or inappropriate). In the first instance, structural conditions, not the individual, establish the range of choices available for the person to choose from; in the second, structural conditions provide the rank order of preferences for the individual. For example, an individual's class circumstances determine what is available to choose from and what *should* be chosen. This starting point suggests that the model is one of downward conflation; however, this is not entirely the case, since as will be discussed, agency enters the model in Box 3.

Class Circumstances

The first category of structural variables in Box 1 is class circumstances, which appears to be the most powerful influence of all on lifestyle forms. Not only is this emphasized by Weber and Bourdieu, but also supported by practically every study. These studies confirm that the lifestyles of the upper and upper-middle classes are the healthiest of any socioeconomic strata and they progressively worsen the lower one descends the social ladder. More affluent classes have the highest participation in leisure-time sports and exercise, healthier diets, moderate or less drinking, little or no smoking, more physical checkups by physicians, and greater opportunities for rest, relaxation, and coping successfully with stress (Antunes 2011; Burdette et al. 2017; Carpiano, Link, and Phelan 2008; Grzywacz and Marks 2001; Margolis 2013; Narcisse et al. 2009; Snead and Cockerham 2002). The upper and upper-middle classes are also the first to have knowledge of new health risks and, because of their greater resources, are most able to adopt new health strategies and practices (Missinne, Daenekindt, and Bracke 2015; Missinne, Neels, and Bracke 2014; Phelan and Link 2013). The advantaged classes have the capability to move in a more fluid fashion to embrace new health behaviors, such as adopting low cholesterol and low carbohydrate diets to collectively reduce their risk of heart disease, or quitting smoking. A decisive component of class standing in the social gradient of health is education (Andrews, Hill, and Cockerham 2017; Clouston et al. 2015; Lawrence 2017; Leopold and Leopold 2018; Margolis 2013; Mirowsky and Ross 2003; Wolfe et al. 2018). Better-educated people are typically healthier because they have the knowledge to help them lead healthier lifestyles and seek medical care when they need it. While education is obviously a critical factor in relation to health, it is nevertheless part of a broader dimension of class membership that enables people in higher social strata to be healthier over the life course. The other factors are income that provides them with the financial resources to live a healthy life and occupational status that provides them with self-esteem and both a sense of responsibility and control over their lives. This view is compatible with fundamental cause theory that maintains that the accumulation and use of flexible resources by more advantaged persons allows them to better avoid health problems (Phelan and Link 2013).

Although it is clear that education plays an especially powerful role in the selection of health lifestyle practices, income and occupational status join education as the major components of socioeconomic status (SES). According to Nancy Adler and her associates (1994), the three SES variables— education, income, and occupation—are interrelated but not identical nor fully overlapping. Since associations between SES and health are found with each of these variables, Adler et al. (1994:15) suggest that a broader underlying dimension of social stratification or social ordering exists that exerts a potent influence on health-related behavior. That is, education is not just a characteristic of individuals, but it can also be viewed in combination with the other components of class to constitute a broad structural variable that produces top-down distinctions in the quality and form of health lifestyles. Moreover, it determines the social context for the practice of such lifestyles. So while education, income, and occupational status are separate individual qualities, collectively they constitute a structural variable whose influence is evident when people express the tastes, distinctions, outlooks, behaviors, and lifestyles common to their class as a whole.

Furthermore, Weber (1946) not only found that lifestyles expressed distinct differences between status groups and their adoption was a necessary feature of successful upward social mobility, he also observed that powerful social strata were "social carriers" of lifestyles. These carrier strata were important causal forces in their own right as they transmitted class-specific norms, values, ethics, and ways of life across generations (Kalberg 1994). In this way, as Bourdieu (1984) observes, patterns of lifestyles in one generation are reproduced over time in successive generations and the powerful influence of class on health lifestyles continues. The upper-middle class typically serves as the most prominent social carrier of positive health lifestyles because its "distance from necessity"—to use Bourdieu's (1984) terminology—allows them the leisure time, access to sources of authoritative knowledge, and resources to learn about and experience health-promoting behavior and adopt such behavior as a public model for other classes.

Age, Gender, Race and Ethnicity

Age. Contemporary empirical studies show that age, gender, and race/ethnicity have their own distinct dynamics that can function as structural variables beyond the individual to configure health lifestyle practices. As people age, they carry their health lifestyles along with them as an age-specific cohort into the next stage of their life, modifying them or keeping them as is while adjusting to an older and physically different self. Several quantitative studies, using latent class analysis, combined with health lifestyle theory and a life course perspective, show that such lifestyles transition from childhood and adolescence with a long reach into adulthood.[1] Life course theory, to be discussed in the next chapter, maintains that social conditions in early life establish "chains of risk" for poor health into adulthood (Burdette et al. 2017; Dannefer, Kelley-Moore, and Huang 2016; Elder, Johnson, and Crosnoe 2006).

As Stefanie Mollborn and Elizabeth Lawrence (2018:134) point out: "A health lifestyle is not just something an adult has." Mollborn and her colleagues (Mollborn et al. 2014) determined that even preschool children have health lifestyles. While young children likely have little agency in their health lifestyles as parents generally make the decisions, they do express judgments over what they will or will not eat, for example, or their preferred physical activities. Mollborn et al. found social background predicts early childhood health lifestyles with those in disadvantaged households likely to have lifestyles with greater health risks. These risks included disadvantages in personal safety, food insecurity, sleep, and exposure to secondhand smoking and violence. Some measures were of the child's behavior and others of parents' management of risks to the child's health. Consistent with health lifestyle theory, primary socialization in the home was a key factor in molding a child's present and future health behavior. The critical variable here is not just age, but class as these findings suggest an intergenerational process in which the parents' social background and resources are reflected in the health lifestyles of their children.

Mollborn et al. (2014) suggested that preschool health lifestyles are precursors to health lifestyles in middle childhood. Various other studies likewise find that childhood and adolescent health lifestyles go on to shape those in adulthood (Burdette et al. 2017; Daw, Margolis, and Wright 2017; Lawrence, Mollborn, and Hummer 2017; Lee et al. 2018; Mize 2017; Mollborn and Lawrence 2018). Adolescent health lifestyles not only reflect family influence but also those of schools and peers, which, in the case of peers, is not necessarily always positive with respect to dietary habits, smoking, and the like as social status (being "cool") in peer groups can outweigh healthy lifestyle practices learned in the home (Mollborn and Lawrence 2018; Stead et al. 2011). Therefore, as Amy Burdette and her colleagues (Burdette et al.

2017) conclude: (1) health lifestyles are socially patterned and (2) adolescent health lifestyles predict health status in adulthood.

Age also affects health lifestyles in later life because people often recognize the need to take better care of their health as they grow older by being more selective about the food they eat, resting and relaxing more, and either reducing or abstaining from alcohol use and smoking. An exception is exercise that declines and is often lost with advancing age because of diminishing strength and energy (Grzywacz and Marks 2001; Rees Jones et al. 2011). Does this mean that, other than exercise, health lifestyles in late-middle age are likely to be on the healthier side? Chrystal Jaye et al. (2018) interviewed a sample of middle-class individuals in late middle age in New Zealand who were recruited because they had reached the point in life where age-related health issues and degenerative physical conditions were likely. The participants recognized that the responsibility for good health through living a healthy lifestyle was under their control and the consequences of the failure to do so. Living such a lifestyle was depicted as a "moral obligation." Even so, some participants felt insecure about their past lifestyles and concern about their health in the next phase of life was common. They acknowledged that healthy living was not easy in that "it required personal sacrifices of enjoyable, but potentially lethal foodstuffs such as butter and fast food, pushing oneself to maintain adequate levels of fitness and resisting indulgent but irresponsible vices such as sunbathing, smoking and alcohol" (Jaye et al. 2018:368). Not all of them expressed a willingness to consistently make such sacrifices, but, nevertheless, did not question whether such an effort was worth it.

While there appears to be a tendency toward healthy lifestyle practices in older ages for many people, especially with respect to drinking, smoking, and diet, this is not the case for everyone. Late-middle age is a critical period in the life course because it not only represents the beginning of the final phase of one's occupational and economic attainment, it is also the last stage of life prior to the onset of old age and inevitable physical decline. Sarah Burgard and her colleagues (Burgard et al. 2018) analyzed alcohol, smoking, and obesity in five waves of the Americans' Changing Lives (ACL) study, covering periods of up to 25 years across middle and late-middle age. They found stability to be more common than change in these health behaviors. Rather than seeing a steady upward arc of continued improvement in health lifestyles as one ages, there is evidence that earlier practices become "locked in" at older ages along class lines (Rees Jones et al. 2011). That is, social-class distinctions seem to retain their significance at older ages with healthier lifestyles remaining typical of people higher on the social scale compared to those toward the bottom (McGovern and Nazroo 2015; Rees Jones et al. 2011; Shaw et al. 2014).

Ian Rees Jones and his colleagues (2011), for example, utilizing multiple correspondence analysis, analyzed data from men in the British Regional

Heart Study through middle age to old age. The participants remained clustered in their usual class-based drinking and smoking patterns at similar levels into old age. Exercise was an exception in that it became minimal for all social classes over time. The findings suggest that class position remains a persistent ("locked-in") influence on smoking and drinking, at least for men. There was not a general coalescing toward a healthier lifestyle as older men higher in the class structure continued to have healthier lifestyles and those lower down tended toward maintaining less healthy practices. Rees Jones et al. conclude that these health lifestyles remain socially structured even in later life. The concept of a lifestyle "lock-in" along class lines illustrates the durability of class influences on health lifestyles over the life course. An exception seen in other research is that of individuals with diagnosed health conditions in late-middle age who tend to adopt healthier lifestyles than previously (Cockerham, Wolfe, and Bauldry 2020).

Gender. As for gender, it likewise serves as a structural variable in health lifestyle theory with its own collective orientation. According to Raewyn Connell and Rebecca Pearse (2015): "Gender is a social structure of a particular kind." They point out men and women wear different types of shoes, button their shirts from opposite sides, get their hair cut in different places, buy pants in separate shops, and take them off in separate toilets—all of which is part of the normative order of everyday life prescribed by society. According to Barbara Risman (1998), gender operates as a structural entity at three distinct levels: (1) the individual level through a person's socialization as a gendered self that is imposed by significant others; (2) the interactional level as men and women interact socially and share mutual expectations on the basis of gender; and (3) the institutional level with respect to differing material resources and opportunities along gendered lines.

Gender also helps provide the social context for the development of health lifestyles during socialization. Beginning in childhood, females visit physicians more often than males and are socialized to take particular care of their bodies as seen in the continuing requirements for breast exams and pap smears that men do not have. The childbearing role is also important in that women often adopt and maintain positive health lifestyles during pregnancy and post-natal care that men do not experience. Since women are typically the caregivers in their families, this means they must maintain their own health in order to care for children and other family members, including the men (Pavalko, Gong, and Long 2007). Being drunk, smoking, eating or serving unhealthy foods, abusing drugs, and similar negative practices jeopardize the health and well-being of their children, others dependent upon them, and themselves, and are therefore less likely behaviors for mothers and women caregivers. All of this suggests a like-minded habitus among many women featuring durable dispositions toward maintaining good health.

Consequently, women generally eat more healthy foods, drink less alcohol, smoke less, visit doctors more often for preventive care, wear seatbelts more frequently when they drive, and, with the exception of exercise, have healthier lifestyles overall than men (Annandale 2016; Cockerham 2018). The often greater feminine concern with health and nurturing is seen in research in Canada showing underprivileged women adapting to the necessity of motherhood and caretaking demands by adopting a healthier lifestyle within the constraints of their living conditions and even sacrificing their own health needs to insure their children are healthy (Dumas, Robitaille, and Jette 2014). This is not to say that all women engage in healthy lifestyle practices as a recent decline in life expectancy among less-educated white women in various low-income rural counties in the U.S. has been associated with smoking and obesity (Cockerham 2014; Cockerham et al. 2017b; Montez and Zajacova 2013).

Compared to women, however, men are generally more likely to drink and smoke, eat less healthy foods, be violent, drive fast, take more health risks, have more accidents, suffer injury, and die younger (Dolan 2011). Having an elevated (hegemonic) sense of masculinity may not necessarily be good for a man's health as men with exaggerated masculinity are less likely to seek preventive care and more likely to engage in risky health behavior (Cockerham 2018; Dolan 2011; Pietilä and Rytkönen 2008; Smith and Dumas 2019; Springer and Mouzon 2011). This seems to be especially the case for working-class men and others further down the social scale who maintain a heightened sense of masculinity and self-control concurrent with a marginal social status. According to a part-time male bus driver in a Canadian study by Adam Smith and Alex Dumas (2019:314)

> The [nurses] tell me to watch my cholesterol; to watch my sugar, and all the things like that. Yes, they say I have to change my habits. That makes me laugh. There is no cutting salt for me ... I like lots of salt. My wife says "watch what you are going to eat there" ... She is always putting her nose in my affairs. She tries to control me ... You want me to eat like a bird? Look at my size; I'm not going to eat like a bird.

Whereas gender is a strong predictor of health lifestyle practices in its own right, its effects can also be moderated by class distinctions, as people higher on the social scale, regardless of gender, visit physicians more for preventive care, eat healthier diets, smoke less, and participate more in leisure-time exercise, and those toward the bottom do less of these things. This is true not just for men, but also women (Audet et al. 2017; Christensen and Carpiano 2014; Saint Onge and Krueger 2017; Smith and Dumas 2019).

Race and Ethnicity. Race and ethnicity are presumed to be important, but there is a paucity of research directly comparing the health lifestyles of different racial and ethnic groups. We do know that blacks have the highest mortality rates of any racial group in the U.S., including mortality from heart disease, cancer, stroke, and diabetes (National Center for Health Statistics 2019). Smoking, poor dietary habits, alcohol abuse, and lack of exercise have a well-established link to these chronic diseases—thereby suggesting unhealthy lifestyle practices are especially prevalent among African Americans. Yet existing studies show an inconsistent pattern. Blacks are not as likely as whites to indulge in heavy episodic drinking (Evans-Polce, Vasilenko, and Lanza 2015; Keyes et al. 2015; Zapolski et al. 2014). Blacks, conversely, are less likely to have a healthy diet (Cockerham et al. 2017a; Hattery and Smith 2011) and participate in health-promoting leisure-time exercise (Grzywacz and Marks 2001; Saint Onge and Krueger 2011). And while proportionately more black men smoke than either white men or white women, black women smoke less than black men and whites generally (Ho and Elo 2013; Pampel 2008). Therefore, both blacks and whites have unhealthy practices, but those of blacks (namely, heavy smoking for men and poor diets and lack of exercise for men and women) seem especially harmful. According to Angela Hattery and Earl Smith (2011:55): "And, just as the poor in other parts of the world are more vulnerable to diseases like malaria and cholera, the poor, and increasingly African Americans, are more vulnerable to the diseases associated with an unhealthy lifestyle."

Research by the author and his associates (Cockerham et al. 2017a) on black–white differences in health lifestyles and cardiovascular disease found that members of both races engaged in a combination of healthy and unhealthy lifestyles, with those in the predominantly latter category showing an elevated risk of coronary heart disease. An important difference was that in each of four lifestyle configurations, blacks showed a higher probability of excessive energy intake than whites—indicative of the potential for obesity. There is also evidence that exercise declines more steeply for blacks than whites across the course of adulthood, yet this pattern may be caused by blacks having more functional health problems and living in less safe neighborhoods (Grzywacz and Marks 2001). Another important factor with regard to race is discrimination whose effects on health lifestyles needs more research. There is evidence that high levels of racial discrimination experienced by blacks is associated with more smoking, consumption of more dietary fat, and less sleep (Sims et al. 2016).

Other research by Jarron Saint Onge and Patrick Krueger (2011, 2017) finds that non-Hispanic whites and more educated individuals exercise more than non-Hispanic blacks, Hispanics, and less-educated persons. Non-Hispanic whites and the educated also disproportionately participate in facility-based exercise (swimming, tennis, golf), while non-Hispanic blacks favor team sports (basketball) and fitness activities (running, walking) and

Hispanics gravitate toward team sports (soccer). Recreational facilities are often absent in low-income areas and the ability to participate in team sports declines much earlier in life than facility-based exercise. This gives non-Hispanic whites and better-educated persons an advantage in exercising longer as they age. Saint Onge and Krueger observe that the type and extent of leisure-time physical activity is shaped by the cultural identities and social circumstances of the participants.

Most studies on health and race compare blacks and whites and there are little data on Hispanic, Asian, or Native American health lifestyle practices. Detailed studies of the health lifestyles of these racial groups is needed before the extent of racial differences in such lifestyles can be fully determined. Research on the health lifestyles of different ethnic groups is also lacking, including how to best conceptualize and measure ethnicity. Existing studies of ethnicity, like those of race, have focused more on the overall health profiles of ethnic groups than on health lifestyles. There is research showing lower-class social status has greater effects on health than ethnic identities, but additional studies are clearly warranted (Karlsen and Nazroo 2002).

Collectivities

Collectivities are collections of actors linked together through specific social relationships and networks, such as kinship, the workplace, religion, and politics. The shared norms, values, ideals, and social perspectives of such collectivities have been held to constitute intersubjective "thought communities" beyond individual subjectivity that reflect a particular collective world view (Zerubavel 1997). The notion of thought communities is akin to Mead's (1934) concept of the generalized other in that both are abstractions of the perspectives of social collectivities or groups that enter into the thinking of the individual. While people may accept, reject, or ignore the normative perspectives of such groups, group views are nonetheless likely to be taken into account when choosing a course of action (Berger and Luckmann 1967). Weber ([1922] 1978) notes that concepts of collective entities have meaning in the minds of individuals, partly as something actually existing and partly as something with normative authority. "Actors," states Weber ([1922] 1978:14), "thus in part orient their action to them, and in this role such ideas have a powerful, often a decisive, causal influence on the course of action of real individuals." This is seen in research on the influence of social networks on obesity and smoking where it was found that obese persons were highly likely to have obese friends, while smokers were in a social network of smokers (Christakis and Fowler 2007, 2008).

Religion and ideology are examples of collective perspectives that also have implications for health lifestyles. This is seen in the usual preference of highly religious persons and groups for positive health lifestyles since their beliefs invariably promote healthy living in the form of good nutrition, exercise, and personal hygiene, while discouraging alcohol use and smoking cigarettes (T. Hill et al. 2007; Idler 2016). However, the full extent of the relationship between religiosity and health lifestyles is not known because of a lack of relevant studies. This is another important area that needs further research.

Little is also known about political ideology and health lifestyles. Research on the effects of the socialist heritage in Russia shows that pro-socialists (those who are in favor of a return to state socialism as it was under communism) have less healthy lifestyles than anti-socialists, even though neither group demonstrated exceptionally positive health practices (Cockerham et al. 2002). Pro-socialists had a particularly passive approach to health lifestyles that seemed left over from Soviet times. The choices of individuals in Soviet society were confined to a single social and political ideology (communism) and expected to conform to it. When a person got sick, the state was responsible for taking care of that person as a benefit of state socialism. Individual incentives in health matters were not encouraged. Thus it could be argued that communism was bad for one's health as it failed to promote healthy lifestyle practices. However, the extent to which ideology generally affects health lifestyles beyond this example has not been determined.

Family and kinship influences on health lifestyle practices can also be powerful (Mollborn et al. 2014). The family typically influences how a particular person perceives his or her health situation beginning in childhood. Most individuals are born into a family of significant others—significant because they provide the child with a specific social identity and sense of self. This identity includes not only an appraisal of physical and intellectual characteristics, but knowledge about the family's social and medical history. In addition to learning the family's social status, perspective, and cultural orientation, the child learns about the health threats most common for the family and the measures needed to prevent them. Children can either accept or reject the perspective of their family as representative of their own social reality. Yet the reality presented to them in the process of primary socialization is set by adults who determine what information is provided and their assessments of the validity of opposing viewpoints.

Although children are not necessarily passive in the socialization experience, they have no choice in their significant others so that identification with them is quasi-automatic (Berger and Luckmann 1967). This means that children's internalization of their family's interpretation of social reality is quasi-inevitable and Bourdieu (1984, 1990) finds this process instrumental in forming the habitus. Although the initial social world presented to children by their significant others may be weakened by later social relationships and views, it can nonetheless be a durable influence. Parental guidance, for example, has been found to be the most important and persistent influence on the preventive health beliefs of their children and significant in shaping their health lifestyles in adulthood (Mollborn et al. 2014; Mollborn and Lawrence 2018). However, the prospect of a healthy lifestyle in later life can be jeopardized when the child's emotional bond with the parents is compromised by physical abuse (Andersson 2015; Lee, Coe, and Ryff 2017).

Living Conditions

Living conditions are a category of structural variables pertaining to differences in the quality of housing and access to basic utilities (e.g., electricity, gas, heating, sewers, indoor plumbing, safe piped water, hot water), neighborhood facilities (e.g., grocery stores, parks, recreation), and personal safety. Such conditions may also apply to other sites where people spend their lives, such as their place of work. The physical environment within which a person lives strongly affects health-related behavior (Fitzpatrick and LaGory 2011; Frohlich and Abel 2014). Health lifestyles are most effective in positive living situations and least effective in unhealthy conditions, such as substandard housing, pollution, lack of public services and medical facilities, poor quality food, sewage and drainage problems, exposure to insects and rodents, and high levels of neighborhood unemployment, crime, alcoholism, and drug abuse.

Socioeconomic circumstances and the living environment can therefore determine the extent to which health lifestyles can be practiced effectively, as the structural conditions of people's lives makes it probable or improbable they can actually achieve a positive health lifestyle. If living conditions are good, healthy behavior appears to have a strong influence on health, but if they are bad, then behavior may make little difference and is often unhealthy. Living a healthy lifestyle is not simply a matter of individual choice, but to a large extent depends upon a person's social and material environment for its success. Several studies in the United States and Canada associate living in disadvantaged neighborhoods with poor health behaviors and unhealthy conditions (Bernard et al. 2007; Browning and Cagney 2002; Fitzpatrick and LaGory 2011; Frohlich and Abel 2014; Grzywacz and Marks 2001), while growing up in affluent neighborhoods has been found to have positive long-term health effects (Vartanian and Houser 2010). Consequently, living conditions can constrain or enhance health lifestyles.

Socialization and Experience

Class circumstances and the other variables shown in Box 1 in Figure 10.1 provide the social context for socialization and experience as depicted by the arrow leading to Box 2. This is consistent with Bourdieu's (1977) view that dispositions to act in particular ways are constructed through socialization and experience, with class position providing the social context for this process. The present model, however, adds the additional structural categories—age, gender, race/ethnicity, collectivities, and living conditions—depicted in Box 1, since they also comprise part of the social environment within which socialization and experience occur.

Whereas primary socialization represents the imposition of society's norms and values on the individual by significant others, and secondary socialization results from later institutional training, experience is the learned outcome of day-to-day activities that comes about through social interaction and the practical exercise of agency. It is through both socialization and experience that the individual acquires reflexive awareness and the capacity to perform agency, but experience—with respect to life choices—provides the essential basis for agency's practical and evaluative dimensions to evolve over time. This is especially the case as people confront new social situations and conditions.

Life Choices (Agency)

Figure 10.1 shows that socialization and experience (Box 2) provides the capacity for life choices (agency) depicted in Box 3. As previously noted, the term "life choices" was introduced by Weber and refers to the self-direction of one's behavior. It is an English-language translation of *Lebensführung*, which in German literally means conducting or managing one's life. Life choices are a process of agency by which individuals critically evaluate and choose their course of action. Weber's notion of life choices accounts for the interpretive process whereby the potential outcomes of choices are imagined, evaluated, and reconstructed in the mind and then selected and acted upon to achieve desired goals. Weber (1949) maintained that individuals have the capacity to interpret their situation, make deliberate choices, and attach subjective meaning to their actions. All social action in his view takes place in contexts that imply both constraints and opportunities, with the actor's interpretive understanding (*Verstehen*) of the situation guiding behavioral choices (Kalberg 1994).

Life Chances (Structure)

Class circumstances, and to a lesser degree the other variables in Box 1, constitute life chances (structure) shown in Box 4. Life chances are the other major component of lifestyles in Weber's model. Weber was ambiguous about what he meant by life chances, but the term is usually associated with the advantages and disadvantages of relative class situations. The higher a person's position in a class hierarchy, the better the person's life chances or probabilities for finding satisfaction. According to Dahrendorf (1979:65): "for Weber, the probability of sequences of action postulated in the concept of chance is not merely an observed and thus calculable probability, but is a probability which is invariably anchored in structural conditions." Thus a person's probabilities for satisfaction that comprise his or her life chances are based on the structural conditions in their life, especially their class position. Weber's thesis is that chance is socially determined and social structure is an arrangement of chances. Therefore, life chances represent the influence of structure in health lifestyle theory.

Choice and Chance Interplay

The arrows in Figure 10.1 indicate the dialectical interplay between life choices (Box 3) and life chances (Box 4). This interaction is clearly Weber's most important contribution to conceptualizing lifestyle construction (Cockerham et al. 1997). Choices and chances operate in tandem to determine a distinctive lifestyle for individuals, groups, and classes. Life chances (structure) either constrain or enable choices (agency); agency is not passive in this process, however. As Margaret Archer (2003) explains, whether or not constraints and enablements are exercised as causal powers is based on agency choosing the practices to be activated. "Constraints," says Archer (2003:4), "require something to constrain, and enablements something to enable." Consequently, people have to consider a course of action if their actions are to be either constrained or enabled. People therefore align their goals, needs, and desires with their probabilities for realizing them and choose a lifestyle according to their assessments of their resources and circumstances. Unrealistic choices are not likely to succeed or be selected, while realistic choices are based upon what is structurally possible.

In this context, choices and chances are not only connected dialectically, but are analytically distinct. As Archer (1998:369) points out: "Because the emergent properties of structures and the actual experiences of agents are not synchronized (due to the very nature of society as an open system), then there will always be the inescapable need for a two-part account." Weber provides such a framework. He conceptualizes choice and chance as separate components in the activation and conduct of a lifestyle and merges the different functions of agency and structure without either losing their distinctiveness.

Up to this point, the health lifestyles paradigm has been an example of Archer's (1995, 1998) notion of downward conflation in which individual behavior is molded by structure in the form of class circumstances, gender, collectivities, etc. However, even though structure is dominant in the beginning because people are socialized and have experiences within the context of the pre-existing social structures that comprise their world, agency enters the model at the mid-point where choices and chances interact and outcomes are chosen from what is available. In this way, the one-dimensional theorizing that the term "conflation" represents in Archer's critique of the macro–micro debate in sociology is avoided. The health lifestyle model presented here seeks to blend agency and structure and be neither fully upward nor downward in its approach. Nevertheless, I recognize that there is an imbalance favoring structure since structure precedes in individuals and subjects them to molding through socialization, even though they are nonetheless able to think for themselves, choose, and be creative in their behavior if they so desire. However, behavior in familiar settings or day-to-day fields is typically routine, and the reality of this situation is that the habitus seems especially powerful in habitually shaping behavioral practices largely along structural lines.

Dispositions to Act (Habitus)

Figure 10.1 shows that the interaction of life choices and life chances produces individual dispositions to action (Box 5). These dispositions constitute a habitus that is a cognitive map or set of perceptions routinely guiding and evaluating a person's choices and options. It is a process of thinking in which social norms and cultural conventions are internalized in the mind, along with the individual's own inclinations, preferences, and interpretations. The habitus produces enduring dispositions toward acting that are normative, habitual, and can be intuitive. One of its principal functions is that of providing a unity of style linking the practices of a single agent to a class of agents that brings together agents or individuals who are very similar to each other but different from members of other classes (Bourdieu 1998). Therefore, Bourdieu finds that the habitus retranslates the relational characteristics of a social position into a lifestyle reflecting a unitary set of choices of practices that differentiates itself from the choices of persons in other classes.

As for health lifestyles, the dispositions that are generated result in practices that are binary. That is, they fall into one or the other of two categories: good or bad. This binary characteristic means that the outcome generated from the interplay of choices and chances have either positive or negative effects on health. Positive health lifestyles are intended to avoid risk and are oriented toward achieving or maintaining one's overall health and fitness. Negative health lifestyles put one at risk for illness and earlier mortality. However, even though health practices have a general binary character, they may not be exclusively one way or the other for some individuals, but a combination of varying degrees of both good and bad in the same lifestyle (Burdette et al. 2017; Cockerham 2005; Cockerham et al. 2017a; Lawrence, Mollborn, and Hummer 2017; Mize 2017; Mollborn et al. 2014). That is, some lifestyles are very healthy and others overwhelmingly unhealthy, whereas others consist of a mixture of both good or bad practices, such as consuming large amounts of alcohol but not smoking or smoking but also exercising. As Amy Burdette et al. (2017:522) observe, "health lifestyle theory suggests that social statuses work to shape qualitatively different patterns of behaviors in individuals that may not be summarized in terms of simple counts of healthy or unhealthy behaviors." This is because health behaviors cluster in varying ways within lifestyle configurations as various social statuses like class, age, gender, and race influence diverse combinations of health practices.

Completing the Model

Figure 10.1 shows that dispositions (Box 5) produce practices (action) that are represented in Box 6. The practices that result from the habitus can be based on deliberate calculations, or habits and intuition. Bourdieu (1984) helps us to realize that practices linked to health lifestyles can be so integrated into routine behavioral repertoires that they can be acted out more or less unthinkingly once established in the habitus. He observes that people tend to adopt generalized strategies (a sense of the game) oriented toward practical ends in routine situations that they can habitually follow without having always to stop to analyze them. As a routinized feature of everyday life, it is therefore appropriate to view health lifestyles as guided more by a practical than an abstract logic (Williams 1995).

The four most common practices measured in studies of health lifestyles are alcohol use, smoking, diet, and exercise. These are shown in Box 7 along with other practices such as physical checkups by physicians and automobile seatbelt use that comprise other typical forms of action taken or not taken. The practices themselves may be positive or negative, but they nonetheless comprise a person's overall pattern of health lifestyles as represented in Box 8. It is important to note that these practices sometimes have a complexity of their own. Smoking tobacco in any form is negative and eating fresh fruits and vegetables is positive, but consuming meat can be either positive or negative depending on how it is cooked, its fat content, and how often it is consumed. Relatively vigorous leisure-time exercise has more health benefits than physical activity at work because the latter is subject to stress from job demands and time schedules, while walking and other everyday forms of exercise have some value. However, measures of leisure-time exercise may not fully represent the physical activities of women who take care of children and do housework (Ainsworth 2000). It is therefore necessary that researchers take the multifaceted features of health lifestyle practices into account when analyzing them.

Action (or inaction) with respect to a particular health practice leads to its reproduction, modification, or nullification by the habitus through a feedback process. This is seen in Figure 10.1 by the arrow showing movement from Box 8 back to Box 5. This is consistent with Bourdieu's (1977, 1984) assertion that when dispositions are acted upon they tend to reproduce or modify the habitus from which they are derived. As conceptualized by Bourdieu, the habitus is the centerpiece of the health lifestyle model.

Summary

This model of health lifestyles states that four categories of (1) structural variables, namely (a) class circumstances, (b) age, gender, and race/ethnicity, (c) collectivities, and (d) living conditions, provide the social context for (2) socialization and experience that influence (3) life choices (agency). These structural variables also collectively constitute (4) life chances (structure). Choices and chances interact and commission the formation of (5) dispositions to act (habitus), leading to (6) practices (action), involving (7) alcohol use, smoking, diets and other health-related actions. Health practices constitute patterns of (8) health lifestyles whose reenactment results in their reproduction (or modification) through feedback to the habitus.

Guide to Critical Thinking

1. What are the major components of Weber's concept of lifestyles and how do they influence each other?
2. Explain Giddens' notion of the duality of structure.
3. Explain what Bourdieu means by the "distance from necessity" and "habitus."
4. Why are class circumstances the most important structural variable in health lifestyle theory?
5. Why do women have healthier lifestyles than men?

Note

1   Latent class analysis (LCA) is a statistical method that offers the advantage of sorting individual health behaviors into categories as indicators of an underlying categorical latent variable (Collins and Lanza 2010). The categories of the latent variable represent distinct health lifestyles (or classes) composed of different combinations of health practices whose number and composition is taken directly from the data. The number of health lifestyles is determined by finding the latent class model that has the best fit with the data based on model

fit statistics, such as the Bayesian Information Criterion (BIC), the chi-square test statistic, or the Lo-Mendell-Rubin test statistic. Based on the overall results of these fit statistics, the preferred latent class model is used to assign respondents to the health lifestyle (latent class) in which they have the highest estimated probability of membership. Invariably one lifestyle is the most healthy, one the least healthy, and any others fit to varying degrees somewhere in-between the most positive and most negative.

Suggested Reading

Burdette, Amy M., Belinda L. Needham, Miles G. Taylor, and Terrence D. Hill. 2017. "Health Lifestyles in Adolescence and Self-rated Health in Adulthood." *Journal of Health and Social Behavior* 58(4):520–36.
An excellent application and discussion of health lifestyle theory.
Mollborn, Stefanie, Laurie James-Hawkins, Elizabeth Lawrence, and Paula Fomby. 2014. "Health Lifestyles in Early Childhood." *Journal of Health and Social Behavior* 55(4):386–402.
Another strong example of the utilization of health lifestyle theory in empirical research.

References

Adler, Nancy E., Thomas Boyce, Margaret A. Chesney, Sheldon Cohen, Susan Folkman, Robert L. Kahn, and S. Leonard Syme. 1994. "Socioeconomic Status and Health: The Challenge of the Gradient." *American Psychologist* 10:15–24.
Ainsworth, Barbara E. 2000. "Issues in the Assessment of Physical Activity in Women." *Research Quarterly for Exercise and Sport* 71:37–50.
Alexander, Jeffrey C. 1983. *Theoretical Logic in Sociology*, vols. 1, 3. Berkeley, CA: University of California Press.
Alexander, Jeffrey C. 1995. *Fin de Siècle Social Theory*. London: Verso.
Andersson, Matthew A. 2015. "Chronic Disease at Midlife: Do Parent–Child Bonds Modify the Effect of Childhood SES?" *Journal of Health and Social Behavior* 57(3):373–89.
Andrews, Hannah, Terrence Hill, and William C. Cockerham. 2017. "Educational Attainment and Dietary Lifestyles," in Sara Shostok (ed.), *Advances in Medical Sociology* (18). Bingley: Emerald, pp. 101–20.
Annandale, Ellen. 2016. "Health Status and Gender," in William Cockerham (ed.), *The New Blackwell Companion to Medical Sociology*. Oxford: Wiley-Blackwell, pp. 97–112.
Antunes, Ricardo Jorge. 2011. "The Social Space of Health Inequalities in Portugal." *Social Theory & Health* 9:393–409.
Archer, Margaret S. 1995. *Realist Social Theory: The Morphogenetic Approach*. Cambridge: Cambridge University Press.
Archer, Margaret S. 1998. "Realism and Morphogenesis," in Margaret Archer, Roy Bhaskar, Andrew Collier, Tony Lawson, and Alan Norrie (eds.), *Critical Realism*. London: Routledge, pp. 356–81.

Archer, Margaret S. 2003. *Structure, Agency, and the Internal Conversation.* Cambridge: Cambridge University Press.

Audet, Melisa, Alex Dumas, Rachelle Binette, and Isabelle J. Dionne. 2017. "Women. Weight, Poverty and Menopause: Understanding Health Practices in a Context of Chronic Disease Prevention." *Sociology of Health & Illness* 39(8):1412–26.

Bauman, Zygmunt. 1999. *In Search of Politics.* Stanford, CA: Stanford University Press.

Berger, Peter L. and Thomas Luckmann. 1967. *The Social Construction of Reality.* New York: Anchor.

Bernard, Paul, Rana Charrafedine, Katherine L. Frohlich, Mark Daniel, Yan Kestens, and Louise Potvin. 2007. "Health Inequalities and Place: A Theoretical Conception of Neighbourhood." *Social Science & Medicine* 65:1839–52.

Blumer, Herbert. 1969. *Symbolic Interaction.* Englewood Cliffs, NJ: Prentice-Hall.

Bohman, James. 1999. "Practical Reason and Cultural Constraint: Agency in Bourdieu's Theory of Practice," in Richard Schusterman (ed.), *Bourdieu: A Critical Reader.* Oxford: Blackwell, pp. 129–52.

Bourdieu, Pierre. 1977. *Outline of a Theory of Practice.* Cambridge: Polity.

Bourdieu, Pierre. 1984. *Distinction.* Cambridge, MA: Harvard University Press.

Bourdieu, Pierre. 1990. *The Logic of Practice.* Stanford, CA: Stanford University Press.

Bourdieu, Pierre. 1996. *The Rules of Art.* Cambridge: Polity.

Bourdieu, Pierre. 1998. *Practical Reason: On the Theory of Action.* Stanford, CA: Stanford University Press.

Bourdieu, Pierre and Loïc J. D. Wacquant. 1992. *An Invitation to Reflexive Modernity.* Chicago, IL: University of Chicago Press.

Browning, Christopher R. and Kathleen A. Cagney. 2003. "Moving Beyond Poverty: Neighborhood Structure, Social Processes, and Health." *Journal of Health and Social Behavior* 44:552–71.

Burdette, Amy M., Belinda L. Needham, Miles G. Taylor, and Terrence D. Hill. 2017. "Health Lifestyles in Adolescence and Self-rated Health in Adulthood." *Journal of Health and Social Behavior* 58(4):520–36.

Burgard, Sarah A., Katherine Y. P. Lin, Brian D. Segal, Michael R. Elliott, and Sarah Seelye. 2018. "Stability and Change in Health Behavior Profiles of U.S. Adults." *The Journals of Gerontology* 75B(3):674–83.

Carpiano, Richard M., Bruce G. Link, and Jo C. Phelan. 2008. "Social Inequality and Health: Future Directions for the Fundamental Cause Explanation," in Annette Lareau and Dalton Conley (eds.), *Social Class.* New York: Russell Sage, pp. 232–63.

Christakis, Nicholas A. and James H. Fowler. 2007. "The Spread of Obesity in a Large Social Network Over 32 Years." *New England Journal of Medicine* 357:370–9.

Christakis, Nicholas A. and James H. Fowler. 2008. "The Collective Dynamics of Smoking in a Large Social Network." *New England Journal of Medicine* 358:2249–58.

Christensen, Vibeke T. and Richard M. Carpiano. 2014. "Social Class Differences in BMI among Danish Women: Applying Cockerham's Health Lifestyles Approach and Bourdieu's Theory of Lifestyle." *Social Science & Medicine* 112:12–21.

Clouston, Sean A. P., Marcus Richards, Dorina Caadar, and Scott M. Hofer. 2015. "Educational Inequalities in Health Behaviors at Midlife: Is There a Role for Early-Life Cognition?" *Journal of Health and Social Behavior* 56(3):323–40.

Cockerham, William C. 1997. "Lifestyles, Social Class, Demographic Characteristics, and Health Behavior," in David S. Gochman (ed.), *Handbook of Health Behavior Research*, Vol. I. New York: Plenum, pp. 253–65.

Cockerham, William C. 1999. *Health and Social Change in Russia and Eastern Europe*. New York: Routledge.

Cockerham, William C. 2000. "Health Lifestyles in Russia." *Social Science & Medicine* 51:1313–24.

Cockerham, William C. 2005. "Health Lifestyle Theory and the Convergence of Agency and Structure." *Journal of Health and Social Behavior* 46:51–67.

Cockerham, William C. 2013a. *Social Causes of Health and Disease*. Cambridge: Polity.

Cockerham, William C. 2013b. "Bourdieu and an Update of Health Lifestyle Theory," in William Cockerham (ed.), *Medical Sociology on the Move: New Directions in Theory*. Dordrecht: Springer, pp. 127–54.

Cockerham, William C. 2014. "The Emerging Crisis in American Female Longevity." *Social Currents* 1(3):220–7.

Cockerham, William C. 2018. "Health Lifestyles and the Search for a Gender-Specific Habitus." *Social Theory & Health* 16(2):142–55.

Cockerham, William C., Thomas Abel, and Günther Lüschen. 1993. "Max Weber, Formal Rationality, and Health Lifestyles." *Sociological Quarterly* 34(3):413–25.

Cockerham, William C., Shawn Bauldry, Bryant W. Hamby, James M. Shikany, and Sejong Bae. 2017a. "A Comparison of Black and White Racial Differences in Health Lifestyles and Cardiovascular Disease." *American Journal of Preventive Medicine* 52(S1):S56–S62.

Cockerham, William C., Bryant W. Hamby, Shawn Bauldry, and Patricia Drentea. 2017b. "Changing Patterns of Female Smoking: A Comparison of Workers and Full-Time Homemakers by Class, Race, and Community Type," in Jennie Kronenfeld (ed.), *Research in the Sociology of Health Care*, Vol. 35. Bingley: Emerald, pp. 279–97.

Cockerham, William C., Brian P. Hinote, and Pamela Abbott. 2006. "A Sociological Model of Health Lifestyles: Conducting a Preliminary Test Using Russian Data." *Kölner Zeitschrift für Soziologie und Sozial Psychologie* [*Cologne Journal of Sociology and Social Psychology*] 46:177–97.

Cockerham, William C., Gerhard Kunz, and Günther Lüschen. 1988. "Social Stratification and Health Lifestyles in Two Systems of Health Care Delivery: A Comparison of the United States and West Germany." *Journal of Health and Social Behavior* 29(2):113–26.

Cockerham, William C., Alfred Rütten, and Thomas Abel. 1997. "Conceptualizing Contemporary Health Lifestyles: Moving Beyond Weber." *Sociological Quarterly* 38(2):321–42.

Cockerham, William C., M. Christine Snead, and Derek F. DeWaal. 2002. "Health Lifestyles in Russia and the Socialist Heritage." *Journal of Health and Social Behavior* 43(1):42–55.

Cockerham, William C., Joseph D. Wolfe, and Shawn Bauldry. 2020. "Health Lifestyles in Late Middle Age." *Research on Aging* 42(1):34–46.

Collins, Linda M. and Stephanie T. Lanza. 2010. *Latent Class and Latent Transition Analysis: With Applications in the Social, Behavioral, and Health Sciences*. New York: Wiley.

Connell, Raewyn and Rebecca Pearse. (2015) *Gender in World Perspective*, 3rd ed. Cambridge: Polity.

Dahrendorf, Ralf. 1979. *Life Chances*. Chicago, IL: University of Chicago Press.

Dannefer, Dale, Jessica Kelley-Moore, and Wenxuan Huang. 2016. "Opening the Social: Sociological Imagination in Life Course Studies," in J. Mortimer and M. Shanahan (eds.), *Handbook of the Life Course*. New York: Springer, pp. 87–110.

Daw, Jonathan, Rachel Margolis, and Laura Wright. 2017. "Emerging Adulthood, Emergent Health Lifestyles: Sociodemographic Determinants of Trajectories of Smoking, Binge Drinking, Obesity, and Sedentary Behavior." *Journal of Health and Social Behavior* 58(2):181–97.

Dolan, Alan. 2011. "'You Can't Ask for a Dubonnet and Lemonade': Working Class Masculinity and Men's Health Practices." *Sociology of Health & Illness* 33(4): 586–601.

Dumas, Alex, J. Robitaille, and S. Jette. 2014. "Lifestyle as a Choice of Necessity: Young Women, Health and Obesity." *Social Theory & Health* 12(2): 138–58.

Elder, Glenn H., Monica K. Johnson, and Robert Crosnoe. 2006. "The Emergence and Development of Life Course Theory," in Jeylan Mortimer and Michael Shanahan (eds.), *Handbook of the Life Course*. New York: Springer, pp. 3–19.

Emirbayer, Mustafa and Ann Mische. 1998. "What is Agency?" *American Journal of Sociology* 103:962–1023.

Evans-Polce, Rebecca J., Sara M. Vasilenko, and Stephanie T. Lanza. 2015. "Changes in Gender and Racial/Ethnic Disparities in Cigarette Use, Regular Heavy Episodic Drinking, and Marijuana Use, Ages 14 to 32." *Addictive Behaviors* 41:218–22.

Fitzpatrick, Kevin and Mark LaGory. 2011. *Unhealthy Cities*. Routledge: New York.

Frohlich, Katherine L. and Thomas Abel. 2014. "Environmental Justice and Health Practices: Understanding How Health Inequities Arise at the Local Level." *Sociology of Health & Illness* 36(2):199–212.

Giddens, Anthony. 1984. *The Constitution of Society: Outline of the Theory of Structuration*. Cambridge: Polity.

Giddens, Anthony. 1987. *Social Theory and Modern Sociology*. Stanford, CA: Stanford University Press.

Giddens, Anthony. 1991. *Modernity and Self-Identity*. Stanford, CA: Stanford University Press.

Grzywacz, Joseph G. and Nadine F. Marks. 2001. "Social Inequalities and Exercise During Adulthood: Toward an Ecological Perspective." *Journal of Health and Social Behavior* 42(2):202–20.

Hattery, Angela and Earl Smith. 2011. "Health, Nutrition, Access to Healthy Food and Well-Being among African Americans," in Anthony Lemelle, Wornie Reed, and Sandra Taylor (eds.), *Handbook of African American Health*. New York: Springer, pp. 47–59.

Hill, Terrence D., Christopher G. Ellison, Amy M. Burdette, and Marc A. Musick. 2007. "Religious Involvement and Healthy Lifestyles: Evidence from a Survey of Texas Adults." *Annals of Behavioral Medicine* 34:217–22.

Hinote, Brian P. 2014. "Habitus, Class, and Health," in William Cockerham, Robert Dingwall, and Stella Quah (eds.), *Wiley-Blackwell Encyclopedia of Health, Illness, Behavior, and Society*. Oxford: Wiley Blackwell, pp. 741–7.

Hinote, Brian P. 2015. "William C. Cockerham: The Contemporary Sociology of Health Lifestyles," in Fran Collyer (ed.), *The Palgrave Handbook of Social Theory in Health, Illness and Medicine*. Basingstoke: Palgrave Macmillan, pp. 471–87.

Hinote, Brian Philip, William C. Cockerham, and Pamela Abbott. 2009. "The Specter of Post-Communism: Women and Alcohol in Eight Post-Soviet Countries." *Social Science & Medicine* 68:1254–62.

Ho, Jessica Y. and Irma T. Elo. 2013. "The Contribution of Smoking to Black–White Differences in U.S. Mortality." *Demography* 50(2):545–68.

Husserl, Edmund. [1952] 1989. *Ideas Pertaining to a Pure Phenomenology and to a Phenomenological Philosophy*. London: Kluwer Academic.

Idler, Ellen L. 2016. "Health and Religion," in William Cockerham (ed.), *The New Blackwell Companion to Medical Sociology*. Oxford: Wiley-Blackwell, pp. 133–58.

Jaye, Chrystal, Jessica Young, Richard Egan, Rebecca Llewellyn, Wayne Cunningham, and Peter Radue. 2018. "The Healthy Lifestyle in Longevity Narratives." *Social Theory & Health* 16(4):361–78.

Joas, Hans and Wolfgang Knöbl. 2009. *Social Theory*. Cambridge: Cambridge University Press.

Kalberg, Stephen. 1994. *Max Weber's Comparative Historical Sociology*. Chicago, IL: University of Chicago Press.

Karlsen, Saffron and James Y. Nazroo. 2002. "Agency and Structure: The Impact of Ethnic Identity and Racism on the Health of Ethnic Minority People." *Sociology of Health & Illness* 24(1):1–20.

Keyes, Katherine M., Thomas Vo, Melanie M. Wall, Raul Caetano, Shakira F. Suglia, Sylvia S. Martins, Sandro Galea, and Deborah Hasin. 2015. "Racial/Ethnic Differences in Use of Alcohol, Tobacco, and Marijuana: Is There a Cross-Over from Adolescence to Adulthood?" *Social Science & Medicine* 124:132–41.

Korp, Peter. 2008. "The Symbolic Power of 'Healthy Lifestyles.'" *Health Sociology Review* 17:18–26.

Lawrence, Elizabeth M. 2017. "Why Do College Graduates Behave More Healthfully Than Those Who Are Less Educated?" *Journal of Health and Social Behavior* 58(3):291–306.

Lawrence, Elizabeth M., Stefanie Mollborn, and Robert A. Hummer. 2017. "Health Lifestyles across the Transition to Adulthood: Implications for Health." *Social Science & Medicine* 193:23–32.

Lee, Chioun, Christopher L. Coe, and Carol D. Ryff. 2017. "Social Disadvantage, Severe Child Abuse, and Biological Profiles in Adulthood." *Journal of Health and Social Behavior* 58(3):371–86.

Lee, Chioun, Vera K. Tsenkova, Jennifer M. Boylan, and Carol D. Ryff. 2018. "Gender Differences in the Pathways from Childhood Disadvantage to Metabolic Syndrome in Adulthood: An Examination of Health Lifestyles." *SSM – Population Health* 4:216–24.

Leopold, Liliya and Thomas Leopold. 2018. "Education and Health across Lives and Cohorts: A Study of Cumulative (Dis)advantage and Its Rising Importance in Germany." *Journal of Health and Social Behavior* 59(1):94–112.

Lüschen, Günther, William Cockerham, Jouke van der Zee, Fred Stevens, Jos Diederijks, Thomas Abel, Manuel Garcia Ferrando, Alphonse d'Houtaud, and Ruud Peters. 1995. *Health Systems in the European Union: Diversity, Convergence, and Integration.* Munich: Oldenbourg Verlag.

Margolis, Rachel. 2013. "Educational Differences in Healthy Behavior Changes and Adherence among Middle-Aged Americans." *Journal of Health and Social Behavior* 54(3):353–68.

McGovern, Pauline and James Y. Nazroo. 2015. "Patterns and Causes of Health Inequalities in Later Life: A Bourdieusian Approach." *Sociology of Health & Illness* 37(1):143–60.

Mead, George H. 1934. *Mind, Self, and Society.* Chicago, IL: University of Chicago Press.

Mirowsky, John and Catherine E. Ross. 2003. *Education, Social Status, and Health.* New York: Aldine de Gruyter.

Missinne, Sarah, Stijn Daenekindt, and Pers Bracke. 2015. "The Social Gradient in Preventive Healthcare Use: What Can We Learn from Socially Mobile Individuals?" *Sociology of Health & Illness* 37(6):823–38.

Missinne, Sarah, Karel Neels, and Pers Bracke. 2014. "Reconsidering Inequalities in Preventive Health Care: An Application of Cultural Health Capital Theory and the Life-Course Perspective to the Take-up of Mammography Screening." *Sociology of Health & Illness* 36(8):1259–75.

Mize, Trenton D. 2017. "Profiles in Health: Multiple Roles and Health Lifestyles in Early Childhood." *Social Science & Medicine* 178:196–205.

Mollborn, Stefanie and Elizabeth Lawrence. 2018. "Family, Peer, and School Influences in Children's Developing Health Lifestyles." *Journal of Health and Social Behavior* 59(1):133–50.

Mollborn, Stefanie, Laurie James-Hawkins, Elizabeth Lawrence, and Paula Fomby. 2014. "Health Lifestyles in Early Childhood." *Journal of Health and Social Behavior* 55(4):386–402.

Montez, Jennifer Karas and Anna Zajacova. 2013. "Explaining the Widening Education Gap in Mortality among U.S. White Women." *Journal of Health and Social Behavior* 54(2):166–82.

Narcisse, Marie-Rachelle, Nicole Dedobbeleer, Andre-Pierre Contandriopoulos, and Antonio Ciampi. 2009. "Understanding the Social Patterning of Smoking Practices: A Dynamic Typology." *Sociology of Health & Illness* 31(4):583–601.

National Center for Health Statistics. 2019. *Health, United States, 2018.* Hyattsville, MD: U.S. Government Printing Office.

Pampel, Fred C. 2008. "Racial Convergence in Cigarette Use from Adolescence to the Mid-Thirties." *Journal of Health and Social Behavior* 49(4):484–98.

Pavalko, Eliza, Fang Gong, and J. Scott Long. 2007. "Women's Work, Cohort Change, and Health." *Journal of Health and Social Behavior* 48(4): 352–68.

Phelan, Jo C. and Bruce G. Link. 2013. "Fundamental Cause Theory," in William Cockerham (ed.), *Medical Sociology on the Move: New Directions in Theory.* Dordrecht: Springer, pp. 105–26.

Pietilä, Ilkla and Marja Rytkönen. 2008. "'Health is not a Man's Domain': Lay Accounts of Gender Difference in Life-expectancy in Russia." *Sociology of Health & Illness* 30(7):1070–85.

Rees Jones, Ian, Olia Papocosta, Peter H. Whincup, S. Goya Wannamethee, and Richard W. Morris. 2011. "Class and Lifestyle 'Lock-in' among Middle-Aged and Older Men: A Multiple Correspondence Analysis of the British Regional Heart Study." *Sociology of Health & Illness* 33(3):399–419.

Risman, Barbara J. 1998. *Gender Vertigo*. New Haven, CT: Yale University Press.

Ritzer, George and William Yagatich. 2012. "Contemporary Theory," in George Ritzer (ed.), *The Wiley-Blackwell Companion to Sociology*. Oxford: Wiley-Blackwell, pp. 98–118.

Saint Onge, Jarron M. and Patrick M. Krueger. 2011. "Education and Racial-Ethnic Differences in Types of Exercise in the United States." *Journal of Health and Social Behavior* 52(2):197–211.

Saint Onge, Jarron M. and Patrick M. Krueger. 2017. "Health Lifestyle Behaviors among U.S. Adults." *SSM—Population Health* 3:89–98.

Scambler, Graham. 2018. *Sociology, Health and the Fractured Society*. London: Routledge.

Shaw, Benjamin A., Kelly McGeever, Elizabeth Vasquez, Neda Agahi, and Stefan Fors. 2014. "Socioeconomic Inequalities in Health After Age 50: Are Health Risk Behaviors to Blame?" *Social Science & Medicine* 101:52–60.

Sibeon, Roger. 2004. *Rethinking Social Theory*. London: Sage.

Sims, Mario, Ana V. Diez-Roux, Samson Y. Gebreab, Allison Brenner, Patricia Dubbert, Sharon Wyatt, Marino Bruce, DeMarc Hickson, Tom Payne, and Herman Taylor. 2016. "Perceived Discrimination is Associated with Health Behaviours among African-Americans in the Jackson Heart Study." *Journal of Epidemiology and Community Health* 70(2):187–94.

Smith, Adam Taylor and Alex Dumas. 2019. "Class-based Masculinity, Cardiovascular Health and Rehabilitation." *Sociology of Health & Illness* 41(2):303–24.

Snead, M. Christine and William C. Cockerham. 2002. "Health Lifestyles and Social Class in the Deep South." *Research in the Sociology of Health Care* 20:107–22.

Springer, Kristen W. and Dawne M. Mouzon. 2011. "'Macho Men' and Preventive Health Care." *Journal of Health and Social Behavior* 52(2): 212–27.

Stead, Martine, Laura McDermott, Anne Marie MacKintosh, and Ashley Adamson. 2011. "Why Healthy Eating is Bad for Young People's Health: Identity, Belonging and Food." *Social Science & Medicine* 72:1121–39.

Swartz, David. 1997. *Culture and Power: The Sociology of Pierre Bourdieu*. Chicago, IL: University of Chicago Press.

Turner, Bryan S. and Steven P. Wainwright. 2003. "Corps de Ballet: The Case of the Injured Dancer." *Sociology of Health & Illness* 25(4):269–88.

Vartanian, Thomas P. and Linda Houser. 2010. "The Effects of Childhood Neighborhood Conditions on Self-Reports of Adult Health." *Journal of Health and Social Behavior* 51(2):291–306.

Veblen, Thorstein. [1899] 1994. *Theory of the Leisure Class*. New York: Dover.

Veenstra, Gerry and Patrick John Burnett. 2014. "A Relational Approach to Health Practices: Towards Transcending the Agency-Structure Divide." *Sociology of Health & Illness* 36(2):187–98.

Wacquant, Loïc. 2016. "A Concise Genealogy and Anatomy of Habitus." *Sociological Review* 64(1):64–72.

Weber, Max. [1922] 1978. *Economy and Society*, Vol. 1. Berkeley, CA: University of California Press.

Weber, Max. 1946. *From Max Weber: Essays in Sociology*. New York: Oxford University Press.

Weber, Max. 1949. *The Methodology of the Social Sciences*. New York: Free Press.

Weber, Max. 1958. *The Protestant Ethic and the Spirit of Capitalism*. New York: Scribners.

Williams, Gareth. 2003. "The Determinants of Health: Structure, Context and Agency." *Sociology of Health & Illness* 25(3):131–54.

Williams, Simon J. 1995. "Theorising Class, Health and Lifestyles: Can Bourdieu Help Us?" *Sociology of Health & Illness* 17(5):577–604.

Wolfe, Joseph D., Shawn Bauldry, Melissa A. Hardy, and Eliza K. Pavalko. 2018. "Multigenerational Attainments, Race, and Mortality Risk among Silent Generation Women." *Journal of Health and Social Behavior* 59(3):335–51.

Zapolski, Tamika C. B., Sarah L. Pederson, Dennis M. McCarthy, and Gregory T. Smith. 2014. "Less Drinking, Yet More Problems: Understanding African American Drinking and Related Problems." *Psychological Bulletin* 140(1):188–223.

Zerubavel, Eviatar. 1997. *Social Mindscapes*. Cambridge, MA: Harvard University Press.

Chapter 11

Life Course Theory

Life course theory in medical sociology is generally used to explain how social experiences and conditions of adversity and inequality in childhood and adolescence impact on health later in life. The theory has been useful in other areas of sociology, especially in criminology linking childhood delinquency to adult criminal behavior (Sampson and Laub 1993). Life course theory is not identified with one particular theorist, as it originated during the 1960s and 1970s as a concept expressed in the work of several scholars in different fields (Alwin 2012; Clausen 1986; Elder, Johnson, and Crosnoe 2006; Halfon et al. 2018). Some trace it in the United States back to Robert Merton's (1968) notion of cumulative advantage—what he called "The Matthew Effect"—in which early recognition in science was depicted as resulting in ever-increasing opportunities and honors for the scientist over the life course. That is, those scientists who are distinguished by achievements early in their careers were described as going on to enjoy ever-greater prominence over time as their honors and rewards accumulated. As Duane Alwin (2012:213) points out, what Merton was illustrating is that in science—as elsewhere in life—"the rich get richer and the poor get poorer."

However, Glen Elder's book, *Children of the Great Depression* ([1974] 1999), is considered a more fundamental contribution to life course theory (Dannefer, Huang, and Estes 2018). This study followed the life situation of people who experienced social and economic hardships in the 1930s during the Great Depression in the U.S. as they moved through the course of their lives. The research revealed the significance of social conditions for the individual at the time of one's growing up and provided a template for research linking earlier life course experiences to later life outcomes, including their effects on physical and mental health (Dannefer et al., 2018:1350).

In Britain, life course research presumably began with what is known as the "Barker hypothesis," based on the work of epidemiologist David Barker

(1995, 1998) who, in the mid-1990s, studied the origins of coronary heart disease (Bury 2004). Barker examined the health records of a sample of men born in two English counties before 1939 and determined that those who were underweight both at birth and one year of age were more likely to die from heart disease later in life. The explanation was that this is the period of life when an infant's cardiovascular and respiratory systems became fully developed and babies who did not wholly undergo this process could not do so later and were more susceptible to heart disease as adults because of it. This led to the hypothesis that health and the onset of chronic disease is biologically programmed at birth.

As Mike Bury (2004) pointed out long ago, not only was the notion of biological programming attractive to medicine, but it also drew the interest of British medical sociologists because the biological deficiencies surrounding birth and the first year of life (especially from undernutrition) were likely triggered by adult social behavior and living conditions promoting smoking, obesity, and other risk factors most common among lower socioeconomic status groups. Consequently, biological factors (i.e., low birth weight) could be connected to social factors (i.e., financial hardship, poor nutrition, unemployment, poverty) in a promising line of inquiry concerning health and the life course.

One view that emerged from the "Barker hypothesis" is the position that there is a critical period in the life course when an adverse biological and social environment (exemplified by undernutrition beginning in the womb) has lifelong health consequences. Although later life circumstances can be important, this perspective maintains early childhood development and circumstances are decisive for the future health of the individual. For example, poor nutrition stemming from conditions of poverty was cited by Barker (1998) as the cause of oxygenated blood in the fetus being redirected to nourish the brain instead of continuing to sustain the growth of the liver. This meant that the body's capacity for blood clotting and cholesterol regulation in the liver relevant for adult cardiovascular functioning could be impaired, even before birth. Low birth weights caused by poor nutrition in particular were seen as major villains. However, Bury (2005) and others (Conley, Strully, and Bennett 2003) suggested that evidence of biological programming has to be met with caution in that low birth weights are not exclusively biological in origin. Smoking, alcohol and drug use, and poor diets as an unhealthy lifestyle on the part of the mother during pregnancy can also produce low birth weights, suggesting that the presumed influence of biological conditions at birth as *the* determinant of poor adult health may be "exaggerated." As Bury (2005:31) noted: "a sociological view would not, in any event, regard low birth weight or conditions in the first weeks and months of life as purely biological in character."

This is because social hardships before birth and early in life stimulate biological programming in the first place, with one major pathway being the dysregulation of stress response systems (Karlamangla et al. 2019). Moreover, socially induced stresses in later life can act as "triggers" to set off biological programming for physical or mental disorders that developed in infancy or were inherited genetically (Bury 2004; Harris and Schorpp 2018; Landecker and Panofsky 2013; Pescosolido et al. 2008; Simons et al. 2011). Without the "triggers," biological programming could remain relatively dormant, or conversely, enhanced socioeconomic resources in later life have been found with the capacity to buffer biological predispositions toward poor health that might exist (Carr 2019; Phelan and Link 2013; Williams et al. 2019). As Ronald Simons et al. (2011:883) put it several years ago, "Rather, genes are turned on (i.e., expressed) and messages they transcribe vary depending on environmental circumstances." Consequently, the relative roles of biological and social factors as part of the critical period of life thesis are intertwined. They still need to be sorted out. Yet it is clear that early childhood adversity is a critical period that promotes severe and lasting poor health in adulthood (Laditka and Laditka 2019).

Another view is that the effects of social adversity are cumulative in that they add up over the life course to build to an unhealthy impact on the adult (Dannefer et al., 2016; Elder et al. 2006). For example, low birth weight is associated with low educational achievement which, in turn, maintains a disadvantaged class position which, based on the adversity associated with it, promotes heavy alcohol use and smoking. The end result is ill health. In the critical period scenario, biology and the social environment set the stage during birth and the first year of life and in the accumulation scenario, biology and socioeconomic influences continue to interact through time to build an outcome. The more bad things happen, the greater the effects on health.

The idea that early life resources and situations carry over to later life circumstances became an appealing concept for medical sociologists investigating why lower-class persons have more health problems and greater mortality over the course of their lives than people in the social classes above them. One way to approach this area of research was to organize the social aspects of aging into stages that denote the life course. Although the stages are based on chronological age and do not account for variations in aging by individuals, they are indicative of the general life cycle most people follow. Implicit in the idea of a life course is a common set of social experiences through which members of a society are expected to pass. For instance, childhood is a time when a person usually receives a primary education, young adulthood is often a time of courtship and marriage, and later maturity a time of retirement.

Table 11.1 The Life Course

Stage	Approximate Age
Infancy	2
Preschool	2–5
Childhood	5–12
Adolescence	12–17
Early maturity	17–25
Maturity	24–40
Middle Age	40–55
Later maturity	55–75
Old Age	75

Age is an important dimension of social organization because the divisions of the life course are those prescribed by a culture to lend stability and predictability to the typical sequence of life events people experience. Also implied in this arrangement is the idea that individuals undergo a change in behavior and roles as they pass from one stage of life into a subsequent stage. People expect infants, children, young adults, middle-aged adults, and older persons to behave in a manner characteristic of their age group; social judgments of their maturity depend on how closely their behavior approximates the corresponding age-related norm. Furthermore, at each stage of the life course, a person takes on new social roles and the responsibilities that accrue to those roles, and the person's status and relationships with other people are modified accordingly. Moreover, the organization of the life course and its social changes are accompanied by physiological changes as people grow to adults and move on to middle and old age in which the stages of their lives are paired with changes in appearance and adjustments to declines in energy, eyesight, hearing, and varying degrees of mental acuity, along with the onset of chronic disease.

The movement of people through time and the changes that occur in and to them all points to the relevance of a life course theory for medical sociology.

The typical stages of the life course and the approximate ages they represent are shown in Table 11.1. A person can be regarded as aging from the moment of conception or moment of birth (depending on one's viewpoint) as part of a distinct age cohort going on to have its particular life experiences through time. Although not everybody necessarily experiences the life course in neatly packaged phases, the division is useful in illustrating the fixed sequence of age-based stages of life.

Age Stratification Theory: A Precursor

An important precursor to life course theory is Matilda White Riley's (1987) age stratification theory that was developed in the 1970s. This theory portrayed society as stratified into different age cohorts, each of which has life course and historical dimensions. The life course dimension refers to shared stages of the life cycle. People belong to a particular age cohort depending on how long they have lived, and, as a result, they share similar social roles and experiences in that they have all been or will be children, students, workers, middle-aged, perhaps parents and grandparents, retired, and so on at approximately the same point in their lives. Thus they have had similar roles in their respective pasts, are occupying similar roles in the present, and are likely to have similar roles in the future as members of the same age cohort moving through the life cycle. As they grow older, everyone else grows older as well, and younger people fill their roles, while they move on with others of their age to assume roles consistent with membership in their cohort. Belonging to a particular age cohort is not only a characteristic of a person beginning at birth but also has consequences for that person at every age.

The historical dimension of age stratification theory pertains to the fact that people experience distinct periods of history together and share the impact of particular historical events on the basis of age. The historical events they experience are unique to their age cohort at the time they experience them and make them different from cohorts yet to come and beyond them. Additionally, the societies they live in change over time because of social and technological developments that cause different age cohorts to age differently. Young people do not become old in the same society in which they began. So while individuals are aging, society is also changing around them. Not only are new patterns of aging caused by social change, age stratification theory claims these patterns also contribute to change as older people now are different from older people in the past.

The link between the aging of individuals and the larger society, in Riley's (1987:4) view, is the flow of age cohorts. Cohort flow affects the numbers and kinds of people in a particular age stratum by way of mortality over time, as well as the capacities, attitudes, and activities of people in that strata. As society moves through time, the age structure and people within that structure are altered as younger cohorts of people replace older ones. Age stratification theory thus provides a perspective that emphasizes a continuing interplay—generated by cohort flow—between social change and individuals as they age. Though interdependent, the process of aging and social change is not synchronized; rather, social change moves along its own axis of historical time and in accordance with its own rhythm. Some periods of history witness greater change than other periods, yet people all follow the same life course. So there is both change and consistency in cohort flows.

Age stratification theory offered an approach in which an age cohort can be seen as a particular generation in relation to other living generations and one that brings its own attitudes, beliefs, and values to bear on situations held in common. Individuals can also be seen as members of a generation living within the context of particular historical circumstances. People can, accordingly, be viewed as experiencing a world already constructed for them and as active participants in further constructing that world. Age stratification theory was attractive to researchers because it is logical, appeared comprehensive, and pointed out a way to analyze the interplay between macro- and micro-level social processes as they related to aging.

However, the theory was difficult to test and put to use in empirical research because of its complexity. Operationalizing the many different variables inherent in cohort flows was a challenge. Moreover, age stratification theory does not consider agency and people do exercise choice in their lives. Nor does the theory take the effects of social inequality into account (Streib and Bourg 1984). Differences within age cohorts, not just between them, especially intracohort socioeconomic disparities, are not given sufficient attention. Besides SES, which is a powerful influence on the aging experience, gender and race also shape how aging is undergone (Carr 2019). But the theory does not address the relevance of these variables and how they function within age cohorts. Life course theory, in contrast, while incorporating the notion of cohort flows, historical events, and transitions into its theoretical repertoire, focuses directly on the effects of social inequalities on people over time and on the significance of class, gender, and race as they affect health over the life span. In doing so, it has become a major theoretical perspective in medical sociology.

Life Course Theory and Health

Life course theory advances the proposition that people go through a sequence of age-based stages and social roles within particular social structures over the course of their lives. It maintains that socioeconomic disadvantages originating in childhood accumulate over the life course to disadvantage health in old age, while socioeconomic advantages over a person's lifetime likewise accumulate but do so to promote relatively good health when elderly. It considers both the early origins of chronic diseases whose symptoms are not obvious until later in life and the social processes and behaviors that promote susceptibility to these diseases until older ages or avoidance of such afflictions. The basic concept underlying life course theory is that:

1. *cohorts* of people born during the same time period experience
2. *transitions* to new roles in the same order or sequence and
3. *life events* (in which earlier events condition later events),
4. which together form *life trajectories* that result in particular outcomes.

Life course researchers concentrate on studying trajectories. These trajectories consist of patterns of behavior that extend through an individual's life, including the transitions and events that affect the direction of the trajectories, in order to determine how later life is affected. The life course can be viewed as an age-based structure within which age cohorts pass through from their beginning on the way to their end. The lives of people in age cohorts are considered shaped by their historical time and places of living, as well as by the transitions and impacts of life events that affect the trajectory of their life course and link them with the trajectories of other people (family, friends, etc.)—giving rise to the notion of "linked lives." As Taylor Hargrove (2018:69) explains: "The life course principle of linked lives posits that relationships are reciprocal and dynamic such that the exposures and events experienced by members of one's social network can have an impact on one's own life trajectory." Thus, events which affect people can also affect others in their social network and, in the case of families, the social circumstances and coping behaviors of parents can have effects on the health of their children for better or worse (Laditka and Laditka 2019).

Similar to age stratification theory, life course theory treats the passage through the life cycle as movement within a structure in which the different time periods are firmly established by both biological and social parameters. "From this perspective," says Dale Dannefer (2012:221), "the problems and 'outcomes' of interest have to do with the life course as a constructed social reality—with historically specific but socially plausible and normative meanings and definitions of the life course as a component of social structure."

Yet to claim that life course theory is exclusively structural in orientation is not accurate. As Dannefer (2012) pointed out, a major conceptual divide in studies of the life course, as in many sociological theories, pertains to the relative influence of agency and structure. While it is clear that the life course is a structure influencing and channeling individuals along its pathways in a top-down fashion as age cohorts irreversibly move on through time, agency nevertheless has an important role in life course theory. As Steven Hitlin and Monica Johnson (2015:1463) explain, individuals do make choices about the direction of their life and "are not simply unconscious carriers of generalized habits or unconscious understandings based on social location, but

[they] actively appraise life conditions and circumstances." In their study that followed the transition of a sample of adolescents into young adulthood over a period of 14 years, they found motivation toward achieving goals that had been set and an optimistic attitude toward the future were features of agency central to constructing a life course. "Agency," according to Hitlin and Johnson (2015:1436), "thus, involves historically embedded individuals contributing to their own life outcomes based on behaviors, dispositions, and preferences, and choices." While the life course itself is a structure, within that structure agency functions to take the individual in a particular direction as opposed to others that are also open. In theorizing about the life course, both structure and agency are relevant. Alwin (2012) points out that life course theory is essentially a theory of lifespan development in which agency is used by individuals to construct their lives through choices and actions within social structures that provide opportunities but also impose constraints.

Life course theory is best tested by the use of longitudinal data that follows individuals and their health or health-related activities over time. Longitudinal data not only can determine *when* changes in health status occur in members of an age cohort, but also allows analysts to account for any attrition in a sample due to loss of participants to mortality or other causes (Lynch 2003). Statistical techniques that can be employed include latent class analysis, hierarchical linear modeling, structural equation modeling, or linear growth curve models applied to data from the cohort or cohorts under investigation at different points in the life course (Brown et al. 2016; Burdette et al. 2017; Umberson et al. 2014; Willson and Shuey 2016; Willson, Shuey, and Elder 2007; Zhang, Hayward, and Yu 2016).

If longitudinal data are not available, other strategies can be used to obtain measures of life course dynamics. For example, Chioun Lee and her colleagues (Lee, Coe, and Ryff 2018) used latent class analysis to identify classes of self-reported child abuse in terms of type and severity in a study of the health effects of childhood trauma. Next they analyzed biomarker data from the adult child abuse survivors to compare present-day adult physiological irregularities with their child abuse profiles. They determined that such abuses were more prevalent in disadvantaged families and that children subjected to the most severe and multifaceted abuse were most likely to have irregular hormone stress reactions, cardiovascular functioning, and blood glucose levels as adults.

Cumulative Advantage/Disadvantage

A subcategory of life course theory that is commonly utilized in medical sociology is the concept of cumulative advantage/disadvantage (Willson et al.

2007; Willson and Shuey 2019). It posits that the initial advantages or disadvantages that people have in life, including health, are typically associated with structural variables—especially SES, but others such as gender and race are also important. The effects of these variables accumulate over time in either positive or negative ways to benefit or increasingly erode health. Kenneth Ferraro and his associates (Ferraro, Schafer, and Wilkinson 2016:108) put it this way: "Whether in sociology or toxicology, a core thesis is that the accumulation of negative exposures raises the risk of subsequent health problems."

While in childhood, adolescence, and young adulthood, both higher and lower SES persons are generally healthy, this does not remain the case. As an age cohort passes through time, lower SES persons in that cohort have greater exposure to health risks, fewer and less quality resources to maintain their health, and engage in less healthy behaviors and lifestyles, thereby making them more susceptible to poor health when older as the disadvantages add up over time. Thus, it is the higher probability of exposure to health risks, reduced ease of access to resources, and greater preponderance of unhealthy behaviors that disadvantages the health of one group in comparison to another over time (Dannefer 2003; DiPrete and Eirich 2006; Ferraro, Shippee, and Schafer 2009). According to Alwin (2012:213):

> Few would on the face of it doubt … [the] observation that the social environment is structured in such a way as to promote the accrual of greater resources to those who already have them—or cumulative advantage—and the withholding of resources from those who begin with less—or cumulative disadvantage. The argument is typically extended further to suggest there is a further compounding, or an accentuation, of the influences of the social environment over time, but this has not been closely examined. Not only do socioenvironmental inequalities affect individual differences at multiple points over the life span, there is considerable theory, suggesting that the residues of these influences in individual differences cumulate over time. Hence, there is a literature that has developed under the topic of "cumulative advantage/disadvantage theory" that fits well within this particular view of the life course.

The focal point of the cumulative advantage/disadvantage perspective is the role of accumulation in analyzing how early life experiences determine later life outcomes (Ferraro et al. 2016). That is, the accumulation of disadvantages over time is the source of enhanced health problems at older ages as negative exposures build up to increasingly negative outcomes. This is seen in past studies where individuals who lived in disadvantaged circumstances in childhood manifested much poorer health as an older adult than those in their age cohort who grew up with more socioeconomic advantages

(Brown et al. 2016; Lynch 2003; Mirowsky and Ross 2008; Willson and Shuey 2019; Willson et al. 2007). Education and income obviously play an important role in this scenario as higher SES individuals have the knowledge and financial resources to better maintain their health and healthy living conditions over the life course (Leopold and Leopold 2018; Lynch 2006; Pudrovska 2014). Generally speaking, studies in this area show health gaps *within* cohorts of socioeconomically advantaged/disadvantaged groups that invariably widen with age. Additionally, it appears that instances of cumulative disadvantage can be transmitted from one generation to the next as seen in research showing that work disabilities in parents increased the probability of work disabilities showing up in their children (Willson and Shuey 2019).

There is also evidence that higher SES in early life is related to lower mortality over the life course with the advantage in mortality increasing with age, especially for women (Pudrovska 2014). An exception for women is obesity, as lower SES women are more likely to gain weight over the life course as seen in research showing significantly higher body mass index (BMI) scores when compared to higher SES women and men generally at age 18 and again at age 54 (Pudrovska et al. 2014). Other research shows low SES black women in particular with increasingly higher BMI scores over the life course (Hargrove 2018). Disadvantaged racial minorities subject to childhood adversities also show greater impaired cognitive functioning in adulthood than non-Hispanic whites (Zhang et al., 2016), while a sample of inner-city African Americans on the south side of Chicago subject to low childhood SES and poor maternal mental health showed an exceptionally high rate of male and female drug use and male psychological distress in mid-adulthood (Fothergill et al. 2016). Debra Umberson and her colleagues (Umberson et al. 2014) observed in a national sample that greater childhood adversity created a "chain of disadvantage" that helped explain why many black men linked to this chain had more strained personal relationships and worse health in adulthood than white men in the study. All of these studies support a cumulative advantage/disadvantage explanation.

Outside of the U.S., in Sweden, with its relatively more homogeneous population and one of the lowest levels of income inequality in the world, there is evidence that the cumulative advantage/disadvantage thesis applies there as well. The gap in self-rated health between higher and lower educational and occupational groups was found to widen between early to middle adulthood and remain constant in old age despite deliberate policies to reduce health disparities (Leopold 2016). In Germany, which also has an extensive system of state-sponsored health benefits, the cumulative advantage/disadvantage hypothesis was found to apply to men but not women (Leopold and Leopold 2018). The reasons for the gender difference could not be determined from the data, but higher-educated German women were in better health than lower-educated women early in life and kept this advantage within their age cohort throughout the life course, suggesting their life course advantage appeared much earlier rather than later and did not change over time.

While the cumulative advantage/disadvantage concept has shown success as an explanatory model of SES, race, and gender differences in health across the life course, some researchers find it is not an entirely satisfying answer to intracohort health differences (DiPrete and Eirich 2006; Ferraro et al. 2016). To say that people of higher social station in an age cohort live increasingly longer than those below them in a class gradient in the same cohort because of accumulated advantages that increase over time may be considered true in many but not all circumstances (Ferraro et al. 2016). Thomas DiPrete and Gregory Eirich (2006) point out that (1) while there may be simple forms of cumulative advantage operating like compound interest in a savings account to increase health and longevity, the relationship between life course development and health is more complex than this and can involve the interaction of several variables (e.g., gender, race); (2) some effects may not have a direct impact on health over time but instead lead to other events or transitions that affect health outcomes instead; and (3) accumulated advantages may not always accumulate over time but be "turned off" at some point and fail to matter, thereby stopping the process prematurely. Consequently, DiPrete and Eirich, along with others (Dannefer 2003; O'Rand 1996), and especially Ferraro (Ferraro et al. 2009, 2016), used life course theory and the accumulative advantage/disadvantage concept to formulate yet another life course theoretical subcategory, that of cumulative inequality theory.

Cumulative Inequality Theory

What primarily distinguishes cumulative inequality theory from the concept of cumulative advantage/disadvantage is that while cumulative inequality likewise maintains that early disadvantage increases the later potential for risks to health and the higher probability of a life filled with hardship over time, it also acknowledges the potential use of mid-life resources to mitigate or eliminate the effects of early life disadvantages before the onset of old age. As Monica Williams et al. (2019:172) note, cumulative inequality theory is useful in studying the life course in four respects: (1) it recognizes the importance of family lineage ("linked lives") and childhood conditions in relation to inequality across families of origin; (2) the theory emphasizes that disadvantage in one domain (family life) diffuses to affect other domains (health), thus misfortune is not a single variable; (3) it notes that early disadvantages do not always accumulate but through agency and resource activation can be reversed; and (4) observes that premature mortality among disadvantaged populations leaving fewer people experiencing adversity does not mean a decrease in inequality.

Cumulative inequality theory begins with an initial position that negative life events and experiences place people at increased risk, positive experiences create opportunities for them, and both can alter life chances for individuals and groups for better or worse (Ferraro, Shippee, and Schafer 2009; Schafer, Ferraro, and Mustillo 2011). Childhood is recognized as the key stage of life for experiencing inequality and a crucial period for adult health. This is because the conditions associated with childhood reflect the influence of genes, the environment, and family background (lineage) on the child. It is the initial step in the child's internalization of status and recognition of growing up in an environment of advantage or disadvantage (Ferraro and Shippee 2009). The SES of a child's parents, for example, signifies the health-related resources the child is socialized to regard as normative (e.g., physician checkups, vaccinations) and indicative of the quality of health lifestyles that are expected on the part of the child by the parents (Mollborn et al. 2014; Mollborn and Lawrence 2018). Stressors that occur during childhood are also considered important with respect to a child's development and social functioning.

Among the existing studies, there is research supporting cumulative equality theory with respect to depression and chronic pain showing low SES persons having more of each over time (Goosby 2013), along with other studies showing elevated cardiovascular risks and less likelihood of being free of chronic diseases in later life (Williams et al. 2019). Ronald Simons and his colleagues (2019) found that early adversity in life predicted accelerated aging in adulthood, and high adult adversity amplified the speed of biological aging. Kristi Williams and Brian Finch (2019) determined that childhood adversity predicted earlier childbearing and greater odds of having nonmarital first births by young women, while Katsuya Oi and Steven Haas (2019) utilized biomarker data indicative of cardiometabolic risk to verify that socioeconomic conditions (good or bad) in childhood predicted cognitive functioning (good or bad) in later life. Higher SES persons had slower cognitive decline in adulthood. Other research by Tyson Brown and his associates utilized hierarchical linear and growth curve models that found a gap between blacks and whites in self-rated health in one study (Brown, O'Rand, and Adkins 2012) and serious health conditions in another (Brown et al. 2016) that increased between middle and late-middle age as suggested by cumulative inequality theory. Whites were more likely to delay but not escape the onset of serious chronic diseases. An anomaly was highly educated black women who showed a steeper decline in health self-ratings than either less-educated black men or whites, that was potentially indicative of greater stress in confronting the challenges in their lives (Brown et al. 2016).

Ferraro and his research team (Ferraro et al. 2016) analyzed data from a national sample and the results supported cumulative inequality theory in finding that childhood disadvantage was connected to adult disadvantage, with those less advantaged as children having more health problems and fewer social psychological resources as adults. Additionally, it was determined that low SES persons who were physically abused at a young age not only had worsening health problems over time but new ones in adulthood that had not previously surfaced. Matthew Andersson (2016), as discussed in the last chapter, reinforces the notion that childhood has a long reach when it comes to health in adulthood. Andersson focused on childhood physical abuse and found that the child–parent bonds compromised by such abuse undermined whatever health protections SES could provide in adulthood for several mid-life diseases.

Life Course and Health Lifestyle Theory

As discussed in Chapter 9, a recent use of life course theory is to combine it with health lifestyle theory to analyze the profile of such lifestyles passing through the life cycle. Stefanie Mollborn et al. (2014), for example, note the relevance of the life course perspective for researching health lifestyles in childhood by observing that children begin life with a *received* health lifestyle from their parents and/or other caregivers and gradually transition to an *achieved* health lifestyle by adolescence. The merit of the life course perspective for these researchers is its theoretical attention to the possibility of differences in health lifestyles at different stages of life. It also points to the relevance of age as an important variable in health lifestyle theory (Cockerham 2005, 2013).

Since life course theory maintains that social conditions in early life affect health in adulthood, then it logically follows that health lifestyles in adulthood also have their origins in childhood and adolescence, which is found to be the case in several studies (Burdette et al. 2017; Lawrence, Mollborn, and Hummer 2017; Mize 2017). In such studies we also usually see an intergenerational process in which the parents' SES and social circumstances are reflected in the health lifestyles of their children. Adolescent health lifestyles, however, are not only connected to family influence but also to those of schools and peers, which may or may not be positive in the case of peers (Mollborn and Lawrence 2018). Overall, the existing research finds that social background predicts early childhood health lifestyles with those in disadvantaged households likely to have lifestyles with greater health risks whose effects are carried over into the next and successive stages of the life course.

Beginning in middle and late-middle age, however, health lifestyles tend to become stable and more positive for many people if this has not already happened (Burgard et al. 2020). Yet as older age approaches, there is evidence that health lifestyle practices become "locked in" along class lines (Rees Jones et al. 2011). That is, social-class distinctions seem to retain their significance at older ages—as they do throughout the life course—with healthier lifestyles remaining typical of people higher on the social ladder compared to those toward or at the bottom (Rees Jones et al. 2011; McGovern and Nazroo 2015). An exception is those persons required to adopt a healthier lifestyle because of a diagnosed health condition (Cockerham, Wolfe, and Bauldry 2020). According to Amy Burdette and her associates (Burdette et al. 2017:522): "The primary implication of the life course perspective and relevant frameworks is that the early adoption of unhealthy lifestyles may play a crucial role in the development of formative challenges and health-related risks in adulthood." Thus the association between life course theory and health lifestyle theory is likely to continue in research on the health practices of age cohorts.

Summary

This chapter discusses life course theory in which social experiences and conditions of adversity and inequality in childhood and adolescence impact on health later in life. Life course theory holds that (1) cohorts of people born during the same time period experience (2) transitions to new roles in the same order or sequence and (3) life events (in which earlier events condition later events), (4) which together form life trajectories that result in particular outcomes. The focus of life course research is on studying trajectories, which consist of patterns of behavior extending through an individual's life, including transitions and events that affect their direction. The life course is viewed as an age-based structure within which age cohorts pass through over time, but agency nevertheless has an important role as individuals make choices and changes about the direction of their life.

Subcategories of life course theory include (1) cumulative advantage/disadvantage, which maintains that the initial advantages or disadvantages that people have in life by way of structural variables, such as SES, gender, and race, accumulate over time to benefit or increasingly erode health. The focal point of the cumulative advantage/disadvantage perspective is the role of accumulation in analyzing how early life experiences determine later life outcomes. Also included as a subcategory is (2) cumulative inequality theory which likewise maintains that early disadvantage increases later life risks to health, but also acknowledges the potential of mid-life resources to mitigate or eliminate the effects of early life disadvantages before the onset of old age. Cumulative inequality theory begins with an initial position that negative life events and experiences place people at increased risk, positive experiences create opportunities for them, and both can alter life chances for individuals and groups for better or worse. This approach recognizes the importance of "linked lives" and adverse childhood conditions in families of origin, disadvantage in one area of life diffuses to affect others, early disadvantages can be reversed, and premature mortality leaving fewer people experiencing adversity does not mean a decrease inequality. A newer development has been to combine life course theory with health lifestyle theory to examine health lifestyle practices among age cohorts.

Guide to Critical Thinking

1. Briefly stated, what is life course theory?
2. Describe the initial thinking that provides the background for life course theory.
3. What is the basic concept underlying the theory?
4. What is the relationship between agency and structure?
5. Name the two major subcategories of life course theory and describe each.

Suggested Reading

Carr, Deborah. 2019. *Golden Years? Social Inequality in Later Life.* New York: Russell Sage. A recent book on social inequality in old age utilizing life course theory.
Shanahan, Michael J., Jeylan T. Mortimer, and Monica Kirkpatrick Johnson (eds.). 2017. *Handbook of the Life Course.* New York: Springer.
Contains several chapters by various authors on the life course.

References

Alwin, Duane F. 2012. "Integrating Varieties of Life Course Concepts." *The Journals of Gerontology* 67B(2):206–20.
Andersson, Matthew A. 2016. "Chronic Disease at Midlife: Do Parent–Child Bonds Modify the Effect of Childhood SES?" *Journal of Health and Social Behavior* 52(3):173–89.
Barker, David J. P. 1995. "Fetal Origins of Coronary Heart Disease." *British Medical Journal* 311:171–4.
Barker, David J. P. 1998. *Mothers, Babies, and Disease in Later Life*, 2nd ed. Edinburgh: Churchill Livingstone.
Brown, Tyson H., Angela M. O'Rand, and Daniel E. Adkins. 2012. "Race-Ethnicity and Health Trajectories: Tests of Three Hypotheses across Multiple Groups and Health Outcomes." *Journal of Health and Social Behavior* 53(3):359–77.
Brown, Tyson H., Liana J. Richardson, Taylor W. Hargrove, and Courtney S. Thomas. 2016. "Using Multiple-hierarchy Stratification and Life Course Approaches to Understand Health Inequalities: The Intersecting Consequences of Race, Gender, SES, and Age." *Journal of Health and Social Behavior* 57(2):200–22.

Burdette, Amy M., Belinda L. Needham, Miles G. Taylor, and Terrence D. Hill. 2017. "Health Lifestyles in Adolescence and Self-rated Health in Adulthood." *Journal of Health and Social Behavior* 58(4):520–36.

Burgard, Sarah A., Katherine Y. P. Lin, Brian D. Segal, Michael R. Elliott, and Sarah Seelye. 2020. "Stability and Change in Health Behavior Profiles of U.S. Adults." *The Journals of Gerontology* 75B(3): 674–83.

Bury, Mike. 2004. "Lifecourse," in Jonathan Gabe, Mike Bury, and Mary Elston (eds.), *Key Concepts in Medical Sociology*. London: Sage, pp. 50–5.

Bury, Mike. 2005. *Health and Illness*. Cambridge: Polity.

Carr, Deborah. 2019. *Golden Years? Social Inequality in Later Life*. New York: Russell Sage.

Clausen, John A. 1986. *The Life Course: A Sociological Perspective*. Englewood Cliffs, NJ: Prentice-Hall.

Cockerham, William C. 2005. "Health Lifestyle Theory and the Convergence of Agency and Structure." *Journal of Health and Social Behavior* 46:51–67.

Cockerham, William C. (ed.). 2013. "Bourdieu and an Update of Health Lifestyle Theory," in William Cockerham (ed.), *Medical Sociology on the Move: New Directions in Theory*. Dordrecht: Springer, pp. 127–54.

Cockerham, William C., Joseph D. Wolfe, and Shawn Bauldry. 2020. "Health Lifestyles in Late Middle Age." *Research on Aging* 42(1):34–46

Conley, Dalton, Kate W. Strully, and Neil G. Bennett. 2003. *The Starting Gate: Birth Weight and Life Chances*. Berkeley, CA: University of California Press,

Dannefer, Dale. 2003. "Cumulative Advantage/Disadvantage and the Life Course: Cross Fertilizing Age and Social Science Theory." *Journals of Gerontology* 58B(6):327–37.

Dannefer, Dale. 2012. "Enriching the Tapestry: Expanding the Scope of Life Course Concepts." *Journals of Gerontology* 67B(2):221–5.

Dannefer, Dale, Wenxuan Huang, and Carroll J. Estes. 2018. "Life Course," in Bryan S. Turner, Chang Kyung-Sup, Cynthia Epstein, Peter Kivisto, William Outhwaite, and J. Michael Ryan (eds.), *The Wiley Blackwell Encyclopedia of Social Theory*. Oxford: Wiley Blackwell, pp. 1349–52.

Dannefer, Dale, Jessica Kelley-Moore, and Wenxuan Huang. 2016. "Opening the Social: Sociological Imagination in Life Course Studies," in J. Mortimer and M. Shanahan (eds.), *Handbook of the Life Course*. New York: Springer, pp. 87–110.

DiPrete, Thomas A. and Gregory M. Eirich. 2006. "Cumulative Advantage as a Mechanism for Inequality: A Review of Theoretical and Empirical Developments." *Annual Review of Sociology* 32:271–97.

Elder, Glen H., Jr. [1974] 1999. *Children of the Great Depression*. Boulder, CO: Westview.

Elder, Glenn H., Jr., Monica K. Johnson, and Robert Crosnoe. 2006. "The Emergence and Development of Life Course Theory," in Jeylan Mortimer and Michael Shanahan (eds.), *Handbook of the Life Course*. New York: Springer, pp. 3–19.

Ferraro, Kenneth F. and Tetyana Pylypiv Shippee. 2009. "Cumulative Inequality: How does Inequality Get Under the Skin?" *The Gerontologist* 49(3):333–43.

Ferraro, Kenneth F., Markus H. Schafer, and Lindsay R. Wilkinson. 2016. "Childhood Disadvantage and Health Problems in Middle and Later Life: Early Imprints on Physical Health?" *American Sociological Review* 81(1):107–33.

Ferraro, Kenneth F., Tetyana Pylypiv Shippee, and Markus H. Schafer. 2009. "Cumulative Inequality Theory for Research on Aging and the Life Course," in V. Bengtson, D. Gans, N. Putney, and M. Silverstein (eds.), *Handbook of Theories of Aging*. New York: Springer, pp. 413–33.

Fothergill, Kate, Margaret E. Ensminger, Elaine E. Doherty, Hee-Soon Juon, and Kerry M. Green. 2016. "Pathways from Childhood Adversity to Later Adult Drug Use and Psychological Distress: A Prospective Study of a Cohort of African Americans." *Journal of Health and Social Behavior* 57(2):223–39.

Goosby, Bridget J. 2013. "Early Life Course Pathways of Adult Depression and Chronic Pain." *Journal of Health and Social Behavior* 54(1):75–91.

Halfon, Neal, Christopher B. Forrest, Richard M. Lerner, and Elaine M. Faustman (eds.). 2018. *Handbook of Life Course Health Development*. New York: Springer.

Hargrove, Taylor W. 2018. "Intersecting Social Inequalities and Body Mass Index Trajectories from Adolescence to Early Adulthood." *Journal of Health and Social Behavior* 59(1):56–73.

Harris, Kathleen Mullan and Kristen M. Schorpp. 2018. "Integrating Biomarkers in Social Stratification and Health Research." *Annual Review of Sociology* 44:361–86.

Hitlin, Steven and Monica Kirkpatrick Johnson. 2015. "Reconceptualizing Agency within the Life Course: The Power of Looking Ahead." *American Journal of Sociology* 120(5):1429–72.

Karlamangla, Arun S., Sharon Stein Merkin, David M. Almeida, Esther M. Friedman, Jacqueline A. Mogle, and Teresa E. Seeman. 2019. "Early-Life Adversity and Dysregulation of Adult Diurnal Cortisol Rhythm." *Journals of Gerontology* 74B(1):160–9.

Laditka, Sarah B. and James N. Laditka. 2019. "An Enduring Health Risk of Childhood Adversity: Earlier, More Severe, and Longer Lasting Work Disability in Adult Life." *Journals of Gerontology* 74B(1):136–47.

Landecker, Hannah and Aaron Panofsky. 2013. "From Social Structure to Gene Regulation, and Back: A Critical Introduction to Environmental Epigenetics for Sociology." *Annual Review of Sociology* 39:333–57.

Lawrence, Elizabeth M., Stefanie Mollborn, and Robert A. Hummer. 2017. "Health Lifestyles across the Transition to Adulthood: Implications for Health." *Social Science & Medicine* 193:23–32.

Lee, Chioun, Christopher L. Coe, and Carol D. Ryff. 2018. "Social Disadvantage, Severe Child Abuse, and Biological Profiles in Adulthood." *Journal of Health and Social Behavior* 58(3):371–86.

Leopold, Liliya. 2016. "Cumulative Advantage in an Egalitarian Country? Socioeconomic Health Disparities Over the Life Course in Sweden." *Journal of Health and Social Behavior* 57(2):257–73.

Leopold, Liliya and Thomas Leopold. 2018. "Education and Health across Lives and Cohorts: A Study of Cumulative (Dis)advantage and its Rising Importance in Germany." *Journal of Health and Social Behavior* 59(1):94–112.

Lynch, Scott M. 2003. "Cohort and Life Course Patterns in the Relationship between Education and Health." *Demography* 40(2):309–31.

Lynch, Scott M. 2006. "Explaining Life Course and Cohort Variation in the Relationship between Education and Health: The Role of Income." *Journal of Health and Social Behavior* 47(4):324–38.

McGovern, Pauline and James Y. Nazroo. 2015. "Patterns and Causes of Health Inequalities in Later Life: A Bourdieusian Approach." *Sociology of Health & Illness* 37(1):143–60.

Merton, Robert K. 1968. "The Matthew Effect in Science." *Science* 159(3810):43–56.

Mirowsky, John and Catherine E. Ross. 2008. "Education and Self-Rated Health: Cumulative Advantage and its Rising Importance." *Research on Aging* 30(1):93–122.

Mize, Trenton D. 2017. "Profiles in Health: Multiple Roles and Health Lifestyles in Early Childhood." *Social Science & Medicine* 178:196–205.

Mollborn, Stefanie and Elizabeth Lawrence. 2018. "Family, Peer, and School Influences in Children's Developing Health Lifestyles." *Journal of Health and Social Behavior* 59(1):133–50.

Mollborn, Stefanie, Laurie James-Hawkins, Elizabeth Lawrence, and Paula Fomby. 2014. "Health Lifestyles in Early Childhood." *Journal of Health and Social Behavior* 55(4):386–402.

Oi, Katsuya and Steven Haas. 2019. "Cardiometabolic Risk and Cognitive Decline: The Role of Socioeconomic Status in Childhood and Adulthood." *Journal of Health and Social Behavior* 60(3):326–43.

O'Rand, Angela M. 1996. "The Precious and the Precocious: Understanding Cumulative Disadvantage and Cumulative Advantage over the Life Course." *The Gerontologist* 36(3):230–38.

Pescosolido, Bernice A., Brea L. Perry, Scott Long, Jack K. Martin, John I. Nurnberger, Jr., and Victor Hesselbrock. 2008. "Under the Influence of Genetics: How Transdisciplinarity Leads us to Rethink Social Pathways to Illness." *American Journal of Sociology* 114:S171–S201.

Phelan, Jo C. and Bruce G. Link. 2013. "Fundamental Cause Theory," in William Cockerham (ed.), *Medical Sociology on the Move: New Directions in Theory*. Dordrecht: Springer, pp. 105–26.

Pudrovska, Tetyana. 2014. "Early-Life Socioeconomic Status and Mortality at Three Life Course Stages: An Increasing Within-Cohort Inequality." *Journal of Health and Social Behavior* 55(2):181–95.

Pudrovska, Tetyana, Eric N. Reither, Ellis S. Logan, and Kyler J. Sherman-Wilkins. 2014. "Gender and Reinforcing Associations between Socioeconomic Disadvantage and Body Mass over the Life Course." *Journal of Health and Social Behavior* 55(3):283–301.

Rees Jones, Ian, Olia Papocosta, Peter H. Whincup, S. Goya Wannamethee, and Richard W. Morris. 2011. "Class and Lifestyle 'Lock-in' among Middle-Aged and Older Men: A Multiple Correspondence Analysis of the British Regional Heart Study." *Sociology of Health & Illness* 33(3):399–419.

Riley, Matilda White. 1987. "On the Significance of Age in Sociology." *American Sociological Review* 52(1):1–14.

Sampson, Robert J. and John H. Laub. 1993. *Crime in the Making: Pathways and Turning Points through Life.* Cambridge, MA: Harvard University Press.

Schafer, Markus H., Kenneth F. Ferraro, and Sarah A. Mustillo. 2011. "Children of Misfortune: Early Adversity and Cumulative Inequality in Perceived Life Trajectories." *American Journal of Sociology* 116(4):1053–91.

Simons, Ronald L., Man Kit Lei, Steven R. H. Beach, Gene H. Brody, Robert A. Philibert, and Frederick X. Gibbons. 2011. "Social Environment, Genes, and Aggression: Evidence Supporting the Differential Susceptibility Perspective." *American Sociological Review* 76(8):883–912.

Simons, Ronald L., Man-Kit Lei, Steven R. H. Beach, Leslie Gordon Simons, Ashley B. Barr, Frederick X. Gibbons, and Robert A. Philibert. 2019. "Testing Life Course Models Whereby Juvenile and Adult Adversity Combine to Influence Speed of Biological Aging." *Journal of Health and Social Behavior* 60(3):291–308.

Stead, Martine, Laura McDermott, Anne Marie MacKintosh, and Ashley Adamson. 2011. "Why Healthy Eating is Bad for Young People's Health: Identity, Belonging and Food." *Social Science & Medicine* 72:1121–39.

Streib, Gordon F. and Carroll J. Bourg. 1984. "Age Stratification Theory, Inequality, and Change." *Comparative Social Research* 7(1):63–77.

Umberson, Debra, Kristi Williams, Patricia A. Thomas, Hui Liu, and Mieke Beth Thomeer. 2014. "Race, Gender, and Chains of Disadvantage: Childhood Adversity, Social Relationships, and Health." *Journal of Health and Social Behavior* 55(1):20–38.

Williams, Kristi and Brian Karl Finch. 2019. "Adverse Childhood Experiences, Early Nonmarital Fertility, and Women's Health at Midlife." *Journal of Health and Social Behavior* 60(3):309–25.

Williams, Monica M., Blakelee R. Kemp, Kenneth F. Ferraro, and Sarah A. Mustillo. 2019. "Avoiding the Major Causes of Death: Does Childhood Misfortune Reduce the Likelihood of Being Disease Free in Later Life?" *Journals of Gerontology* 74B(1):170–80.

Willson, Andrea E. and Kim M. Shuey. 2016. "Life Course Pathways of Economic Hardship and Mobility and Midlife Trajectories of Health." *Journal of Health and Social Behavior* 57(3):407–22.

Willson, Andrea E. and Kim M. Shuey. 2019. "A Longitudinal Analysis of the Intergenerational Transmission of Health Inequality." *The Journals of Gerontology* 74B(1):181–91.

Willson, Andrea E., Kim M. Shuey, and Glen Elder, Jr. 2007. "Cumulative Advantage Processes as Mechanisms of Inequality in Life Course Health." *American Journal of Sociology* 112(6):1886–924.

Zhang, Zhenmel, Mark D. Hayward, and Yan-Ling Yu. 2016. "Life Course Pathways to Racial Disparities in Cognitive Impairment among Older Americans." *Journal of Health and Social Behavior* 57(2):184–99.

Chapter 12

Fundamental Cause Theory

Fundamental cause theory is one of the best-known contemporary theories in medical sociology. It was initially conceptualized by Bruce Link and Jo Phelan in 1995 and provides a theoretical explanation for the persistent effects of one of the most basic variables in sociology—socioeconomic status or class position—on health and mortality. Link and Phelan had observed that SES is associated with multiple diseases in a relationship reproduced in multiple contexts through successive historical periods. Even though the level of threats from these diseases and their modes of treatment changed over time, the association with SES remained constant. Link and Phelan wanted to account theoretically why this is the case.

They began by incorporating sociologist Stanley Lieberson's (1985) notion of causation into their model. Lieberson maintained that the "basic causes" of social phenomena have enduring effects on dependent variables because when the effects of one cause or mechanism decline or end, the effects of another become more prominent or emerge. Thus, multiple factors or mechanisms can be involved in contributing to a lasting or persistent relationship between a basic cause such as SES and its effects. What this signals for the health–SES relationship is that even though diseases ebb and flow and treatments come and go, the effects of SES on that disease remain the same. James House and his colleagues (1990) went on to suggest that the idea of a basic cause might explain the persistent connection between SES and mortality.

Link and Phelan therefore proposed that SES is a "fundamental cause" of health, illness, disability, and death (Link 2008; Link and Phelan 1995, 2000; Phelan et al. 2004; Phelan and Link 2013, 2015; Phelan, Link, and Tehranifar 2010). While it is clear there is a connection between SES and health, it was not widely considered up until then that SES could be causal. What this proposition signified is that society, or rather the structure of society, could make people sick. Perhaps even hasten their death. This was a bold assertion at the time because many researchers in the past, especially those outside of medical sociology, viewed SES as simply "background." Diseases were invariably seen as biologically driven regardless of the social context of a person's life. SES contributed only indirectly, if at all, to health and mortality, not as a direct cause. It put people in a position to become sick because low SES meant greater exposure to unhealthy conditions, not make them sick with its own properties. Some epidemiologists, as reported by Karen Lutfey and Jeremy Freese (2005), had declared that SES was "causally related to few if any diseases" but instead was "a correlate of many diseases" (Rothman 1986:90).

However, Link and Phelan (1995) had identified the persistent association of SES with a variety of diseases throughout different periods of history which increasingly pointed toward SES as having a causal role. For example, diseases such as the plague, cholera, and typhoid go back centuries and invariably it is the poor who suffered much more so than the affluent. This connection continues today as seen in diseases like cancer and heart disease, as well as newly emerging ones like Ebola and COVID-19. We have not witnessed communicable illnesses where the affluent get sick first and then spread to the poor, or chronic diseases where the prevalence is greater among the financially secure than the insecure. In the mid-twentieth century, coronary heart disease was not uncommon among wealthy men because of rich diets, smoking cigars and cigarettes, heavy drinking, lack of exercise and relaxation, and job-related stress. This changed with the widespread and quicker adoption of healthier lifestyles by such men, along with the more rapid use of statin drugs to reduce cholesterol, other drugs to control blood pressure, heart rate, and the risk of stroke, and various medical procedures (i.e., stents, bypass surgery, artificial heart valves, and pace-makers). Mortality from heart disease became more prevalent among those lower on the social scale (Chang and Lauderdale 2009).

Several studies have consistently linked low SES with poor health and higher mortality (Carpiano, Link, and Phelan 2008; Cockerham 2013; Herd, Goesling, and House 2007; Link and Phelan 1995; Lutfey and Freese 2005; Olafsdottir 2007; Warren and Hernandez 2007). Even though the poor live longer now than the wealthy in past periods of history, people in the upper social stratum still live the longest on average than people in the stratum just below them and so on down the social ladder until the bottom of society is reached where the greatest health disparities reside. If biology was the sole story, this would not always be the case and class boundaries would not matter. But the fact is, class does matter when it comes to health and longevity. Fundamental cause theory addresses the dynamics of this situation.

Fundamental Cause Theory

Fundamental cause theory maintains that in order for a social variable to qualify as a cause of sickness and mortality, and by extension, health inequalities, it must meet four basic criteria: First, it must influence multiple disease outcomes. Thus, the association is not limited to affecting only one or a few diseases but many. The evidence shows that SES is related to virtually all major causes of death from disease (Phelan and Link 2013). Second, it must impact the onset and outcomes of diseases through multiple risk factors, not just one or two. So there have to be more than a few ways it can cause people to become sick. Also, there are several means by which SES causes sickness, such as its ties to stress, smoking, inadequate diets, poor housing, obesity, drug and alcohol abuse, lack of exercise, insufficient preventive health care, and the like. Third, it involves access to resources that can be used to avoid risks or minimize the consequences of a disease if a person does become ill. This is relevant because SES is a determinant of such resources. And fourth, the connection with health is reproduced over time. The historical connection of SES with many health problems is well-documented. The effects persist despite changes in risks, protective factors, and diseases which led Link and Phelan (1995:87) to call them "fundamental" in the first place. In order to test the theory, empirical validation of these four core features is required (Link and Phelan 1995). In sum, the four qualifying criteria for a fundamental cause are that it:

1. must influence multiple diseases;
2. must affect these diseases through multiple pathways of risks;
3. must involve access to resources that can be used to avoid risks or minimize the consequences of disease if it occurs; and
4. must be reproduced over time.

SES meets all four of these criteria because a person's class position influences the risk and outcome of multiple diseases in multiple ways, higher SES persons have the resources to better avoid health problems or minimize them when they occur, and the association has endured for centuries. The reason that SES is related to multiple disease outcomes through multiple pathways that change over time is that individuals and groups use their resources to avoid risks and adopt protective strategies. Consequently, the theory's basic principle is that a superior assortment of flexible resources permits higher SES persons to avoid disease and death in widely divergent conditions. This "leads to the prediction," state Phelan and Link (2013:), "that, at any given time, greater resources will produce better health, and consequently, inequalities in health and mortality will persist as long as resource inequalities do."

The socioeconomic resources a person has or does not have are money, knowledge, status, power, and beneficial social connections. These resources are flexible because they can be used in varied circumstances. Their availability is central to understanding the operation of the theory at both individual (micro) and contextual (macro) levels because the deployment of resources is critical to health. At the individual level, Phelan, Link, and Parisa Tehranifar (2010:S30) consider flexible resources as the "causes of causes" or "risks of risk" that influence individual health behaviors with respect to whether people know about, have access to, can afford, and are motivated to engage in health-promoting practices, as well as determining access to jobs, neighborhoods, and social networks that vary dramatically in the amount of risk and protection they provide. Resources and the ability to use them are most effective for preventable causes of mortality and less so or ineffective for those that are not preventable, such as diseases and disabilities associated with growing old.

Contextual-level resources pertain to access to broad social contexts that also vary significantly in levels of risk or protection, such as living in pleasant or unpleasant neighborhoods, having a job with or without health benefits, or working in healthy or unhealthy job conditions. As Phelan and Link (2013:107) state:

> For example, a person with many resources can afford to live in a high SES neighborhood where neighbors are also of high status and where, collectively, substantial clout is exerted to ensure that crime, noise, violence, pollution, traffic and vermin are kept at a minimum and that the best health-care facilities, parks, playgrounds, and food markets are located nearby. Once a person has used SES-related resources to locate in an advantaged neighborhood, a host of health-enhancing circumstances comes along as a "package deal." Similarly, a person who uses educational credentials to procure a high-status occupation inherits a package deal that is more likely to include excellent health benefits and less likely to involve dangerous conditions and toxic exposures.

There is also easier access by the more affluent to the $25 billion annual market in the U.S. for health-enhancing products, in addition to the better availability of quality health care and the healthiest living conditions. Phelan et al. (2010) also point out the much healthier lifestyles of high-status groups and note the author's (Cockerham 2005) health lifestyle theory illustrates the influence of such groups on healthy behavior. "In these instances," says Phelan et al. (2010:S30), "status groups do not explicitly advocate for health-enhancing conditions, but rather members form cultural practices around food, exercise, and other health-related circumstances that influence the behavior of status-group members." People thus benefit in many ways from membership in the healthiest higher SES groups which can be an "add on" contextual-level benefit.

Box 12.1 Bruce G. Link and Jo C. Phelan

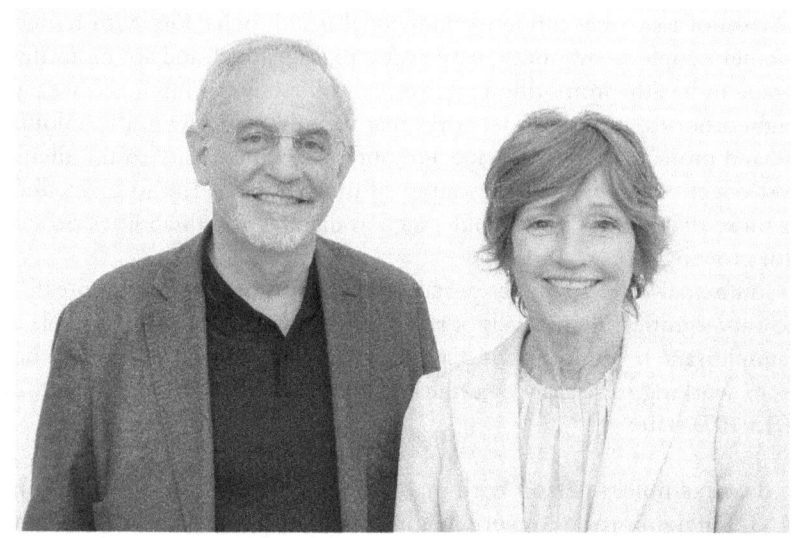

Image 12.1 Bruce Link and Jo Phelan

Bruce Link received his Ph.D. from Columbia University and was a Professor of Epidemiology and Sociomedical Sciences at Columbia and Research Scientist at the New York State Psychiatric Institute when he formulated fundamental cause theory in 1995 with Jo Phelan. She received her Ph.D. from SUNY-Albany and was Special Research Scientist in Sociomedical Sciences at Columbia. They moved to Riverside, California where he is a Distinguished Professor of Sociology and Public Policy at the University of California at Riverside and she is retired after an outstanding career. They provide the following account about what led them to devise their theory:

> The sociological theory of fundamental causes was developed in the early to mid-1990s at the peak of the risk-factor approach to population health. The risk-factor approach held that the way to address social inequalities in health was to identify the intervening risk-factor mechanisms linking social inequalities to health, to use public health principles to intervene on those mechanisms, thereby addressing the health inequalities. In this framework, a social epidemiology was essentially unnecessary because the behavioral risk factors were what mattered most. Fundamental-cause theory

countered this explanation with the insight that socioeconomic related resources of knowledge, money, power, prestige, and beneficial social connections were *flexible resources* that could be used in different places and at different times to avoid risks and adopt protective factors no matter what those factors happened to be in a particular place or time. The theory explained enduring associations between SES and health even as risk factors, protective factors, and diseases changed, thereby supporting the need for a robust social epidemiology to understand population health.

Among the various mechanisms linking socioeconomic status with health and mortality, there is also a greater sense of personal control over one's life because people with such control typically feel good about themselves, handle stress better, and have the capability and living situations to adopt healthy lifestyles. This circumstance may especially apply to people in powerful social positions. "Social power," state Link and Phelan (2000:37), "allows one to feel in control, and feeling in control provides a sense of security and well-being that is [health-promoting]." Persons at the bottom of society, in contrast, are less able to control their lives, have fewer resources to cope with problems, live in more unhealthy situations, face powerful constraints in choosing a healthy way of life, and tend to die earlier.

This not a new situation as inequalities in health and mortality have persisted throughout history; even though older diseases become largely eradicated, newer ones appear, and the mechanisms for causing them and resources for dealing with them change. What the theory of fundamental causes seeks to explain is the persistence of health inequalities across time. Phelan and Link (2013:106)

> reasoned that we cannot claim to understand why health inequalities exist if we cannot explain why they persist under conditions that should eliminate or reduce them, and if we can understand why they persist, this may provide clues to the more general problem of the causes of health inequalities.

Racism

Although fundamental cause theory was developed to explain the lasting effects of SES on health and mortality, Phelan and Link (2013) note that it is likely other social statuses, such as race, ethnicity or gender, also may function as a fundamental cause although the case for these possibilities has yet to be fully made. An exception is racism. In a subsequent paper, Phelan and Link (2015) argued that racism should be considered a fundamental cause of health inequalities. They made three logical deductions—all based on research evidence and each linking into the other—to support their contention: (1) racism is a fundamental cause of racial differences in SES; (2) SES is a fundamental cause of health inequalities; and (3) racism is a fundamental cause of racial differences in health and mortality independent of SES. They (Phelan and Link 2015:311) "conclude that racial inequalities in health endure primarily because racism is a fundamental cause of racial differences in SES and SES is a fundamental cause of health inequalities." Therefore, racism, SES, and health are all connected.

Phelan and Link also added "freedom" to their list of flexible socio-economic resources with respect to race in that freedom refers to the ability to control one's own actions and circumstances in life, which is curtailed in racist environments. Examples from the past in this regard cited by Phelan and Link were slavery and more recently the disproportionate arrest rates and imprisonment of African American men. But constraints on freedom could also apply to situations in which racism acted to limit or deny decision-making, opportunities to act freely, and to participate fully in activities on the basis of race. A particular feature of the harmful effects of racism on health stems from racism's creation of stressful situations causing adverse physiological reactions within the body.

Yet is racism a fundamental cause in its own right or because racial patterns in health and mortality are largely determined by SES? Phelan and Link recognize that much of the enduring relationship between race and health is based on inequalities in SES and the resources associated with class position in which racism is a major underlying factor. But while most of the effects of racism on health are linked to differences in SES, they find that racism does have some independent effects on health that operate through multiple mechanisms, namely racial discrimination as a stressor (i.e., "weathering") and residence in racially segregated neighborhoods with less healthy housing and sources of water, air, and food, and greater exposure in these locales to crime, the availability of harmful substances, and less optimal medical care. To this list could be added the lessened availability of quality dental and vision care, opportunities for good jobs, and substandard neighborhood schools.

In formulating their conceptual framework for establishing racism as a fundamental cause of health disparities, Phelan and Link utilized the socio-historical experience and health profile of black Americans in relation to whites to make a well-reasoned theoretical case. As noted in Chapter 8, U.S. data clearly show that blacks are the most disadvantaged segment of the American population with respect to health and this has been the situation for many years as blacks continue to have the highest rates of mortality for all causes of death and specifically for deaths from heart disease, stroke, cancer, diabetes, AIDS, and homicide (National Center for Health Statistics 2019). However, what about Hispanics? When it comes to theorizing generally in medical sociology about race, racism, and health, Hispanics—whose health indicators are typically better than that of non-Hispanic blacks and whites (National Center for Health Statistics 2019)—are usually absent although they are the largest U.S. racial/ethnic minority. An important next step on examining racism as a fundamental cause would be to apply it to an Hispanic population.

Modifications to Fundamental Cause Theory

While primarily developed by Link and Phelan, there have been efforts to supplement fundamental cause theory with additional contributions on the part of Karen Lutfey Spencer and Jeremy Freese (Freese and Lutfey 2011; Lutfey and Freese 2005), Jonathan Daw (2015), and Sean Clouston and his colleagues (2016). Freese and Lutfey (2011:68) argued that to proclaim SES is a fundamental cause of health is not especially interesting if it means simply that SES causes health. To be a "fundamental" cause means that it must provide something especially meaningful to the process of causality. In their view, a fundamental cause implies a systematic asymmetry by which the relevant mechanisms overwhelmingly exert their influence in one direction and when new mechanisms emerge, they more often than not, preserve the relationship.

Freese and Lutfey proposed that SES operates as a fundamental cause through a "massive multiplicity of mechanisms" that they call "metamechanisms." The term "metamechanisms" appears to refer to causal mechanisms whose effects persist over time, even though they may have transitioned from one form into another. Lutfey and Freese (2005:1326–7) maintained that fundamental cause theory does not imply "a theory of the *specific proximate mechanisms* responsible for a persistent association, but rather that some *metamechanism(s)* are continuously generated over historical time in such a way that the direction of the enduring association is preserved." So while the metamechanisms that put people at risk may change over time, the overall relationship remains the same as replacement metamechanisms keep the association alive. Lutfey and Freese (2005:1331) thus suggest that fundamental cause processes are "holographic" in that "just as each piece of a broken hologram retains a reasonable and whole replication of the original image," so does SES as a fundamental cause of health disparities. This is because its general effects remain operational despite changes in diseases and their treatments, and the appearance of replacement mechanisms.

Freese and Lutfey (2011) condensed their menu of applicable metamechanisms into four general categories: (1) *means* (flexible resources, such as money, power, knowledge, prestige, and beneficial social connections) in which an individual purposefully uses his or her resources to maintain or improve his or her health; (2) *spillovers* (contextual resources) occur when people in an individual's social network or the network itself use their resources and in doing so produce health benefits for the person without any purposeful action on the individual's part; (3) *habitus*, where different norms, dispositions, and lifestyles are adopted by different social classes and groups, with those of higher status groups more beneficial for the person's health. In the case of habitus, unlike spillovers, the individual's health-related behavior does play a role in his or her own health outcomes, but unlike the "means" metamechanism, these actions are not necessarily consciously aimed at improving one's health. They are preferences (or "tastes") resulting from socialization experiences in different social classes as originally depicted by Pierre Bourdieu (1984). Finally, (4) *institutions*, which refers to the actions of institutions that treat people differentially, according to their SES and do so in a way that causes health inequalities.

Lutfey and Freese (2005), for example, used an ethnographic analysis to determine that two diabetes clinics, one serving higher and the other lower SES patients, differed in certain aspects of the care each provided. These differences included being a regular patient of a particular physician at the higher SES clinic who was familiar with their case in order to provide better continuity of care as compared to seeing whoever was on rotating duty at the time at the low SES clinic. The educational resources available at the two clinics also contributed to SES differences in diabetic control of blood sugar levels. The higher SES clinic had better educational services for the self-management of diabetes. Thus, features of institutions themselves could be characterized as metamechanisms promoting class disparities in diabetes. Phelan and Link (2013) observed that a contribution of Freese and Lutfey's description of metamechanisms to their theory was to extend awareness of the different processes, especially the institutional metamechanism, that link SES as a fundamental cause to health inequalities.

However, Daw (2015) claimed that the metamechanisms hypothesized thus far are inadequate to explain many health disparities, which he illustrated in a study of kidney transplantation. He found that the two major metamechanisms of the persistent relationship between social class and health, based on higher status persons making better use of health information and having greater access to health care technology to prevent or treat disease, were not directly applicable to obtaining kidney transplants in an allegedly equitable system of racial selection. The kidney transplantation allocation system in the U.S. is organized to be equitable in that it features universal, single payer health insurance (Medicare) and is administered with an organizational commitment to distributive fairness. Yet racial minority recipients on the waiting list were not as likely as whites to receive transplants from deceased or live kidney donors.

Why the disparity? Daw found that it was because of what he called the efficiency-equity trade-off metamechanism that consisted of a scarcity of living-donor kidneys (occurring most often when a close relative needed a transplant), the probability of a genetic match with the donor pool, the potential recipient's degree of immunological presensitization, and geographic place of residence. All except residence promoted higher rates of transplantation among whites. The efficiency-equity trade-off metamechanism may apply to other health situations involving scarcity in which non-social, namely biological, factors outweigh social equity. Another implication of this study is that there may be other fundamental cause metamechanisms yet to be determined.

The Clouston et al. (2016) paper, which includes Phelan and Link among its co-authors, suggested that social inequalities in health rise and fall according to a predictable process, which they call the "unnatural history of disease." They characterize the history of a disease as progressing through four stages: (1) The *Natural Mortality Stage* which consists of a general lack of knowledge about prevention or effective types of treatment. No one group shows an advantage in avoiding the particular disease which is either randomly distributed or non-randomly distributed because of differential exposure. (2) The *Producing Inequalities Stage* is next in which populations develop new methods to avoid or reduce the burden of a disease's impact on mortality and the benefits are unevenly distributed on a socioeconomic basis, producing health inequalities.

Fundamental cause theory is focused primarily on the transition from the first to the second stage, but Clouston et al. add two more stages. Next is (3) the *Reducing Inequalities Stage*, which begins when health-beneficial innovations to treat a disease become more evenly distributed throughout the population. This can occur if the innovation saturates the advantaged group, making further reduction impossible, or if diffusion efforts are sufficiently focused and the innovation is made widely accessible. In this stage, inequalities stabilize or shrink. (4) The *Reduced Mortality and Disease Death Stage* occurs when a specific health innovation becomes universal and no more gains can be made, regardless of socioeconomic status. Either a treatment is effective (Reduced Mortality) or a disease is eradicated (Disease Death). Whether and when a disease transitions from one stage to another is influenced by social and political efforts to reduce the mortality in disadvantaged groups.

The Clouston et al. analysis suggests that the association of SES with mortality from a particular disease changes in each stage, but nonetheless supports fundamental cause theory that predicts that SES inequalities in mortality from a disease will persist as long as innovations at controlling a disease's inequalities are not spread throughout society. The study concluded that the more rapid the proliferation of methods of prevention and treatment, the less time each stage may take, and the quicker inequalities can be controlled.

Research Applications of Fundamental Cause Theory

Several studies have successfully used fundamental cause theory. Among them is that of Phelan et al. (2004) who investigated causes of death data on 370,930 people in the U.S. National Longitudinal Mortality Study. They found a strong relationship between SES and deaths from preventable causes. Persons with higher SES had significantly higher probabilities of survival from preventable causes because they were able—consistent with the theory—to utilize their resources (money, knowledge, connections, etc.) to obtain what they needed to live longer. Conversely, the lower the SES, the more likely the person was to die from something that could have otherwise been prevented. The deliberate use of flexible socioeconomic resources was found to be a critical factor in maintaining the differences in mortality.

The Lutfey and Freese (2005) study discussed in the previous section not only emphasized the relevance of the institutional metamechanism, but the means metamechanism likewise had powerful effects according to their research. The low SES diabetic patients had financial and job-related constraints. Although the cost of their care was subsidized by the state, they nevertheless did not have the financial resources or health insurance to pay for insulin pumps that higher SES patients could purchase when needed. They were less likely to have jobs where they had access to refrigerators for storing insulin. Some worked as manual laborers and others had night shifts that interfered with medication schedules. Those taking state-subsidized medications were required to get their prescriptions refilled in person at their clinic pharmacy, which was time-consuming and took them away from their jobs. The low SES patients had less family support, particularly single mothers with children, less motivation to take responsibility for their treatment regimens, longer waits for their doctor appointments, more transportation problems in getting to the clinic, and knew less about diabetes. They were much less likely to have access to gym facilities for exercise, and healthy diets. The role of SES as a fundamental cause is shown in the significantly better glucose management of the higher SES patients than the less affluent in the other clinic for reasons that were primarily socioeconomic.

Virginia Chang and Diane Lauderdale (2009) found in a nationwide study that individuals with high socioeconomic status were significantly more likely to have reversed their formerly high levels of cholesterol through the use of statin drugs to the point that low SES persons are now more likely to have high cholesterol and be at greater risk for heart disease. Previously, more affluent persons, especially overachieving men, with rich diets who smoked and drank heavily, were especially prone to heart attacks. This study likewise points to the relevance of SES as a fundamental cause in which flexible resources influence the diffusion of innovations in treatment.

Marcie Rubin, Clouston, and Link (2014) examined how the association between SES and lung and pancreatic cancer mortality changed over time in the U.S. Their data consisted of county-level mortality records for cancer deaths matched with ratings of a county's socioeconomic characteristics. Their findings supported the fundamental cause hypothesis for lung cancer in that class-based resources affected the lowering of mortality rates by way of preventive knowledge. People living in higher SES-ranked counties were quicker and more thorough in both stopping or not starting smoking as information about tobacco's carcinogenic properties became more fully known. Mortality rates from lung cancer were significantly greater in lower SES counties than higher SES counties over time. The conversion was so complete that smoking became identified as a characteristic lower-class behavior and lung cancer as a cause of mortality associated more with deaths of lower SES persons (Pampel 2009).

Whereas lung cancer became increasingly preventable through the widespread dissemination of information about the effects of smoking cigarettes, there were no major prevention or treatment innovations for pancreatic cancer. Rubin et al. therefore found no substantive effect of SES having any causal effects on pancreatic cancer mortality over time. Fundamental cause theory provided an explanation for the existence of class disparities in lung cancer as health-promoting information was not acted on uniformly throughout the class structure. Those with greater access to flexible resources (knowledge, money, power, prestige, and beneficial social connections) and/ or living in a contextual environment of higher SES, disproportionately benefited from the innovation. But for pancreatic cancer, a disease lacking major innovations in prevention and treatment, fundamental cause theory's emphasis on SES was not sustained. This does not diminish fundamental cause theory's explanatory power with respect to diseases with preventable causes, but supports the earlier findings of Phelan et al. (2004) that the theory does not fully explain the association of SES with diseases lacking cures or preventive measures.

In a later study using the same research method, Clouston et al. (2017) determined that improvements in colorectal cancer mortality rates, associated with more widespread use of colonoscopies, were influenced by SES and race, as higher SES groups and whites as compared to lower SES and blacks were more likely to have a colonoscopy showing the presence or absence of polyps in the colon. Although an overall decline in colorectal cancer mortality did occur over time, whites experienced this decline some four years earlier than blacks, and people in higher SES counties, some 23 years earlier than those in lower SES counties.

Other findings supporting fundamental cause theory in the U.S. also analyzed colorectal cancer mortality (Saldana-Ruiz et al. 2013), as well as the effects of SES or its components on health disparities (Herd et al. 2007; Link 2008; Masters, Link, and Phelan 2015; Miech, Pampel, Kim, and Rodgers 2011; Warren and Hernandez 2007), vaccination (Polonijo and Carpiano 2013), and HIV/AIDS (Rubin, Colen, and Link 2010). Elsewhere, fundamental cause theory was applied to the use of welfare state benefits to equalize health resources in Iceland (Olafsdottir 2007) and declines in mortality in some 20 European countries (Mackenbach et al. 2017). The enduring outcome of better health at the top of society and worse health in descending order toward the bottom over the years marks SES as a fundamental cause of health inequalities, disease, and death.

Discussion and Summary

Fundamental cause theory has worked best to date in studies of preventable health problems that can be caused, avoided, or remedied by the level of resources linked to an individual or a larger social entity's (i.e., counties) socioeconomic ranking. It applies particularly to situations in which SES causes people to be exposed to and contract a disease by way of less privileged circumstances (i.e., poverty, unhealthy living conditions or lifestyle, stress) or exposure on the job to a toxic environment. An inability or an absence of resources to escape the situation would be causal. Variables other than SES and racism may also be found to be fundamental causes. Gender, for example, has been identified by Phelan and Link (2013) as a possible fundamental cause of health inequalities. They pointed out that men have historically been accorded higher status than women who report worse health in a manner consistent with fundamental cause theory, yet women live longer on average than men which the theory thus far does not explain.

There have been few critiques of fundamental cause theory to date, but a critical review comes from Gerry Veenstra (2018) who finds that much of the theory lacks specificity. Veenstra maintains that: (1) the components of SES (income, education, and occupation) in the theory do not blend together in a straightforward or clear-cut way; (2) the notion of flexible resources is insufficiently theorized in that there is no clear separation between money, knowledge, power, prestige, and beneficial social connections which can all be considered forms of power or in some cases, prestige, making it difficult to determine the effects of any one specific resource on health; and (3) the distinction between SES and resources is ambiguous. Veenstra (2018:50) suggests that Pierre Bourdieu's (1977, 1998) idea of symbolic power is better suited than SES to informing fundamental cause theory. This is because Bourdieu offers a broad conceptualization of class in which resources are inherent in forms of social, economic, and symbolic capital that play out in fields or social settings through relationships of power expressed by way of differing class positions.

Veenstra's (2018:51) concept of what fundamental cause theory would look like if based on Bourdieu's notion of symbolic power unfolds as follows: (1) resources such as money, knowledge, etc. are all manifestations of power unequally distributed in society; (2) these resources are configured in particular ways that minimize the risk of disease or curtail the negative consequences of a disease once it occurs; and (3) these resources affect multiple diseases through multiple mechanisms linking them to disease change over time as the proximal (closest) factors that affect the disease are replaced. This restatement of fundamental cause theory is similar to the original and the extent to which it is an improvement has yet to be determined through empirical research. Whether Bourdieu's concepts of capital can improve the level of specificity being sought about the meaning of resources awaits verification, as does whether the concept of symbolic power is a better explanatory vehicle than SES for representing a fundamental cause. But for the time being, this remains an alternative approach to conceptualizing SES in the theory.

Phelan and Link (2013:114) themselves observed that "empirical tests of fundamental cause theory are not obvious or straightforward." The theory is broad in scope and complex as it tries to account for a changing landscape of shifting metamechanisms, threats of disease, and treatments, with SES a constant presence. Separating a fundamental cause from proximate causes can also be difficult. In order to test the theory as noted earlier in this chapter, Phelan and Link (2013:114) state that its four core features, namely that "(1) SES influences multiple disease outcomes; (2) SES is related to multiple risk factors for disease and death; (3) the deployment of resources plays a critical role in the association between SES and health/mortality; and (4) the association between SES and health/mortality is reproduced over time via the replacement of intervening mechanisms"—must be investigated empirically. Several studies have done just this and show that class position is a fundamental cause of both good and bad health.

Fundamental cause theory is a theory of the middle range that resides a notch below "grand theory" and is intended to generate empirical predictions that can provide evidence bearing on the theory's utility, not offer a general philosophical statement. This would apply to any other theory associated with the processes explained by fundamental cause theory. Phelan and Link (2013:121) point out that "implicit in the idea that fundamental cause theory is a theory of the middle range is that it must join with other theories to account for the social distribution of health and illness." Fundamental cause theory could potentially be enhanced by joining with other theories that, in turn, could likewise benefit from fundamental cause theory to more fully explain the SES-health connection. Applicable theories in medical sociology include other middle-range theories such as the stress process model, health lifestyles theory, and life course theory to name but a few candidates. Stress is already a feature of fundamental cause theory, which could integrate with the stress process model by bringing its focus on SES as a fundamental cause of stress. The most important structural variable in health lifestyle theory is class circumstances whose relevance could be supported by adding in the notion of SES as a fundamental cause and likewise transferring its emphasis on a class-based habitus as a determinant of specific forms of health behavior to reinforce the causal nature of SES. As for life course theory, fundamental cause theory could contribute to understanding the manner in which the relationship between SES and health vary over time as earlier periods of life influence later periods (Kail, Spring, and Gayman 2019).

It is clear that fundamental cause theory has "legs" into the future as a major sociological theory of health and illness addressing the connection between social class and health—a relationship that has attracted the attention of medical sociologists since the beginning of the subdiscipline, and the notice of physicians before the field existed. Fundamental cause theory lays out the basic stipulations for analyzing this connection. Theories tend to come and go, but as fundamental cause theory continues to develop, it appears likely to be a fixture in other theories, as well as a theory in its own right, for years to come.

Guide to Critical Thinking

1. Explain why SES was conceptualized as a fundamental cause of health and mortality.
2. What are the four core features of fundamental cause theory?
3. How is racism able to qualify as a fundamental cause of health?
4. Explain the role of metamechanisms in fundamental cause theory.
5. What are the four general categories of metamechanisms?
6. Summarize what fundamental cause theory explains and how it explains it.

Suggested Reading

Phelan, Jo C. and Bruce G. Link. 2013. "Fundamental Cause Theory," in William Cockerham (ed.), *Medical Sociology on the Move: New Directions in Theory.* Dordrecht: Springer, pp. 105–26.
A follow-up account of fundamental cause theory by the original theorists.
Phelan, Jo C. and Bruce G. Link. 2015. "Is Racism a Fundamental Cause of Inequalities in Health?" *Annual Review of Sociology* 41:311–30.
Explains why racism qualifies as a fundamental cause of health.

References

Bourdieu, Pierre. 1977. *Outline of a Theory of Practice.* Cambridge: Cambridge University Press.

Bourdieu, Pierre. 1984. *Distinction: A Social Critique of the Judgment of Taste.* Cambridge, MA: Harvard University Press.

Bourdieu, Pierre. 1998. *Practical Reason.* Stanford, CA: Stanford University Press.

Carpiano, Richard M., Bruce G. Link, and Jo C. Phelan. 2008. "Social Inequality and Health: Future Directions for the Fundamental Cause Explanation," in Annette Lareau and Dalton Conley (eds.), *Social Class.* New York: Russell Sage, pp. 232–63.

Chang, Virginia W. and Diane S. Lauderdale. 2009. "Fundamental Cause Theory, Technological Innovation, and Health Disparities: The Case of Cholesterol in the Era of Statins." *Journal of Health and Social Behavior* 50: 245–60.

Clouston, Sean A. P., Marcie S. Rubin, David H. Chae, Jeremy Freese, Barbara Nemesure, and Bruce G. Link. 2017. "Fundamental Causes of Accelerated Declines in Colorectal Cancer Mortality: Modeling Multiple Ways that Disadvantage Influences Mortality Risk." *Social Science & Medicine* 187:1–10.

Clouston, Sean A. P., Marcie S. Rubin, Jo C. Phelan and Bruce G. Link. 2016. "An Unnatural History: Contextualizing the Rise and Fall of the Social Inequality in Mortality." *Demography* 53(5):1631–56.

Cockerham, William. 2005. "Health Lifestyle Theory and the Convergence of Agency and Structure." *Journal of Health & Social Behavior* 46(1):51–67.

Cockerham, William C. 2013. *Social Causes of Health and Disease,* 2nd ed. Cambridge: Polity.

Daw, Jonathan. 2015. "Explaining the Persistence of Health Disparities: Social Stratification and the Efficiency-Equity Trade-off in the Kidney Transplantation System." *American Journal of Sociology* 120(6):1595–640.

Freese, Jeremy and Karen Lutfey. 2011. "Fundamental Causality: Challenges of an Animating Concept for Medical Sociology," in Bernice A. Pescosolido, Jack K. Martin, Jane McLeod and Anne Rogers (eds.), *The Handbook of the Sociology of Health, Illness, and Healing.* New York: Springer, pp. 67–83.

Herd, Pamela A., Brian Goesling, and James S. House. 2007. "Socioeconomic Position and Health: The Differential Effects of Education versus Income on the Onset versus Progression of Health Problems." *Journal of Health and Social Behavior* 48(2):223–38.

House, James S., Ronald C. Kessler, A. Regula Herzog, Richard P. Mero, Ann M. Kinney, and Martha J. Breslow. 1990. "Age, Socioeconomic Status, and Health." *Milbank Quarterly* 68(3):383–411.

Kail, Ben Lennox, Amy Spring, and Matt Gayman. 2019. "A Conceptual Matrix of the Temporal and Spatial Dimensions of Socioeconomic Status and Their Relationship with Health." *Journals of Gerontology* 74B(1):148–59.

Lieberson, Stanley. 1985. *Making it Count: The Improvement of Social Research*. Berkeley, CA: University of California Press.

Link, Bruce G. 2008. "Epidemiological Sociology and the Social Shaping of Population Health." *Journal of Health and Social Behavior* 49(4):367–84.

Link, Bruce G. and Jo C. Phelan. 1995. "Social Conditions as Fundamental Causes of Disease." *Journal of Health and Social Behavior* (extra issue):80–94.

Link, Bruce G. and Jo C. Phelan. 2000. "Evaluating the Fundamental Cause Explanation," in Chloe Bird, Peter Conrad, and Allen Fremont (eds.), *Handbook of Medical Sociology*, 5th ed. Englewood Cliffs, NJ: Prentice-Hall, pp. 33–46.

Lutfey, Karen and Jeremy Freese. 2005. "Toward Some Fundamentals of Fundamental Causality: Socioeconomic Status and Health in the Routine Clinic Visit for Diabetes." *American Journal of Sociology* 110(5):1326–72.

Mackenbach, Johan P., Caspar W. N. Looman, Barbara Artnik, Matthias Bopp et al. 2017. "'Fundamental Causes' of Inequalities in Mortality: An Empirical Test of the Theory in 20 European Populations." *Sociology of Health & Illness* 39(7):117–33.

Masters, Ryan K., Bruce G. Link, and Jo C. Phelan. 2015. "Trends in Education Gradients of 'Preventable' Mortality: A Test of Fundamental Cause Theory." *Social Science & Medicine* 127:19–28.

Miech, Richard, Fred Pampel, Jinyoung Kim, and Richard G. Rodgers. 2011. "The Enduring Association between Education and Mortality: The Role of Widening and Narrowing Disparities." *American Sociological Review* 76(6): 913–34.

National Center for Health Statistics. 2019. *Health, United States, 2018*. Hyattsville, MD: U.S. Department of Health and Human Services.

Olafsdottir, Sigrun. 2007. "Fundamental Causes of Health Disparities: Stratification, the Welfare State, and Health in the United States and Iceland." *Journal of Health and Social Behavior* 48(2):239–53.

Pampel, Fred C. 2009. "The Persistence of Educational Differences in Smoking." *Social Problems* 56(3):526–42.

Phelan, Jo C. and Bruce G. Link. 2013. "Fundamental Cause Theory," in William Cockerham (ed.), *Medical Sociology on the Move: New Directions in Theory*. Dordrecht: Springer, pp. 105–26.

Phelan, Jo C. and Bruce G. Link. 2015. "Is Racism a Fundamental Cause of Inequalities in Health?" *Annual Review of Sociology* 41:311–30.

Phelan, Jo C., Bruce G. Link, Ana Diez-Roux, Ichiro Kawachi, and Bruce Levin. 2004. "Fundamental Causes of Social Inequalities in Mortality: A Test of the Theory." *Journal of Health and Social Behavior* 45(3):265–85.

Phelan, Jo C., Bruce G. Link and Parisa Tehranifar. 2010. "Social Conditions as Fundamental Causes of Health Inequalities: Theory, Evidence, and Policy Implications." *Journal of Health and Social Behavior* 51(extra issue):S28–S40.

Polonijo, Andrea N. and Richard M. Carpiano. 2013. "Social Inequalities in Adolescent Human Papillomavirus (HPV) Vaccination: A Test of Fundamental Cause Theory." *Social Science & Medicine* 82:115–25.

Rothman, Kenneth. 1986. *Modern Epidemiology*. Boston, MA: Little, Brown.

Rubin, Marcie S., Sean Clouston, and Bruce G. Link. 2014. "A Fundamental Cause Approach to the Study of Disparities in Lung Cancer and Pancreatic Cancer Mortality in the United States." *Social Science & Medicine* 100:54–61.

Rubin, Marcie S., Cynthia G. Colen, and Bruce G. Link. 2010. "Examination of Inequalities in HIV/AIDS Mortality in the United States from a Fundamental Cause Perspective." *American Journal of Public Health* 100(6):1053–9.

Saldana-Ruiz, Nallely, Sean A. P. Clouston, Marcie S. Rubin, Cynthia G. Colen, and Bruce G. Link. 2013. "Fundamental Causes of Colorectal Cancer Mortality in the United States: Understanding the Importance of Socioeconomic Status in Creating Inequality in Mortality." *American Journal of Public Health* 103(1):99–104.

Veenstra, Gerry. 2018. "Infusing Fundamental Cause Theory with Features of Pierre Bourdieu's Theory of Symbolic Power." *Scandinavian Journal of Public Health* 46:49–52.

Warren, John Robert, and Elaine M. Hernandez. 2007. "Did Socioeconomic Inequalities in Morbidity and Mortality Change in the United States over the Course of the Twentieth Century?" *Journal of Health and Social Behavior* 48(4): 335–51.

Chapter 13

The Medical Profession and Medicalization

Three professions—medicine, law, and the clergy—occupy an especially privileged position in society because of special forms of expertise unique to them. Bernice Pescosolido (2013) and others (Freidson 1970a) find, however, that medicine is the most powerful of all professions. A major reason is that medicine has the power to heal or repair people and extend life if possible. Also, medicine determines whether someone should or should not be prosecuted for committing a crime if insanity or an impaired mental condition is claimed as a legal defense. Medicine is *the* authority on what does or does not constitute a physical or mental affliction and what to do about it, while most types of health procedures are based on a doctor's "orders." In some patients medicine is able to prolong life through drug regimens or life-saving surgeries, giving it an especially prominent place among the professions. Yet in recent decades medicine's status and authority have declined somewhat in a process some sociologists have called "deprofessionalization" (Ritzer and Walczak 1988). The purpose of this chapter, accordingly, is to review the sociological theories of professionalization that apply to medicine and then extend that discussion to medicalization—one of the most widely cited concepts in medical sociology today.

Sociological Theories of the Medical Profession

As Eliot Freidson (1970a:71) noted long ago in his seminal study of the American medical profession, "a profession is usually taken to be a special kind of occupation, so that it is necessary to develop analytically useful distinctions between the profession and other occupations." The most strategic distinction, in Freidson's view, is a profession's right to control its own work. Some occupations like circus jugglers and magicians, says Freidson (1970a:71–2), may have autonomy, but, in the case of professions, that autonomy is *deliberately* granted by society and includes "the exclusive right to determine who can legitimately do its work and how the work should be done." Professions, unlike occupations, are therefore able to claim exclusive mastery over a particular body of knowledge and use that knowledge to engage in complex and authoritative judgments about the subject matter.

An early analysis in Britain shows that a profession can be distinguished from an occupation not only because of expert knowledge, but also formal university training and the establishment of a professional association providing an enforceable code of ethics and licensing requirements (Carr-Saunders and Wilson 1933). In the United States, William Goode (1957) followed up with a theory of professional status based on two basic qualifications, namely that members of a profession are characterized by: (1) prolonged specialized training in a body of abstract knowledge and (2) an orientation toward providing a service. These two conditions remain basic components of any definition of a profession.

Goode maintained that once a profession meets these two criteria, its next steps are to gain autonomy and control over its work by (1) determining its own standards of education and training, along with (2) requiring high-caliber students and (3) some form of legally recognized licensure from (4) boards staffed by the profession. It also needs to (5) demonstrate competence in order to gain public acceptance of its claims of expertise. Members also (6) assume the identity of their profession; that is, they are known as a doctor, dentist, lawyer, sociologist, or whatever their profession happens to be. And as practitioners, they become (7) relatively free of evaluation and control by laypersons.

Goode's framework fits the early development of the medical profession in the U.S. While physicians have historically shared a service orientation, the second requirement, that of lengthy training in a specialized and abstract body of knowledge, was initially lacking. In the colonial period and the aftermath of the American Revolution, few physicians had been educated at a medical school or even attended a university. Ship surgeons, barbers, apothecaries, clergy, and anyone with some rudimentary medical knowledge could be a "doctor." The most distinguished early American physicians had trained in Britain and members of this group were instrumental in establishing the first medical schools, beginning in 1765 at the College of Philadelphia (later the University of Pennsylvania). By the 1800s, there was virtually a flood of new medical schools, many of which had been established outside of universities as a private business to make money. These for-profit (proprietary) schools had low admission standards and a questionable quality of education (Porter 1997). Anyone able to pay the fees could obtain a medical degree and practice medicine. Not surprisingly, physicians collectively had little prestige until the late nineteenth century.

But this changed in 1878–1879 with Louis Pasteur's germ theory of disease that revolutionized medicine and provided a scientific basis for the discovery, classification, and successful treatment of many communicable diseases. The growth of clinics and university-affiliated research laboratories multiplied in response. At the beginning of the twentieth century, the impressive advancements in medical science allowed physicians to fully claim the other core characteristic of a profession as outlined by Goode— prolonged specialized training in a body of abstract knowledge. Mastery of this knowledge was the medical profession's monopoly. Moreover, at this time, medical discoveries in the U.S. began to surpass those of Europe, as scientific medicine attracted large sums of research money from private American philanthropic foundations to eradicate diseases. Additionally, the Flexner Report of 1910, a landmark survey of all U.S. medical schools, resulted in a thorough reorganization of medical education. Better schools improved their programs and lesser schools closed because of bad publicity, financial adversity, and failure to meet the requirements of state licensing boards. Many states refused to certify the graduates of low-grade medical schools and financial support from various levels of government and private foundations was usually provided only to those schools with good reputations. Other important measures included the organization of the American Medical Association (AMA) in 1847, which eventually became a powerful organization with respect to protecting the professional interests of medical doctors and shaping health policy at the national and state levels, along with the AMA's establishment of the Council on Medical Education in 1904 to monitor the quality of medical education. The professionalization of medicine would not have been possible without control over standards for medical education (Ludmerer 1999).

Talcott Parsons, in his book *The Social System* (1951), provided a structural-functionalist analysis of the medical profession that accompanied his concept of the sick role. It was the first conceptualization of the medical profession in sociology. Physicians were of particular interest in the sociological study of professions because the welfare of its clients came before self-interest and the pursuit of profits (Timmerman and Oh 2010). What separated professions in the division of labor, in Parsons' view, was their particular specialization of technical competence. In the continuum of professional specialties, the physician ranked highest. Parsons depicted the medical role as a patterned form of social action whose specific components, as clarified by Pescosolido (2013:176–7), are the following: (1) medicine has an *achievement orientation*, in that it is a learned profession requiring lengthy and rigorous training; (2) it is *functionally specific* to health; (3) physicians are expected to have an *affective neutrality* in that illnesses and patients are treated objectively; and (4) it has a *collectivity orientation*, meaning that physicians are obligated to put the welfare of patients above all else and reject the profit motive. As Parsons (1951:435) explains this latter orientation:

The "ideology" of the profession lays great emphasis on the obligation of the physician to put the "welfare of the patient" above his [or her] personal interests, and regards "commercialism" as the most serious and insidious evil with which it has to contend.

Parsons' concept of the medical profession came to be seen in sociology as an "ideal type" along the lines suggested by Max Weber [(1922) 1978), rather than an operational theory (Pescosolido 2013). An ideal type is an abstract model of the essence of some particular and unique form of human interaction intended as an analytic tool against which reality can be compared (Kalberg 1994). But even though it had merit as an ideal type, Parsons' concept of the medical profession has generally faded from the literature in medical sociology. This outcome is likely due more to structural-functionalism's disappearance as a major sociological theory than any inherent weakness or error in the concept itself. It may have simply gotten old.

The leading theory, for a while, was Freidson's (1970a, 1970b) professional dominance thesis. This approach held that a profession is an occupation that assumes a dominant position in a division of labor at the point it gains control over its work. Therefore, unlike an occupation, a profession is autonomous and self-directing under society's umbrella. In the case of medicine, it has the authority to direct and evaluate the work of others in the health field without being subject to direction and formal evaluation by them in response. Freidson (1970a:5) states:

If we consider the profession of medicine today [it was the 1970s], it is clear that its major characteristic is preeminence. Such preeminence is not merely that of prestige but also of expert authority. This is to say, medicine's knowledge about illness and its treatment is considered to be authoritative and definitive ... there are no representatives of occupations in direct competition with medicine who hold official policy-making positions related to health affairs. Medicine's position today is akin to state religions yesterday—it has an officially approved monopoly of the right to define health and illness and to treat illness.

By the mid-1950s, the medical profession stood at the height of its professional power and prestige. There was unprecedented professional control by doctors over health care delivery to a degree that no longer exists. Yet it was also a period of rising costs, overcharging to a level previously unknown, an expansion of medical facilities, and a proliferation of unnecessary tests, hospitalizations, prescriptions, and surgical operations (Light 2000:202). Private health insurance companies tended to pay whatever was charged and the federal government had to intervene to assist disadvantaged segments of society by establishing government-sponsored health insurance for the elderly (Medicare) and the poor (Medicaid) in 1965. Historian Roy Porter (1997:658) observed that health had become a major growth industry in America. In the 1960s, health costs were approaching 15 percent of the Gross Domestic Product (in 2017 it was 17.9 percent of GDP, reflecting a slowing of the rising costs for health care since that time). Costs were generally unchecked as insurers boosted them as high as the market could bear, physician incomes were seven times higher than the national average, and hospitals added costly technology that was often duplicated in nearby facilities. Donald Light (2004:15) referred to this "Golden Age of Medicine" as the "Age of Gold."

A weakness of the professional dominance thesis is that it did not allow for decline. Instead, dominance had nowhere else to go except toward greater dominance in which a profession theoretically became even more powerful over time without taking into account the possibility that it could become less powerful (Hafferty and Light 1995; Light 1993, 2000; Light and Hafferty 1993). But decline did come to the medical profession and professional dominance is no longer an adequate theory (McKinlay and Marceau 2002). A new term emerged in sociological theories of the medical profession— that of "countervailing power" (Light 2000; Light and Hafferty 1993). This phrase signified that the medical profession was but one of many influential groups in society staking claims to controlling its interests in health care. In establishing its control over health care, the medical profession had left the medical marketplace open and as costs rose, other powerful entities entered the health field (Starr 1982). Over time, the medical profession's level of dominance gave way as these countervailing powers established powerful positions of their own and ended its monopoly. "Dominance," states Light (2000:204), "slowly produces imbalances, excesses, and neglects that offend or threaten other countervailing powers and alienate the larger public." And this is what occurred.

The countervailing powers external to medicine included: (1) the federal government and its efforts to control costs through public insurance programs and set fee schedules (diagnostic-related groups or DRGs) for those programs; (2) the rise and expansion of managed care systems that manage the cost of care by monitoring treatment decisions and requiring physicians as employees to follow its guidelines; (3) the emergence of large health care corporate conglomerates expanding into the health care marketplace to compete for patients in which medical doctors become employees and subject to corporate policies; and (4) the changing doctor–patient relationship in which patients pushed for a greater role in decision-making about their health and developed more consumer-oriented attitudes by shopping for the doctors and insurance coverage that best suited their needs and was more affordable. Private health insurance companies were also important players in the marketplace as they determined the costs, eligibility, and extent of coverage of their product.

All of these factors produced a decline in the authority and professional status of physicians. The AMA, the medical profession's protective trade association, which had historically opposed reforms in health care delivery, lost both importance and membership. The direction for the profession was away from being the absolute authority in medical matters toward having lessened authority as many physicians became employees in managed care systems instead of independent, solo practitioners who had dominated health care delivery in the past. Marie Haug (1976), along with George Ritzer and David Walczak (1988), described the medical profession as undergoing a process of "deprofessionalization." Ritzer and Walczak (1988:6) define deprofessionalization as "a decline in power which results in a decline in the degree to which professions possess, or are perceived to possess, a constellation of characteristics denoting a profession." Deprofessionalization did not mean physicians were becoming less professional in their work; rather, they were experiencing decreased autonomy and control over patients. They still retained the greatest authority in clinical matters but that authority was no longer unconditional and subject to greater external scrutiny by patients, health care delivery corporations, health insurance companies, and government agencies.

Utilizing a Weberian interpretation, Ritzer and Walczak argued that the rise of a profit orientation in medicine pointed to a trend in medical practice away from substantive rationality (stressing ideals like serving the patient) toward greater formal rationality (stressing efficiency) leading to greater profit. Formal rationality is defined by Weber ([1922] 1978) as the purposeful calculation of the most efficient means to reach goals, while substantive rationality is an emphasis on ideal values. Ritzer and Walczak claim that formal rationality has become dominant in medical practice. The decline of the substantive element signaled a loss of public support and an invitation to countervailing powers to enter into an open market that the medical profession had previously kept for itself.

An update on theories of the professional status of medicine is lacking. Interest in this topic began to slow in medical sociology in the 1980s and has not revived (Mechanic 1989; Pescosolido 2006, 2013). No new theories rose to replace those of the past. Medical sociologists seemed to generally accept the status quo, namely the notion of deprofessionalization as theoretically representative of medicine's ongoing professional status.

However, although weakened, the medical profession nevertheless retains much of its power (Timmermans and Oh 2010). As Pescosolido (2013:188) makes clear: "As long as the profession is relatively free of technical evaluation and control by other occupations in the medical division of labor, intrusions that change the socioeconomic terms of modern medical work do not significantly change medicine's professional character." Consequently, theorizing about the medical profession remains dormant at present and theoretical restatements about the current situation have yet to appear.

Medicalization

Medicalization is a product of medical power. The leading proponent of the medicalization concept in sociology is Peter Conrad (2007, 2013) who graciously provided much of the material in the following pages. His contribution of a first-person account provides a window into his thinking. Conrad says that medicalization in its simplest form means "to make medical." More broadly, the term "medicalization" refers to how previously nonmedical conditions become defined and treated as a medical problem, typically as a disease or disorder. A similar definition of medicalization comes from Joseph Davis (2016:211) who states, it "is the name for the process by which medical definitions and practices are applied to behaviors, psychological phenomena, and somatic experiences not previously within the conceptual or therapeutic scope of medicine."

Sociologists who study medicalization are usually not interested in whether a condition is "really" a medical problem, since that is a medical decision, but rather focus on how a problem becomes defined as medical and what the social consequences are of doing so. Conrad notes that many examples of medicalization exist, such as alcoholism, drug addiction, attention deficit hyperactivity disorder (ADHD), normal sadness, premenstrual syndrome (PMS), sleep disorders, childbirth, aging, obesity, infertility, learning disabilities, erectile dysfunction, gender dysphoria, cosmetic surgery, and baldness among others. Medicalization can be viewed as operative in several broad categories of social life, such as deviance (e.g., mental disorder, addiction), normal life events (e.g., menopause, aging), and personal enhancement (e.g., breast enlargements, weight-loss surgery).

The origins of the issues surrounding medicalization can be found in the works of the notable mid-twentieth-century sociological thinkers Talcott Parsons, Erving Goffman, and Michel Foucault. However, with an occasional exception, these theorists didn't use the term "medicalization," although they analyzed phenomena that would later be known as medicalization. For example, implicit in Parsons' (1951) concept of sickness as a form of deviance is the idea that medicine is an institution for the social control of deviant behavior by medical means on behalf of society. Goffman (1961) described the medical control of mental patients as inmates in total institutions, while Foucault (1975) analyzed medicine's gaze and surveillance as forms of biopower and biopolitics.

The first sociological use of the term can be attributed to Jesse Pitts, in his 1968 *International Encyclopedia of the Social Sciences* article on "Social Control: The Concept," where he discussed the medicalization of certain forms of deviant behavior by redefining them as illnesses instead of crime and utilizing medicine as a means of social control along the lines suggested by Parsons (1951). The responsibility for a crime in this instance is deflected from the individual to the illness as an excusing condition, which could make medicalization a more humane and forgiving approach but also more relentless and pervasive throughout society (Pitts 1968:381). Next was Irving Zola's (1972) often-cited article "Medicine as an Institution of Social Control." He saw the origins of medicalization in the expansion of the medical profession's extended jurisdiction over normal conditions such as aging and human weaknesses like drug addiction and alcoholism. Conrad's (1976) research on what is now called ADHD followed and he focused on how the condition was increasingly medicalized by doctors. Similar to Zola, Conrad viewed illness as socially constructed. Since the 1970s, scholars in multiple disciplines have gone on to conduct research on various aspects of medicalization and its use appears frequently in the literature (see Bell and Figert 2015; Busfield 2017; Clarke et al. 2010; Conrad 1992, 2007, 2013).

Conrad (2007), for example, found hyperactivity in children at school was defined by the medical profession as attention deficit hyperactivity disorder (ADHD), which requires the use of the drug Ritalin to treat it; menopause was made subject to estrogen replacement therapy, whose side effects were determined a few years later to promote even greater risk from blood clots, stroke, heart disease, and breast cancer; being short in stature necessitates growth hormones for people with below average height; and male baldness slowed or prevented by using Propecia and lost hair is restored by surgical transplants. There was a time when hyperactivity, menopause, shortness, and baldness were not medical conditions. A similar trend is seen in studies of mental health showing psychiatry transforming normal sorrow into clinically treated depression and natural anxiety into an anxiety disorder (Horwitz and Wakefield 2007, 2012).

Box 13.1 Peter Conrad

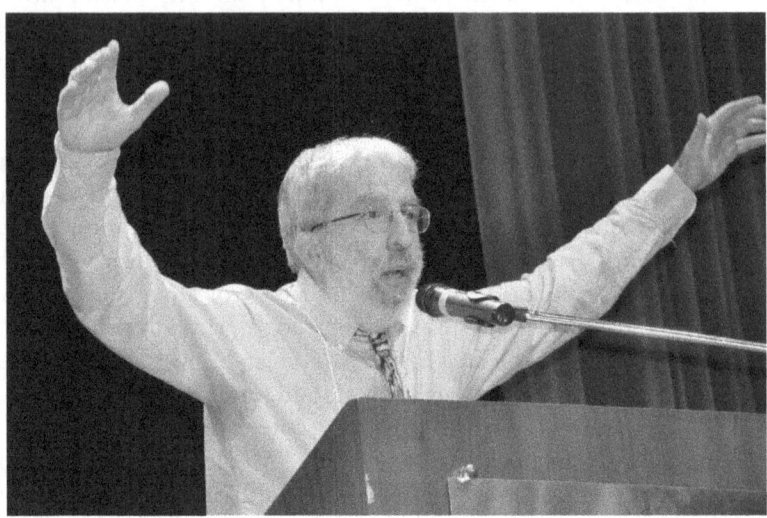

Image 13.1 Peter Conrad

I became interested in medicalization as I was researching my Ph.D. dissertation in Sociology, "Factors in the Identification of Hyperactive Children," at Boston University (1976). At its start it was framed as a deviance and "labeling theory" study. As I was collecting my observation and interview data, I came across an article by Irving Zola "Medicine as an Institution of Social Control" and was introduced to the concept of medicalization and that changed the frame of my study. I now saw my study as focusing on the medicalization of deviance, with hyperactivity (now called ADHD) as my case. This not only changed the focus of my dissertation; it changed the direction of my career (toward medical sociology) and the direction of much of my research for decades.

After completing my dissertation and publishing it as a book, along with a few related articles, I took a job at Drake University in Des Moines, Iowa (why Iowa? my wife had been accepted to medical school in Des Moines). There I had the good fortune to meet a colleague, Joseph W. Schneider, who had an interest in deviance and in our regular lunches we discussed mutual sociological interests. We talked frequently about issues related to deviance and medicalization. At that point I felt I knew a lot about the medicalization of hyperactive children, but much less about medicalization as a social process. We decided to (take on) writing a more historical and comparative study of medicalization, focusing on several major deviant categories (mental illness, alcoholism, homosexuality, opiate addiction, and childhood deviance). A few years later we published *Deviance and Medicalization: From Badness to Sickness* (1980). This book (Conrad and Schneider 1980) helped to make medicalization a more central concern in sociology and has been cited more than a thousand times.

At this point I had come to a place of saturation on medicalization and turned my attention to other research (experience of illness, wellness in the workplace, social meanings of genetics). I didn't publish anything of significance on medicalization for more than a decade until "Medicalization and Social Control" in the *Annual Review of Sociology* (1992). This article expanded the framework of medicalization to beyond deviance on to larger medical sociological issues and more examples of medicalization and its consequences (e.g., aging, childbirth, erectile dysfunction, sadness among many others). Writing this article refocused my research back on medical sociological aspects and culminated with the publication of *The Medicalization of Society: The Transformation of Human Conditions into Treatable Disorders* (2007). I still consider this my key book on medicalization. While I have published about a dozen articles related to aspects of medicalization since on issues like demedicalization, the promotion of the pharmaceutical industry, the role of consumers, and the medical profession, that volume provides a solid basis for the breadth, understanding and utility of medicalization. I recently retired after 37 years on the faculty of Brandeis University, and continue to explore further aspects of the origins and consequences of medicalization, such as the migration of medicalized categories from the U.S. to other countries (see Conrad and Bergey 2014).

Along with medicalization, there are examples of demedicalization. The most often mentioned is the demedicalization of homosexuality. From the mid-nineteenth century through the mid-twentieth century, homosexuality was seen as a form of mental illness that required treatment. After several years of protest by gay activists, the American Psychiatric Association voted in 1973 to remove homosexuality as a diagnosis from the official diagnostic compendium, which eventually led to a virtually complete demedicalization of homosexuality. There are a few other examples of efforts at demedicalization, such as masturbation, which was considered a disease (as onanism) through the early twentieth century and the recent attempts to reconceptualize some types of autism as "neurodiversity." However, there is far more medicalization than demedicalization.

At least five characteristics of medicalization exist (see Conrad 2013). First, and of central importance, is the *definitional* issue. How a problem is defined medically is key to what is done about it. Second, there are *degrees* of medicalization. Some conditions are fully medicalized (e.g., schizophrenia, epilepsy) while others are marginally medicalized (e.g., sexual addiction, Internet addiction), and still others are contested or in the initial steps of medicalization (e.g., obesity). Thus, medicalization is not binary (either yes or no) but part of a continuum. Third, medicalized categories are *elastic* and can expand or contract. When ADHD emerged in the 1970s, it was limited to children in primary school between ages 6–12. But at present it has expanded to include adolescent and adult ADHD, with a focus on inattention more than hyperactive behavior. Hysteria, a popular medical diagnostic category for women in the late nineteenth century, has largely disappeared. So the process of medicalization can have an elastic composition. Fourth, physician involvement in medicalization is *variable* and sometimes only marginally necessary. Alcoholism, for example, was medicalized largely through the efforts of Alcoholics Anonymous, with little participation on the part of the medical profession. And fifth, medicalization is *bi-directional* in that the process is typically that of medicalization but on occasion may consist of demedicalization.

Do these five characteristics constitute a theory? While there are some references in the medical sociology literature to medicalization as a theory and some aspects of the medicalization concept can be converted into theoretical propositions, Conrad (2013) does not call it a theory. He notes that he hasn't consistently presented it as a theory and that most papers on medicalization are cases studies or analyses of some part of the medicalization process. Rather, he sees medicalization as similar to labeling theory as it is more of a conceptual framework than a full-blown theory. Nevertheless, medicalization is one of the most cited "conceptualizations" in contemporary medical sociology because it illustrates a modern tendency to view social problems as medical problems.

As originally presented, medicalization was subject to a few criticisms, namely that (1) patients seem to have a passive role, (2) medicine is depicted as actively "imperialistic," and (3) medicine's value is downplayed. British medical sociologist Joan Busfield (2017) examined these criticisms and determined that if patients were passive in the past, this was not the situation today for patients generally. Many have used the Internet and other sources to become more knowledgeable and have turned into informed "consumers," actively participating in decisions about their own health care.

Moreover, Busfield observed that the term "medicalization" does not necessarily in and of itself imply "medical imperialism" as medicine is only one
of several groups (i.e., patients, governments, insurance companies, corporations) involved in health care and that medicalization has positive benefits
for many people. She also rejects the idea that "pharmaceuticalization" is
an alternative or even a complementary form of medicalization (Williams,
Coveney, and Gabe 2017). In Busfield's view, pharmaceuticalization does
not seem as pertinent or illuminating for describing the process of making
things medical, as does the concept of medicalization. Rather, as will be
discussed, the challenge to medicalization's conceptual role comes from
biomedicalization theory.

The Shifting Engines of Medicalization

As a social process, Conrad finds the "drivers" of medicalization, namely the
forces or "engines" that push it into existence, are varied and shifting. Yet
even though the "engines" of medicalization shift, Conrad (2005:5) holds
that "the definitional center of medicalization remains constant" (namely,
making things medical). Conrad says that the ascending engines currently
are (1) biotechnology, especially the pharmaceutical industry and possibly
genetics in the future, (2) consumers, and (3) managed care. Physicians are
considered a likely fourth engine because their mission is to reduce human
suffering and in this endeavor Conrad (2013) finds they still contribute
to medicalization by providing medical treatments for problems that have
questionable medical origins, such as shyness, sadness, sleep issues, and some
forms of ADHD. If problems can be connected to the body in some way,
they are open to being treated medically (Zola 1972).

Up until the 1980s, most medicalization studies focused on the role of
the medical profession in expanding its jurisdiction over problems that
were not necessarily medical (Clarke et al. 2003, 2010; Conrad 2007, 2013).
Conrad (2013:199) points out that because of this, medicalization is sometimes referred to as a form of "medical imperialism" in which physicians
are still seen as expanding the profession's power by taking control of and
treating previously nonmedical problems. That is, acts that might have been
defined as sin or crime in the past and addressed by the church or the law
became increasingly regarded as illnesses to be controlled through medical
treatment. Although this happens, the blame cannot be assigned solely to
the medical profession because patients as consumers come to physicians
requesting or demanding services. These requests may well include treatment for nonmedical concerns about what their body is experiencing that
is causing them concern or discomfort, such as conditions like short stature,
small female breasts, and male baldness. When it comes to aberrant behavior,

there may be few problems that some group does not think of as a medical problem. Therefore, Conrad (2013) assigns shared responsibility for medicalization to both physicians for expanding their services and consumers as their patients requesting those services.

As for managed care, Conrad (2013:205) maintains that he uses the term to refer to all types of health insurance in that insurance fuels medicalization for conditions that it covers and slows it for those that it does not. In this way, health insurance "manages care" by approving or disapproving payments for the health care services of providers. For example, he notes that the lack of insurance coverage for infertility and transgender surgery has slowed medicalization of those procedures, while coverage for gastric bypass surgery for obesity has accelerated its medicalization. Health insurance also does not cover expenses for health conditions that do not have a diagnosis from a doctor and this requirement is relevant for channeling people toward medicalizing their problems.

The other major engine is biotechnology, especially the pharmaceutical industry as it markets its drugs not only directly to doctors but increasingly to the general public through mass media advertising campaigns as an effective way to solve various medical conditions, including drug treatments for newly medicalized conditions. The clear intent is to influence people to request pharmaceutical products from their doctor. This is why sociologists have broadened their analysis and identified the "shifting engines of medicalization" in which biotechnology (especially the pharmaceutical industry and its marketing apparatus) has emerged in greater strength (Clarke et al. 2003, 2010; Conrad 2007).

Conrad notes that, for sociologists, medicalization is not necessarily a good or bad thing. For some patients, it can be a good thing that helps them and for others potentially harmful through side effects or perhaps being useless. Regardless, it should be studied like any other social process (e.g., industrialization, secularization). The question to be asked in his view is: "What are the origins and consequences of medicalization for society?" Some consequences of concern are that medicalization leads to (1) the *pathologization* of everything by turning human differences into some form of medical pathology. Another is (2) that *medical definitions of normality* become social norms; that is, medicine creates what is supposed to be normal in society by determining what people should act and look like, which is especially evident in the use of pharmaceutical drugs for treating increasing numbers of newly medicalized behavioral conditions and various types of cosmetic surgery. A related concern is that (3) medicalization increases *medical control over social behavior* through expanded methods of surveillance—thereby establishing medicine as an "overseer" or supervisor of behavior. There is also (4) *the individualization of social problems* in medicine that converts complex social problems like alcoholism, obesity, and ADHD into an individual clinical problem to be treated with a medical solution that ignores the social contexts in which the problems originate and persist. Finally, there is (5) *the consumerization of medicine* in which medical procedures and treatments become consumer items, subject to trends in the marketplace that can affect costs and access to quality care.

Biomedicalization versus Medicalization

However, as medical sociology moved into the twenty-first century, not all sociologists saw the medicalization concept keeping pace with the spread of biotechnology. This led Adele Clarke and her colleagues (Clarke 2014; Clarke et al. 2003, 2010; Clarke and Shim 2011) to provide an alternative view of medicalization. They see the expansion of medical jurisdiction over social problems as one of the most potent recent transformations taking place in Western society. Whereas medicalization has traditionally been a means by which professional medicine acquired increasingly more problems to treat, Clarke et al. (2003, 2010) find that major technological and scientific advances in biomedicine are taking this capability even further and producing what she and her colleagues refer to as "biomedicalization."

Theoretically, biomedicalization is seen as part of a broader shift from Michel Foucault's (1975) notion of the "clinical gaze" in the eighteenth century to Nikolas Rose's (2007) concept of the "molecular gaze" in the twenty-first century. Foucault saw the past as the beginning of "biopower" in which medicine subjected bodies and populations to its surveillance and control, while Rose notes the current extension of medicine's gaze even further into the replacement, engineering, or regeneration of human cells and tissues. Rose (2007:700) thus finds medicalization to be an outmoded concept that has evolved into "a cliché of critical social analysis." Because of the innovations coming from molecular biology, genetics, biotechnologies, and the like, Clarke and her associates (2003) therefore decided to add "bio" to the term "medicalization." Their thesis was that medicalization had become more complex and extended through technology, thereby transforming it into biomedicalization. This occurred around 1985. Accordingly, Clarke et al. (2003:162) define biomedicalization as "the increasingly complex, multi-sited, multi-directional processes of medicalization that today are being reconstituted through the emergent social forms and practices of a highly and increasingly technoscientific medicine."

Biomedicalization consists of the capability of computer information and new technologies to spread medical surveillance and treatment interventions well beyond past boundaries by the use of genetics, bioengineering, chemoprevention, individualized designer drugs, multiple sources of information, patient data banks, digitized patient records, and other innovations. Also important in this process is the Internet making it easier to get medicalized information and merchandise, advertising, consumerism, and the role of pharmaceutical companies in marketing their products. Clarke et al. (2010:48) find that "clinical innovations are at the heart of biomedicalization" and at "the beginning of the twenty-first century, such technoscientific innovations are the jewels in the clinical crown of biomedicine and vectors of biomedicalization in the West and beyond."

They advance what they call biomedicalization theory, which consists of five interactive processes: (1) the rise of a new biopolitical economy of medicine, health, illness, living, and dying in which biomedical knowledge, technologies, services, and capital are increasingly constituted; (2) a new and intensive focus on health enhancement and optimization by technoscientific means and surveillance of risks; (3) interventions for treatment increasingly based on science and technology; (4) transformations of biomedical knowledge production, information management, distribution, and consumption; and (5) transformations in bodies and the production of new technoscientific identities among individuals, groups, and populations. Examples of the latter are medical measures that transform the body and cause adjustments in personal identities, such as promoting anti-aging, manipulating the "biological clock" in women to achieve pregnancy, sex-change surgeries or treating sexual dysfunctions, infertility, and breast cancer. Biomedicalization is therefore not only a comprehensive new theory, but also points to an historical change in the development of medicine.

Busfield (2017), however, finds two difficulties with biomedicalization as a replacement for medicalization. One problem is that she finds it debatable that a major transformation in American medicine occurred around 1985 whose changes were so sweeping or sufficient that a "bio" needed to be linked to medicalization. Second, while medicalization is conceptualized by Conrad as a process that continues over time, it is limited to being representative of a single historical era of medicine by Clarke et al. (2010). That is, the rise of medicine (1890–1945) is followed by medicalization (1940–1990) which is followed by biomedicalization (1985–present). Busfield (2017:768) claims, in rebuttal, that medicalization "is not intended as a label for a particular period in American medicine." It is an ongoing social process, not a specific era. Alternately, Clarke et al. see medicalization having been transformed into biomedicalization, leaving medicalization behind in the rear view mirror.

Yet Conrad (2005, 2007, 2013; Conrad and Waggoner 2014) maintains biomedicalization theory covers such a broad range of developments that what is meant by medicalization seems to get lost. Instead of a transformation of medicalization into biomedicalization, he believes that the process of medicalization became instead more intensified and widespread in the twenty-first century than it was in the late twentieth century. While recognizing some merits of the biomedicalization concept, Conrad nevertheless takes the position that the "engines" of medicalization have simply shifted, with the ascendance of certain influences (consumers, drug companies, health insurance as a form of managed care) and the diminution of others (the medical profession).

Busfield (2017) clearly comes down on the side of medicalization in this dispute, while others (Rose 2007) do not. Susan Bell and Anne Figert (2015), however, present yet another viewpoint when they question whether medicalization fully captures what is meant by biomedicalization, pharmaceuticalization, or geneticization. Pharmaceuticalization "is the process by which social, behavioral or bodily conditions are treated or deemed to be in need of treatment, with medical drugs by doctors or patients" (Abraham 2010:604). Geneticization is the process by which "differences between individuals are reduced to their DNA codes, with most disorders, behaviors, and physiological variations defined, at least in part, as genetic in origin" (Lippman 1991:19).

Bell and Figert (2015:2) conclude that medicalization alone is not an adequate concept for understanding these new "izations" or the globalized changes taking place in medicine in the twenty-first century. This is because the medicalization concept is grounded in an earlier version of modernity, yet they also recognize that the concept is worth keeping because sometimes it is precisely "the right tool to get the job done." It can explain how medical phenomena are produced, utilized, expanded, and transformed. On the other hand, biomedicalization might be better equipped in their estimation to study some aspects of pharmaceuticalization and new developments in genetic medicine.

Where does this leave us with respect to theory? Whether medicalization or biomedicalization is most accurate in explaining medicine's ever-increasing acquisition of problems to heal has not been determined. Either may apply, depending on the afflictions and treatments to be explained. This may be why some medical sociologists use the term "[bio]medicalization" (i.e., Bell and Figert 2015), perhaps as a compromise to capture the strengths of each approach. Although not a full-fledged theory, medicalization has nevertheless served in that role for decades and, with the incorporation of biotechnology as a component, it extends into ongoing medical techniques. Given that the concept of medicalization has also been widely accepted by both scholars and the general public (Bell and Figert 2015), it would appear that medicalization is the dominant approach to its subject matter at present.

Yet biomedicalization theory has its merits with respect to representing the transformations of bodies by genetics, pharmacological interventions, and other clinical procedures. Of particular relevance is that research on the human genome is expected to revolutionize the treatment of gene-based diseases and behavioral affliction. In doing so, medicine's boundaries will be expanded even further. Italian bio-sociologist Maurizio Meloni (2019:131) points out, for example, that what is new in human genome research is the scale of analysis and level of integration between epigenetic and post-genomic lines of enquiry. He notes these research programs have the potential to change the ways in which we understand the management of bodies and the reproduction of social norms. It may be that as medicalization ages as a concept, biomedicalization may be its replacement or the two perspectives may merge, as medical sociology and biology draw closer to each other through epigenetics and the use of biological measures like biomarkers. Regardless, this area in medical sociology is likely to become an exceptionally active area of theory construction, research, and debate.

Summary

This chapter reviews sociological theories pertaining to the medical profession and medicalization. The rise of medicine as a profession is traced by way of Goode's (1957) theory that holds all professions are characterized by two basic qualifications: (1) prolonged specialized training in a body of abstract knowledge and (2) an orientation toward providing a service. Medicine was able to meet these criteria and others as they gained control over medical education and organized the American Medical Association, which became a powerful influence on health policy. Featured is Freidson's (1970a) professional dominance theory, which is no longer applicable but was the leading theoretical perspective until countervailing powers intervened to produce a level of deprofessionalization.

The second part of the chapter discusses medicalization as a product of medical power. Medicalization in its simplest form means "to make medical." It refers to how previously nonmedical conditions become defined and treated as a medical problem, typically as a disease or disorder. Conrad (2007, 2013) finds the engines of medicalization that push it into existence are varied and shifting, currently consisting of (1) biotechnology, (2) consumers, and (3) managed care. Physicians are considered a likely fourth engine. Medicalization is challenged by biomedicalization theory formulated by Clarke et al. (2010) as the leading theoretical concept in this area.

Guide to Critical Thinking

1. What are the two basic criteria of a profession?
2. Describe deprofessionalization.
3. What does medicalization explain? What are its shifting engines?
4. What does biomedicalization explain? Compare it to medicalization.

Suggested Reading

Clarke, Adele, Laura Mamo, Jennifer Ruth Fosket, Jennifer R. Fishman, and Janet K. Shim (eds.). 2010. *Biomedicalization: Technoscience, Health and Illness in the U.S.* Durham, NC: Duke University Press.
A thorough introduction to biomedicalization.

Conrad, Peter. 2007. *The Medicalization of Society: On the Transformation of Human Conditions into Treatable Disorders.* Baltimore, MD: Johns Hopkins University Press.
Conrad's seminal work on medicalization.

Conrad, Peter. 2013. "Medicalization: Changing Contours, Characteristics and Contexts," in William Cockerham (ed.), *Medical Sociology on the Move: New Directions in Theory.* Dordrecht: Springer, pp. 195–214.
An update of Conrad's perspective on medicalization.

References

Abraham, John. 2010. "Pharmaceuticalization of Society in Context: Theoretical, Empirical and Health Dimensions." *Sociology* 44(4):603–22.

Bell, Susan E. and Anne E. Figert (eds.). 2015. *Reimagining (Bio)medicalization, Pharmaceuticals, and Genetics.* New York: Routledge.

Busfield, Joan. 2017. "The Concept of Medicalisation Reassessed." *Sociology of Health & Illness* 39(5):759–74.

Carr-Saunders, Alexander Morris and Paul A. Wilson. 1933. *The Professions.* London: Cass.

Clarke, Adele E. 2014. "Biomedicalization," in William Cockerham, Robert Dingwall, and Stella Quah (eds.), *The Wiley Blackwell Encyclopedia of Health, Illness, Behavior, and Society,* vol. I. Oxford: Wiley Blackwell, pp. 137–42.

Clarke, Adele E. and Janet Shim. 2011. "Medicalization and Biomedicalization Revisited: Technoscience and Transformations of Health, Illness and American Medicine," in Bernice Pescosolido, Jack Martin, Jane McLeod, and Anne Rogers (eds.), *Handbook of the Sociology of Health, Illness, and Healing.* New York: Springer, pp. 173–99.

Clarke, Adele, Laura Mamo, Jennifer Ruth Fosket, Jennifer R. Fishman, and Janet K. Shim (eds.). 2010. *Biomedicalization: Technoscience, Health and Illness in the U.S.* Durham, NC: Duke University Press.

Clarke, Adele E., Janet K. Shim, Laura Mamo, Jennifer Ruth Fosket, and Jennifer R. Fishman 2003. "Biomedicalization: Technoscientific Transformation of Health, Illness, and U.S. Biomedicine." *American Sociological Review* 68(2):161–94.

Conrad, Peter. 1976. *Identifying Hyperactive Children: The Medicalization of Deviant Behavior.* Boston, MA: Heath.

Conrad, Peter. 1992. "Medicalization and Social Control." *Annual Review of Sociology* 18:209–32.

Conrad, Peter. 2005. "The Shifting Engines of Medicalization." *Journal of Health and Social Behavior* 46(1):3–14.

Conrad, Peter. 2007. *The Medicalization of Society: On the Transformation of Human Conditions into Treatable Disorders.* Baltimore, MD: Johns Hopkins University Press.

Conrad, Peter. 2013. "Medicalization: Changing Contours, Characteristics and Contexts," in William Cockerham (ed.), *Medical Sociology on the Move: New Directions in Theory*. Dordrecht: Springer, pp. 195–214.

Conrad, Peter and Meredith Bergey. 2014. "The Impending Globalization of ADHD: Notes on the Expansion and Growth of a Medicalized Disorder." *Social Science & Medicine* 122: 31–43.

Conrad, Peter and Joseph W. Schneider. 1980. *Deviance and Medicalization: From Badness to Sickness*. St. Louis, MO: Mosby.

Conrad, Peter and Miranda Waggoner. 2014. "Medicalization," in William Cockerham, Robert Dingwall, and Stella Quah (eds.), *The Wiley Blackwell Encyclopedia of Health, Illness, Behavior, and Society*, vol. III. Oxford: Wiley Blackwell, pp. 1448–52.

Davis, Joseph E. 2016. "Medicalization, Social Control, and the Relief of Suffering," in William Cockerham (ed.), *The New Blackwell Companion to Medical Sociology*. Oxford: Wiley Blackwell, pp. 211–41.

Foucault, Michel. 1975. *The Birth of the Clinic*. New York: Vintage Books.

Freidson, Eliot. 1970a. *Profession of Medicine: A Study of the Sociology of Applied Knowledge*. New York: Dodd, Mead, and Co.

Freidson, Eliot. 1970b. *Professional Dominance: The Social Structure of Medical Care*. New York: Atherton Press.

Goffman, Erving. 1961. *Asylums*. New York: Anchor.

Goode, William J. 1957. "Community within a Community." *American Sociological Review* 22(2):194–200.

Hafferty, Frederic W. and Donald W. Light. 1995. "Professional Dynamics and the Changing Nature of Medical Work." *Journal of Health and Social Behavior* 36:132–53.

Haug, Marie R. 1976. "The Erosion of Professional Authority: A Cross-Cultural Inquiry in the Case of the Physician." *Milbank Memorial Fund Quarterly* 54(1):83–106.

Horwitz, Allan V. and Jerome C. Wakefield. 2007. *The Loss of Sadness: How Psychiatry Transformed Normal Sorrow into Depressive Disorder*. New York: Oxford University Press.

Horwitz, Allan V. and Jerome C. Wakefield. 2012. *All We Have to Fear: Psychiatry's Transformation of Natural Anxieties into Mental Disorder*. New York: Oxford University Press.

Kalberg, Stephen. 1994. *Max Weber's Comparative Historical Sociology*. Chicago, IL: University of Chicago Press.

Light, Donald W. 1993. "Countervailing Power: The Changing Character of the Medical Profession in the United States," in Frederic Hafferty and John McKinlay (eds.), *The Changing Medical Profession: An International Perspective*. New York: Oxford University Press, pp. 69–79.

Light, Donald W. 2000. "The Medical Profession and Organizational Change: From Professional Dominance to Countervailing Power," in Chloe Bird, Peter Conrad, and Allen Fremont (eds.), *Handbook of Medical Sociology*, 5th ed. Upper Saddle River, NJ: Prentice Hall, pp. 201–16.

Light, Donald W. 2004. "Introduction: Ironies of Success—A New History of the American Health Care 'System.'" *Journal of Health and Social Behavior* 45(extra issue):1–24.

Light, Donald W. and Frederic W. Hafferty (eds.). 1993. *The Changing Medical Profession: An International Perspective.* New York: Oxford University Press.

Lippman, Abby. 1991. "Prenatal Genetic Testing and Screening: Constructing Needs and Reforming Inequities." *American Journal of Law & Medicine* 17:15–50.

Ludmerer, Kenneth. 1999. *Time to Heal.* New York: Oxford University Press.

McKinlay, John, and Lisa Marceau. 2002. "The End of the Golden Age of Doctoring." *International Journal of Health Services* 32:379–416.

Mechanic, David. 1989. "Medical Sociology: Some Tensions among Theory, Method, and Substance." *Journal of Health and Social Behavior* 30(2):147–60.

Meloni, Maurizio. 2019. *Impressionable Biologies.* New York: Routledge.

Parsons, Talcott. 1951. *The Social System.* New York: Free Press.

Pescosolido, Bernice A. 2006. "Professional Dominance and the Limits of Erosion." *Society* 43(6):21–9.

Pescosolido, Bernice A. 2013. "Theories and the Rise and Fall of the Medical Profession," in William Cockerham (ed.), *Medical Sociology on the Move: New Directions in Theory.* Dordrecht: Springer, pp. 173–94.

Pitts, Jesse R. 1968. "Social Control: The Concept," in D. Sills (ed.), *International Encyclopedia of Social Sciences,* vol. 14. New York: Macmillan, pp. 381–96.

Porter, Roy. 1997. *The Greatest Benefit to Mankind: A Medical History of Humanity.* New York: W. W. Norton.

Ritzer, George and David Walczak. 1988. "Rationalization and the Deprofessionalization of Physicians." *Social Forces* 67(1):1–22.

Rose, Nikolas. 2007. *The Politics of Life Itself: Biomedicine, Power, and Subjectivity in the Twenty-First Century.* Princeton, NJ: Princeton University Press.

Starr, Paul. 1982. *The Social Transformation of American Medicine: The Rise of a Sovereign Profession and the Making of a Vast Industry.* New York: Basic Books.

Timmermans, Stefan, and Hyeyoung Oh. 2010. "The Continued Social Transformation of the Medical Profession." *Journal of Health and Social Behavior* 51(extra issue):S94–106.

Weber, Max. [1922] 1978. *Economy and Society,* vol. 1, Guenther Roth and Claus Wittich (trans. and eds.). Berkeley, CA: University of California Press.

Williams, Simon J., Catherine Coveney, and Jonathan Gabe. 2017. "The Concept of Medicalisation Reassessed: A Response to Joan Busfield." *Sociology of Health & Illness* 39(5):775–80.

Zola, Irving K. 1972. "Medicine as an Institution of Social Control." *Sociological Review* 20: 487–504.

Chapter 14

Theories of Social Capital

Social capital refers to "the social investments of individuals in society in terms of their membership in formal and informal groups, networks, and institutions" (Turner 2004:13). It consists of cooperative relationships between people, featuring strong levels of interpersonal trust, norms of reciprocity, and mutual aid. It reflects a supportive social atmosphere where people look out for one another and interact with a sense of belonging. While social capital is a characteristic of the social networks from which individuals are able to draw psychological and material benefits, it is also a property of individuals who have access to it through their investment in it. The basic idea is that people invest in social relationships as a form of capital and draw a return from it as they would other types of capital they might invest in, but in this case the investment and return are both social and the health benefits provided are associated with sociability.

Social capital can therefore be considered a positive product of social interaction and good for one's physical and mental health. A person's level of social capital is determined (measured) by the degree to which an individual is socially integrated into his or her family, neighborhood, community, groups, places of worship, clubs, voluntary service organizations, and the like. People in highly supportive social relationships are predicted to have better health and longevity than those who are not. The concept of social capital, however, has been subjected to criticism on various methodological and theoretical grounds, causing some researchers to question its effectiveness as a social determinant of health (Carpiano 2006). While there may be questions about the extent to which feelings of belonging and supportive social environments have positive effects on health, theories of social capital have nonetheless become popular in medical sociology and public health as findings emerged that health benefits from social capital may indeed exist, although more research is needed. As Spanish public health researchers Elena Álvarez and Jordi Romaní (2017:60) advise:

While designing research to study this topic, it is essential to consider the theory behind social capital, its different dimensions and their relationship to health at every level. In this way, before choosing any measure of social capital one should consider the level at which variables will be measured and inferences wanted to be made; as well as through which mechanisms are thought to mediate these influences.

Gerry Veenstra and his colleagues (2005) suggest that social capital has the potential to affect health in three major ways. First, it may influence health directly through the extension of a community's or social network's resources to an individual who needs help, such as caregiving or through the provision of medical services. Second, it may influence health indirectly through its effects on the larger social, economic, political, and physical environments that serve as health determinants for the population. And third, social capital may interact with other health determinants at the individual or group level to promote health. For example, education may promote healthy lifestyles more readily in communities with high levels of social capital as compared to locales lacking such capital. There is also the notion that simply feeling good about one's self and being loved, supported, and nurtured in a caring environment is positive for health and well-being. As Bryan Turner (2003:14) explains, "one can reasonably assume that a sense of self-worth is a consequence of supportive social environments that have beneficial consequences for the human body."

The notion of capital, especially nonhuman capital (assets that can be owned and exchanged in the marketplace) and human capital (labor power, skills, training, and abilities) is a concept with a long history (Piketty 2014:46). It was present in sociology at its inception in the writings of Karl Marx. But when it comes to social capital, the origins of the concept, as for many theories in sociology, can be traced back to the classical theorists, which in this instance is Émile Durkheim. It can be found in Durkheim's ([1897] 1951) theory of suicide in which individuals were protected from self-harm by their close integration into society. Durkheim had discovered that suicide rates were low when social integration was strong and high when social ties were weak. Social relationships were what kept people from feeling alone and isolated, and consequently vulnerable to suicide—thereby highlighting the relevance of close companionship. Turner (2004) noted that Durkheim never used the term "social capital," but maintained that his concept of social solidarity is similar and still valid as an example of how social capital is protective of the health of the individual.

The modern concept of social capital originated in the 1980s and 1990s in the work of several theorists, including sociologists Pierre Bourdieu

([1983] 1986) and James Coleman (1990). Thus, it is obviously a more recent development when compared to Durkheim, but no longer a new concept. Three theorists have been particularly influential in medical sociology, so their work will be featured in this chapter. One is Bourdieu, whose ideas have been noted in other chapters. Another is a political scientist, Robert Putnam (1995, 2000), who has been especially prominent in social capital studies in public health (Song 2013), while the third is Nan Lin (1982, 2001) who previously conducted research in medical sociology.

Bourdieu: Social Capital as Structure

Bourdieu presented his concept of social capital in 1983 in a chapter published in an edited volume in Germany that was subsequently translated into English and reprinted for a handbook on the sociology of education. In it, Bourdieu ([1983] 1986:248) defines social capital as

> the aggregate of the actual or potential resources which are linked to possession of a durable network of more or less institutionalized relationships of mutual acquaintance and recognition—or in other words, to membership in a group—which provides each of its members with the backing of the collectively owned capital, a "credential" which entitles them to credit, in the various senses of the word.

His concept did not gain much recognition until he made references to different forms of capital in his better-known work *Distinction* (1984). Bourdieu ([1983] 1986:243) said that capital can present itself in three fundamental forms: (1) *economic capital*, which can be converted into money and institutionalized in property rights; (2) *cultural capital*, which exists in an embodied state (dispositions of mind and body), an objectified state (i.e., cultural goods), and an institutionalized state (i.e., schooling), which can be converted, in certain situations, into economic capital and institutionalized in educational credentials; and (3) *social capital*, which consists of social obligations (connections), convertible in certain conditions to economic capital, and institutionalized in formal titles (like doctor, general, president/prime minister, or those of the nobility).

Bourdieu also added the notion of *symbolic capital* to refer to the symbolic forms of legitimate power derived from the successful use of the other capitals (Swartz 1997). Symbolic capital and social capital are inextricably linked, as Bourdieu ([1983] 1986: 257) notes, in that "social capital is so totally governed by the logic of knowledge and acknowledgment that it always functions as symbolic capital." Yet much of Bourdieu's (1984) interest in capital was to show how cultural resources arbitrate class differences, particularly in relation to tastes and lifestyles. In this regard, economic and especially cultural capital takes up most of his attention on the topic of capital (Swartz 1997). Nevertheless, in recent years, as medical sociologists have turned their attention increasingly toward the relationship between social capital and health, his concept of social capital has received greater scrutiny.

Box 14.1 Pierre Bourdieu

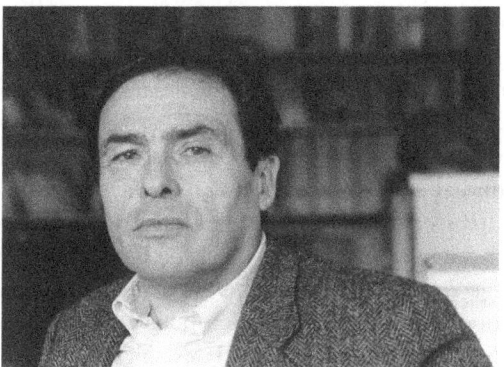

Image 14.1 Pierre Bourdieu

Pierre Bourdieu (1930–2002) was born on August 1, 1930 in Denguin, in southwest France. He grew up in the small and remote mountain village of Béarn. His grandfather had been a peasant sharecropper and his father, according to Bourdieu's description in a *Sketch for a Self-Analysis* (2008), was a postman and later a postal clerk. His mother, who came from a "great family of peasants," was a housewife. Both parents had left school in their teens. Bourdieu was sent to be educated as a boarding student at a *lycée* (secondary school) in Pau, 20 miles away from his home before moving on to the *Lycée Louis-le-Grand* in Paris after being recognized for his scholastic promise. He then attended university at the prestigious *École normale supérieure* in Paris, where he studied philosophy. After passing his examination (*agrégation*), he worked for a year as a *lycée* teacher before being conscripted into the French Army in 1955. He was sent to Algeria and served there for a year, mostly as a clerk, during the Algerian War of Independence.

Following his Army service he took a lecturer position at the University of Algiers and undertook fieldwork in the countryside described as "intense" (Heilbron 2015), including a study of the Kabyle people of the Berber tribe, which helped him formulate his notion of habitus and develop his own distinctive research style. He also published his first book, *Sociologie de l'Algérie* (The Sociology of Algeria) in 1958, based on his fieldwork. Bourdieu observed he had arrived in Algeria as a philosopher but left it as a sociologist (Lane 2000:9).

He returned to Paris in 1960 to become a research assistant to Raymond Aaron while he worked on his Ph.D. at the University of Paris. Shortly thereafter he accepted a teaching position at the University of Lille, publishing several books and articles on his Algerian research. In 1962, he married Marie-Claire Brizard and they had three sons Jérôme, Emmanuel, and Laurent. Next, in 1964, he was back in Paris as Director of Studies at the *École Pratique des Hautes Études* and, in 1968, he became head of the *Centre de Sociologie Européenne*, founded by Aaron, and remained in that position until his death. While there, in 1975, he founded the journal *Actes de la recherche en sciences sociales* (Social Science Research Acts), which became a major scientific journal for French sociologists. And in 1981, he became Chair of Sociology at the *Collège de France*. Many of his theories are contained in the pages of this book, as Bourdieu went on to become recognized as France's leading intellectual. He died of cancer in Paris on January 23, 2002 at the age of 71 years. He never completed his Ph.D.

Bourdieu views economic and cultural capital as property of the person; social capital is a resource that accrues to individuals through their membership in particular groups or networks. Consequently, social capital is a characteristic of social networks or social structures from which individuals draw benefits. As Bourdieu (1993:32) states: "Take social capital, for example: one can give an intuitive idea of it by saying that it is what ordinary language calls 'connections.'" Bourdieu also recognizes class disparities in social capital with more of it accruing to higher classes and maintains that the amount of social capital a person possesses depends on (1) the size of the network whose connections the person can effectively mobilize and (2) the volume of capital possessed by the person that he or she can claim through connections to those networks.

Richard Carpiano (2006:167) points out that it is this twofold feature of social capital that makes Bourdieu's theory useful for studying health. This is because Bourdieu requires us to consider not only the existence of community networks, but also the type and volume (amount) of resources possessed by that network and the individual's ability to draw on those resources. Not all networks and individuals are equal in this process, as some networks have better resources than others and certain individuals may be excluded from particular networks. However, Bourdieu takes an extra step by linking social capital to economic (financial) and cultural (education, taste) capital, showing how they are all interrelated—with economic capital the basis of all other types of capital. The different forms of capital can be used in concert or separately. One type can also be converted into another. In *Distinction*, Bourdieu (1984:122) refers to social capital as a "capital of social connections, honourability and respectability" that can be changed into economic, political, and social advantages. For example, people with economic capital can convert that capital into social and cultural capital. Social capital, in turn, may enhance cultural or economic capital and vice versa. Bourdieu says that the convertibility of the different types of capital is the basis of strategies aimed at ensuring the reproduction of that capital. He also maintains that the existence of a social network of connections outside the family is not a natural given, but must be cultivated and developed so that it contains social relationships that are durable and directly usable in either the long or short term.

Bourdieu did not address health concerns in his discussion of social capital and translations of his work from French into English are often difficult to read because of his writing style, so his writings have often required careful analysis to figure out what he really means. Many studies of social capital and health have instead relied more on Putnam or Lin. Moreover, Bourdieu did not specify how his notion of social capital could be measured. What Bourdieu does provide, however, is a concept of social capital that some researchers have described as having considerable potential and led them to adapt various statistical measures to test it (Carpiano 2006; Christensen and Carpiano 2014; Pinxten and Lievens 2014). For example, there is research showing that Bourdieu's concept of social capital can be used to examine how such capital affects bodyweight (Christensen and Carpiano 2014) and how it functions as a neighborhood-based health resource (Carpiano 2006; Carpiano and Kimbro 2012; Stephens 2008; Ziersch et al. 2005). In Latin America, collective (country-level) social capital was found to be more effective than individual social capital in explaining class-based health inequalities (Vincens, Emmelin, and Stafström 2018). Therefore, as Anna Ziersch and her colleagues (2005:2130) observed in Australia: "Bourdieu's notion [of social capital] is clearly part of the jigsaw puzzle of health inequities in the way it links the everyday social lives of individuals to the broader structural factors that have an impact on health."

Consequently, Bourdieu's concept of social capital appears to be more applicable to studies of social structures than those of agency, as he views such capital exclusively as a resource of social networks, not a property of individuals (Carpiano 2006). Social capital is drawn from and used by individuals from the structures in their lives, not the reverse. There are claims, accordingly, that because of the strong emphasis on structure, Bourdieu's notion of social capital cannot be quantified at the individual level (Stephens 2008). Yet subsequent work by Carpiano and Rachel Kimbro (2012) based on Bourdieu's theory of social capital shows that individual-level quantitative measures can be employed with his theoretical scheme. This is seen, for example, in the use of scales in their research that measured a sense of personal mastery, strain from parenting, neighborhood attachment, and neighborhood social cohesion in determining how strong ties with neighbors moderated strain among female primary caregivers (Carpiano and Kimbro 2012). Other scales exist on similar topics providing individual-level measures supplementing structural indicators of social capital (Álvarez and Romaní 2017).

Putnam: Bowling Alone

Robert Putnam deserves credit for popularizing the concept of social capital both in and outside of academia. In his seminal book, *Bowling Alone*, Putnam (2000:19) points out that: "Whereas physical capital refers to physical objects and human capital refers to properties of individuals, social capital refers to connections among individuals—social networks and the norms of reciprocity and trustworthiness that arise from them." To him, social capital is both a "private good" and a "public good." He goes on to suggest there are two types of social capital: bonding and bridging. Bonding social capital ties people together from the same social background and examples range from fraternal organizations and church-based women's groups to fashionable country clubs. Bonding tends to create in-group loyalty, but has a dark side in that it also can promote out-group antagonism. That is, the social bonds may be strengthened internally by united opposition to other groups. In this instance, one group's social capital may have negative consequences for another group. Bridging social capital, in contrast, links people of different social backgrounds together. Examples of bridging social capital include the civil rights movement, youth service groups, and ecumenical religious organizations.

Each type of social capital has its own particular social function. Putnam (2000:23) says that "bonding social capital constitutes a kind of sociological superglue, whereas bridging social capital provides a sociological WD-40 [a lubricant]." That is, bonding causes social reciprocity and solidarity to be stronger, while bridging links communities and individuals to resources and information. Individuals or communities may possess both types of social capital but usually do so in varying amounts. This means that the social networks providing social capital are not solely bonding or bridging; rather, they reflect more or less of each type of capital. "In short," states Putnam

(2000: 23), "bonding and bridging are not 'either-or' categories into which social networks can be neatly divided, but 'more or less' dimensions along which we can compare different forms of social capital."

Putnam also suggests various ways to measure social capital. Bonding social capital can be determined by the extent of a person's (1) religious involvement, (2) group participation or civic engagement, and (3) social trust and reciprocity. In the United States, religious social capital is particularly important because of its history of religious activity. Putnam estimates that approximately one-half of all group memberships, as well as charitable donations and volunteer work, are church-related. Churches and other religious organizations in his view are incubators for civic norms, skills, and recruitment, along with influencing community interests. Religious affiliations and levels of participation in its activities therefore constitute an important source of social capital. Next is group participation or what Putnam calls "civic engagement," which is determined by affiliations with groups like the PTA (Parent-Teacher Association), National Wildlife Federation, Junior League, and other voluntary organizations. Those groups that have regular face-to-face contact provide significantly greater social capital than groups that never bring its members together—so such groups vary in the amount of social capital they produce. Nevertheless, they provide a useful indicator of community social integration.

Finally, there is social trust and reciprocity that represents normative rather than behavioral standards. Putnam believes that a generalized sense of reciprocity is the benchmark of social capital. Social reciprocity is the sense of obligation to help others with the understanding that they or someone else will help you at some point in the future. Raking one's leaves before they blow into a neighbor's yard, giving coins to a stranger for a parking meter, buying a round of drinks at a local bar, keeping an eye on a friend's house, and taking snacks to a gathering are all examples of a generalized sense of reciprocity. Social trust is the expectation that such reciprocity is generally available. Social trust, however, is trust in other people, and is different from trust in institutions or politicians, which is why it is a measure of social capital.

While the specific mechanisms by which reciprocity and trust are measured are not fully detailed, Putnam makes several suggestions about how they operate in relation to health:

- social networks furnish tangible assistance to people like money, convalescent care, and transportation that reduces stress and provides a safety net;
- social networks reinforce healthy norms with respect to smoking, drinking alcohol, diet, and the like that promote health;
- socially cohesive communities are most able to organize quality medical services; and

- especially intriguing in Putnam's view, is his assertion that social capital may serve as a physiological triggering mechanism stimulating the immune systems of individuals to block stress and fight disease.

Social connectedness, Putnam claims, is one of the most powerful determinants of an individual's health. "Of all the domains in which I have traced the consequences of social capital," states Putnam (2000:236), "in none is the importance of social connectedness so well established as in the case of health and well-being." Beginning with Durkheim's ([1897] 1951) study of suicide, Putnam reviewed the health-related research literature on social solidarity, finding that several studies, including the once well-known Alameda County study in California that was under way in the 1960s (Berkman and Breslow 1983), demonstrated the importance of social integration for health. Social networks of families and friends were found to provide important resources and reinforce healthy behavior, while rejecting unhealthy practices. Later, in a nine-year follow-up study of Alameda County residents (Berkman and Syme 2017:1070), the findings at that time showed "that people who lacked social and community ties were more likely to die in the follow-up period than those with extensive [social] contacts."

Putnam used this and other data to estimate that people who are socially disconnected are between two to five times more likely to die from various causes when compared with similar individuals having close ties to family, friends, and community. He concludes that the more people are socially integrated, the better their health and longevity. As Putnam (2000:289) puts it: "Mounting evidence suggests people whose lives are rich in social capital cope better with traumas and fight illness more effectively."

Kimberly Lochner and her colleagues (2003) investigated whether the social organization of neighborhoods—not just their physical environment—affected mortality rates. They constructed a hierarchical linear model to examine the association of social capital with race and gender in Chicago's neighborhoods. The analysis showed that high neighborhood social capital as measured by reciprocity, trust, and civic engagement was linked to lower neighborhood death rates after adjusting for neighborhood material deprivation. Thus social capital affected mortality rates even after the effects of run-down, physically dilapidated neighborhood environments were taken into account. An exception was cancer mortality, which was not associated with social capital for gender or race. Other than cancer, this study produced evidence of the relatively strong effects of social capital on mortality at the neighborhood level.

However, some criticisms about Putnam's approach have been issued. One is that his notions of bonding and bridging can be seen to be properties of social networks instead of two different types of social capital (Lin 2008;

Song 2013). This is because bonding and bridging are what happens inside social networks, which in this context makes them processes, not resources. Yet resources (hence the term "capital") is how social capital is usually described. Another problem is that quantitative measures of social capital and its components, such as trust and reciprocity, have been a challenge to many researchers, although over time more precise measures have emerged that can be used (see Álvarez and Romaní 2017).

Lin: Social Structure and Capital

Nan Lin's (2001) concept of social capital begins with classical Marxist theory and highlights Marx's analysis of how capital emerges from social relations between capitalists and workers through the process of commodity production and consumption. He observes how the formation of economic capital in Marx's view results from the production and exchange of commodities as a process that entails social activity on the part of all concerned. He notes the manner in which workers in capitalist societies evolved into investors in the companies they worked for through stock options. This led Lin to characterize social capital as relationships embedded in social structures. Lin (2001:19) says that the premise underlying "the notion of social capital is relatively simple and straightforward: *investment in social relations with expected returns in the marketplace* or community, politics, etc." Thus social capital is formed through social relations and is seen as an asset by virtue of the connections between people and access to resources in the group or social network to which they belong. People are viewed as actively engaging in specific activities intended to increase their level of social capital received from their networks for the purpose of achieving their targeted goals. People in isolated situations have little or no social capital because they lack the social networks providing such capital.

Social capital in Lin's view consists of three components: structure, opportunity, and action. Social capital is seen as a product of positions within a hierarchical social structure that stretches beyond the individual. Individuals may change positions within this structure, but social capital remains associated with the position rather than the person. Individuals do have capital, what Lin calls human capital, that they have the freedom to use as they will, but social capital consists of resources entrenched in networks and associations. As Lin (2001:41) indicates, "social capital is rooted in social networks and social relations and is conceived as resources embedded in a social structure that are accessed and/or mobilized in purposive actions." Opportunity is also related to positions in a social structure, with persons in higher social positions having an advantage in accessing and mobilizing social ties with better resources. Consequently, social capital is not uniformly distributed in society, as certain groups have access to more and better capital than others. They are more able to take action with the opportunities they have. Obviously, people in lower social-class positions have less access to social capital and the capital that might be available has less resources. Differences may also exist between men and women and racial groups if their respective social positions are unequal.

Lin's emphasis on socioeconomic differences in social capital differs from Putnam who does not consider this type of variation (Song, Son, and Lin 2016). Whereas Putnam concentrates on how group participation and civic engagement build social capital at the community level, which individuals can draw on, Lin is more concerned with explaining the relationship between social structure and social capital. In doing so, Lin applies more of a sociological perspective to the social capital phenomenon than Putnam. Putnam, however, provides a more extensive consideration of the effects of social capital on health, which might be considered surprising given Lin's publications in medical sociology. His work on social capital represented a departure from his usual focus, although much of his past research is somewhat related as it dealt with the role of social support (feelings of being loved, accepted, cared for, and needed by others) as a buffer against stress, feelings of tension, and depression (Lin, Ye, and Ensel 1999). Lijun Song and Lin (2009) have found, however, that social capital contributes to health beyond and independently of social support as a more inclusive concept of the collective resources that benefit health.

Contrary to both Bourdieu and Lin, however, British psychologist Wouter Poortinga (2006) argues that variables at the individual level are more important than structural variables when it comes to the effects of social capital on health. The research suggests that social capital is more embedded in individuals than social structures. This finding, however, is likely due to the way social capital was measured. The average scores of individuals on questionnaire items about trusting other people (social trust) and their total number of memberships in voluntary organizations (civic participation) were aggregated (added together) to represent collective level social capital. Consequently, the collective measures were derived from summing up individual characteristics and were therefore not the properties of collectivities whose strength he was allegedly testing. Other researchers have done the same.

The effects of structures are best determined by measuring characteristics that are direct measures of the structures themselves and independent of the characteristics of individuals. As Álvarez and Romaní (2017:57) correctly point out, the existing research has investigated the effects of social capital on health in several different contexts, such as families, neighborhoods, workplaces, counties, states, or countries; however, these different levels are not the same and the measures used should not be the same either. Given the variety of measures of social capital that have been employed in the past and a lack of consensus about its precise meaning, it is clear that exact concepts and measurement strategies having general applicability are required in future research.

Among the studies that have successfully used the social capital concept is that of Patricia Drentea and Jennifer Moren-Cross (2005) who investigated an Internet site for young mothers that served as a virtual online community for support and the exchange of information about taking care of babies and young children. They agreed with the theoretical line advanced by Lin (2001) who maintained cybernetworks constitute a form of social capital. They found that the website they studied created a source of feminine thinking, thereby establishing a circle of women that took the power to influence them away from an exclusive reliance on the masculine medical establishment and placed it in a realm of women. The Internet helped young mothers establish links with other women like themselves, as urban neighborhoods are often empty of working mothers and their offspring during the workday. "In this case," state Drentea and Moren-Cross (2005:939), "we find a virtual community of mothers with young children increases social capital during a time when women are [often socially] isolated as new mothers." This was one of the first studies supporting Lin's (2001) contention that social networks in cyberspace signal a new era in the construction and development of the concept of social capital. As Lin (2001:257) states:

> No longer is social capital constrained by time or space; cybernetworks open up the possibility of global reaches in social capital. Social ties can now transcend geopolitical boundaries, and exchanges can occur as fast and as willingly as the actors care to participate.

What this indicates is an extension of social capital theory into the online world of social media in cyberspace. This is made possible by the Internet, which connects people globally through digital technology. In this context, health benefits from social capital are not limited to face-to-face encounters or relationships with local organizations, but can be derived through various electronic, wireless, and optical networking technologies providing access to information, social support, and other resources. As these technological developments play out over time, not only continuing but expanding, any forecasts of social capital theory being in decline and fading from use are not only premature but false (Lin 2001:237). Adjustments or refinements to the theory are likely because of its applicability to cyber-based relationships.

Summary

Despite the obvious difficulty in measuring a variable like social capital that operates at multiple (i.e., individual, group, neighborhood, community) conceptual levels, the general concept has grown in popularity as an explanation for structural influences on health outcomes. This is likely to continue as the theory is adjusted to account for relationship benefits in cyberspace. At present, there are different versions of social capital and even some subtheories, such as collective efficacy theory that applies to the capacity of neighborhoods to mobilize social action for positive outcomes that in some instances include health concerns (Sampson, Morenoff, and Earls 1999). Nevertheless, there is a general understanding that social capital is a feature of social structures consisting of networks of cooperative relationships between people in communities involving high levels of interpersonal trust and strong norms of reciprocity and mutual aid that facilitate action for shared benefits.

The social capital concept has both subjective and objective components, or what some might call cognitive and structural elements. Its subjective aspect is the positive feeling stemming from awareness of belonging to a community that offers social support for problems. Such feelings promote a sense of well-being. The objective component is the actual provision of assistance when in need, such as advice, looking out for one another, help when sick, law enforcement, options for emergency financial support, and community medical and social welfare services. Social capital thereby consists of resources embedded in a neighborhood or community (that can include cyberspace) structure beyond the level of the individual that the person can draw on to improve his or her life situation, including health.

Most researchers use Putnam's work as their starting point, but in sociology others favor Lin or Bourdieu. Both of these theorists emphasize social capital as a structural phenomenon that individuals can draw on, rather than a characteristic of individuals themselves. Part of its popularity may be due to it allowing researchers to construct more complete and thorough explanations of the social determinants of health. Yet full acceptance of the role of social capital in causing health outcomes is not universal in medical sociology, as not all studies find its effects to be strong. But some do and so its use as a major theory not only continues, but is likely to expand because of its potential for accounting for online social relationships. The basic message of social capital research is that structural variables like neighborhoods and communities can have a causal impact on health. The extent to which this is precisely the case still needs to be determined. It is clear, for example, that we do not fully understand the connection between health and well-being in individuals with social capital in relation to their feelings of trust, social support, happiness, confidence, self-esteem, and sense of belonging (Turner 2003). So although considerable work needs to be done, the relationship between social capital and health is another promising avenue of research showing how social factors cause health and illness.

Guide to Critical Thinking

1. Define social capital.
2. How does social capital provide health benefits?
3. Compare the theoretical viewpoints of Bourdieu, Putnam, and Lin. How are they different? How are they the same?

Suggested Reading

Lin, Nan. 2001. *Social Capital: A Theory of Social Structure and Action*. Cambridge: Cambridge University Press.
An introduction to social capital theory by one of the leading theorists.

References

Álvarez, Elena Carrillo and Jordi Riera Romaní. 2017. "Measuring Social Capital: Further Insights." *Gaceta Sanitaria (Health Gazette)* 31(1):57–61.

Berkman, Lisa F. and Lester Breslow. 1983. *Health and Ways of Living: The Alameda County Study*. Fairlawn, NJ: Oxford University Press.

Berkman, Lisa F. and Leonard Syme. 2017. "Social Networks, Host Resistance, and Mortality: A Nine-Year Follow-up Study of Alameda County Residents." *American Journal of Epidemiology* 185(11):1070–88.

Bourdieu, Pierre. [1983] 1986. "The Forms of Capital," in J. G. Richardson (ed.), *Handbook of Theory and Research for the Sociology of Education*. Westport, CT: Greenwood Press, pp. 241–58.

Bourdieu, Pierre. 1984. *Distinction: A Social Critique of the Judgment of Taste*. Cambridge, MA: Harvard University Press.

Bourdieu, Pierre. 1993. *Sociology in Question*. London: Sage.

Busfield, Joan. 2017. "The Concept of Medicalisation Reassessed." *Sociology of Health & Illness* 35(4):759–74.

Carpiano, Richard M. 2006. "Toward a Neighborhood Resource-based Theory of Social Capital for Health: Can Bourdieu and Sociology Help Us?" *Social Science & Medicine* 62:165–75.

Carpiano, Richard M. and Rachel T. Kimbro. 2012. "Neighborhood Social Capital, Parenting Strain, and Personal Mastery among Female Primary Caregivers of Children." *Journal of Health and Social Behavior* 53(2):323–47.

Christensen, Vibeke T. and Richard M. Carpiano. 2014. "Social Class Differences in BMI among Danish Women: Applying Cockerham's Health Lifestyles Approach and Bourdieu's Theory of Lifestyle." *Social Science & Medicine* 112:12–21.

Coleman, James S. 1990. *Foundations of Social Theory*. Cambridge, MA: Belknap Press of Harvard University Press.

Drentea, Patricia and Jennifer L. Moren-Cross. 2005. "Social Capital and Social Support on the Web: The Case of an Internet Mother Site." *Sociology of Health & Illness* 27(7):920–43.

Durkheim, Émile. [1897] 1951 *Suicide: A Study in Sociology*. New York: Free Press.

Heilbron, Johan. 2015. *French Sociology*. Ithaca, NY: Cornell University Press.

Lane, Jeremy F. 2000. *Pierre Bourdieu: A Critical Introduction*. London: Pluto.

Lin, Nan. 1982. "Social Resources and Instrumental Action," in P. V. Marsden and Nan Lin (eds.), *Social Structure and Network Analysis*. Beverly Hills, CA: Sage, pp. 131–45.

Lin, Nan. 2001. *Social Capital: A Theory of Social Structure and Action*. Cambridge: Cambridge University Press.

Lin, Nan. 2008. "A Network Theory of Social Capital," in Dario Castiglione, Jan van Deth, and Guglielmo Wolleb (eds.), *Handbook on Social Capital*. Oxford: Oxford University Press, pp. 50–69.

Lin, Nan, Xiaolan Ye, and Walter W. Ensel. 1999. "Social Support and Depressed Mood: A Structural Analysis." *Journal of Health and Social Behavior* 40(3):344–59.

Lochner, Kimberly A., Ichiro Kawachi, Robert T. Brennan, and Stephen L. Buka. 2003. "Social Capital and Neighborhood Mortality Rates in Chicago." *Social Science & Medicine* 56:1797–805.

Piketty, Thomas. 2014. *Capital in the Twenty-First Century*, Arthur Goldhammer (trans.). Cambridge, MA: Belknap Press of Harvard University Press.

Pinxten, Wouter and John Lievens. 2014. "The Importance of Economic, Social, and Cultural Capital in Understanding Health Inequalities: Using a Bourdieu-based Approach in Research on Physical and Mental Health Perceptions." *Sociology of Health & Illness* 36(7):1095–110.

Poortinga, Wouter. 2006. "Social Capital: An Individual or Collective Resource for Health?" *Social Science & Medicine* 62:292–302.

Putnam, Robert D. 1995. "Bowling Alone: America's Declining Social Capital." *Journal of Democracy* 6:65–78.

Putnam, Robert D. 2000. *Bowling Alone: The Collapse and Revival of American Community*. New York: Simon and Schuster.

Sampson, Robert J., Jeffrey D. Morenoff, and Felton Earls. 1999. "Beyond Social Capital: Spatial Dynamics of Collective Efficacy for Children." *American Sociological Review* 64(4): 633–60.

Song, Lijun. 2013. "Social Capital and Health," in William Cockerham (ed.), *Medical Sociology on the Move: New Directions in Theory*. Dordrecht: Springer, pp. 233–58.

Song, Lijun and Nan Lin. 2009. "Social Capital and Health Inequality: Evidence from Taiwan." *Journal of Health and Social Behavior* 50(2):149–63.

Song, Lijun, Joonmo Son, and Nan Lin. 2016. "Social Capital and Health," in William Cockerham (ed.), *The New Blackwell Companion to Medical Sociology*. Oxford: Wiley-Blackwell, pp. 184–210.

Stephens, Christine. 2008. "Social Capital in Its Place: Using Social Theory to Understand Social Capital and Inequalities in Health." *Social Science & Medicine* 66:1174–84.

Swartz, David. 1997. *Culture and Power: The Sociology of Pierre Bourdieu.* Chicago, IL: University of Chicago Press.

Turner, Bryan. 2003. "Social Capital, Inequality, and Health: The Durkheim Revival." *Sociology of Health & Illness* 1(1):4–20.

Turner, Bryan. 2004. *The New Medical Sociology: Social Forms of Health and Illness.* New York: W. W. Norton.

Veenstra, Gerry, Isaac Luginaah, Sarah Wakefield, Stephen Borch, John Eyles, and Susan Elliott. 2005. "Who You Know, Where You Live: Social Capital, Neighbourhood and Health." *Social Science & Medicine* 60:2799–818.

Vincens, Natalia, Maria Emmelin, and Martin Stafström. 2018. "Social Capital, Income Inequality and the Social Gradient in Self-Reported Health in Latin America: A Fixed Effects Analysis." *Social Science & Medicine* 196:115–22.

Ziersch, Anna M., Fran E. Baum, Colin MacDougall, and Christine Putland. 2005. "Health Implications of Access to Social Capital: Findings from an Australian Study." *Social Science & Medicine* 60:71–86.

Subject Index

Name Index